Thrombosis and Thromboembolism

FUNDAMENTAL AND CLINICAL CARDIOLOGY

Editor-in-Chief

Samuel Z. Goldhaber, M.D.

*Harvard Medical School
and Brigham and Women's Hospital
Boston, Massachusetts*

Associate Editor, Europe

Henri Bounameaux, M.D.

*University Hospital of Geneva
Geneva, Switzerland*

ADDITIONAL VOLUMES IN PREPARATION

Thrombosis and Thromboembolism

edited by
Samuel Z. Goldhaber
Paul M. Ridker

Brigham and Women's Hospital
and Harvard Medical School
Boston, Massachusetts

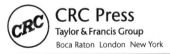
CRC Press
Taylor & Francis Group
Boca Raton London New York

CRC Press is an imprint of the
Taylor & Francis Group, an **informa** business

CRC Press
Taylor & Francis Group
6000 Broken Sound Parkway NW, Suite 300
Boca Raton, FL 33487-2742

First issued in paperback 2019

© 2002 by Taylor & Francis Group, LLC
CRC Press is an imprint of Taylor & Francis Group, an Informa business

No claim to original U.S. Government works

ISBN-13: 978-0-8247-0646-3 (hbk)
ISBN-13: 978-0-367-39652-7 (pbk)

Visit the Taylor & Francis Web site at
http://www.taylorandfrancis.com

and the CRC Press Web site at
http://www.crcpress.com

For our children and the children of those
lost on September 11, 2001

Series Introduction

For the past decade, I have had the good fortune of serving as Editor-in-Chief of the Fundamental and Clinical Cardiology series of books published by Marcel Dekker, Inc. These books have delved into the many basic and clinical subjects within the field of cardiovascular medicine. They have facilitated the compilation and integration of rapidly evolving knowledge for both the clinician and the research scientist. This series is composed of books that have received lavish critical acclaim because they adhere to the imperative of academic excellence. The publisher and I take pride in selecting topics that are timely, relevant, and insightful and in choosing book editors who are devoted and committed to perfecting every aspect of their work.

It is a special treat for me to wear two hats with the publication of *Thrombosis and Thromboembolism*. As co-editor of this book, I am pleased to be contributing the forty-sixth volume to this series, which provides me with the opportunity to reminisce pleasantly about my previous contribution, *Prevention of Venous Thromboembolism*, published in 1993, as the twelfth volume in this series. In both cases, I felt privileged to work with such a dedicated and top-of-the-line publisher. I do believe that *Thrombosis and Thromboembolism* will fulfill an otherwise unmet need within the community of physicians and scientists with particular interest in this field.

Samuel Z. Goldhaber

Foreword

Few areas of medicine have evolved as quickly on so many fronts as the field of thrombosis and thromboembolism. The underlying science continues to progress, with the discovery of the genetic bases of the thrombophilias, exemplified by the characterization of mutations in Factor V, furnishing but one example. The intriguing links between the coagulation and fibrinolytic pathways and inflammation are gaining increased recognition.

Progress in the clinic in regard to thrombosis and thromboembolism has evolved apace. Within this volume, individual chapters illustrate these clinical advances in many ways. Large observational studies and pools of data emerging from international cooperation have afforded much new insight into the natural history and outcomes of thromboembolic diseases. For example, diagnosis of thromboembolic disease has progressed biochemically, with the increased use of the D dimer as a first-line screening test for pulmonary embolism. Advances have also come from application of cross-sectional imaging techniques, such as computed tomography or magnetic resonance imaging, and have found increasing application in the diagnosis of pulmonary embolism.

Perhaps therapeutic innovation has proven most promising. The introduction into daily clinical practice of low-molecular-weight heparins, novel thienopyridine antagonists of the platelet ADP receptor, and several varieties of inhibitors of glycoprotein IIb/IIIa has provided a dizzying array of therapies. The interventional approaches to thromboembolic disease have gained new life in recent years. Catheter-directed thrombolysis, percutaneous clot extraction, and surgical embolectomy are finding their way into clinical practice.

For the clinician, this perplexing array of diagnostic and therapeutic possibilities presents a daily challenge. The contributors to this volume, assembled by Drs. Goldhaber and Ridker, provide a roadmap for the practitioner, guiding application of these diagnostic and therapeutic tools. The practical clinical information conveyed in this timely compilation rests on a firm scientific foundation.

Yet the very success and rapid pace of clinical science in the area of thrombosis and thromboembolism have bred controversy and confusion in many areas.

A number of important questions remain outstanding. The clinical application of markers of hemostatic function and long-term risk for thromboembolism and other vascular diseases remains controversial. How do we apply emerging markers of inflammation, related to risk of arterial thrombosis, in daily practice? Should we routinely measure novel markers of risk such as C-reactive protein? If so, in what populations and with what clinical consequences? These issues are considered in Chapters 1 and 2. What is the place of hormone replacement therapy in light of continued concerns regarding increased thrombotic risks? Chapter 4 considers this quandary in some detail. In the patient undergoing coronary intervention, our pharmacological tools have become so effective that we risk paying the price of increased bleeding complications. The optimal deployment of antithrombotic strategies in the context of acute vascular interventions engenders much discussion. Chapters 5, 6, and 10 address this quickly changing field. The role of antiplatelet therapy is expanding to new patient populations, including those with peripheral vascular disease. What patient populations should we target for chronic thienopyridine use? What are the benefits versus costs for expanded preventive therapy with antiplatelet agents? Chapter 7 grapples with these difficult issues. Recently, concerns have emerged regarding diminished benefits of angiotensin-converting-enzyme inhibition in individuals receiving antiplatelet therapy with aspirin, and Chapter 8 reviews this clinically important issue critically and provides a "bottom line" for daily practice. The failure of the oral antiglycoprotein IIb/IIIa antagonists in clinical trials, discussed in Chapter 6, still seeks an adequate mechanistic explanation. Several chapters address the appropriate deployment of diagnostic and treatment strategies for venous thromboembolism and pulmonary embolism. Practitioners will find the straightforward algorithms, such as those provided in Chapter 15, of daily utility.

In sum, Drs. Goldhaber and Ridker have provided us with a "catalogue raisonée" of current practice and controversies. Given the pace of innovation and clinical experience, one anticipates the need for a renewed look at these issues in the coming years.

Peter Libby

Preface

Thrombosis and Thromboembolism serves the medical and scientific community by compiling a timely and comprehensive update on this rapidly evolving field. Our contribution covers fundamental and clinical aspects of this broad topic and focuses on both arterial and venous disease, ranging from acute coronary syndromes to acute pulmonary embolism.

Vascular medicine is now recognized as a crucially important component of cardiovascular medicine, which is no longer confined to the study of acute myocardial infarction. Multiple sessions on peripheral arterial disease, pulmonary embolism, and deep venous thrombosis are now included at the three major cardiovascular meetings: the American Heart Association, the American College of Cardiology, and the European Society of Cardiology. Attendance is often "standing room only." Despite keen interest by cardiovascular physicians and scientists, the field is interdisciplinary and is shared by internists, hematologists, angiologists, pulmonologists, epidemiologists, vascular radiologists, and cardiovascular surgeons. The interdisciplinary involvement in thrombotic problems is perhaps exemplified by the soaring membership in the International Society on Thrombosis and Haemostasis, which celebrated an all-time high in registration at its most recent meeting in Paris.

Our book is written to assist the practicing physician, clinical investigator, and scientist dedicated to translational research. We have devoted Part I to fundamental issues of hypercoagulability, including the pivotal role of inflammation, several crucial hypercoagulable states, and the topic of hormone replacement therapy. Part II updates the therapy of acute coronary syndromes, including acute myocardial infarction (both ST-segment and non-ST-segment elevation) and unstable angina. We focus on novel approaches using low-molecular-weight heparins, direct thrombin inhibitors, and platelet inhibitors. Part III provides a contemporary update of the miraculous interventions that have occurred in the treatment of arterial thrombosis in the catheterization laboratory. These successes are due, in part, to adjunctive antithrombotic and antiplatelet therapy. Part IV focuses on venous thromboembolism, an area that for decades has been neglected, but which is now being recognized as "the other half" of the key to managing thrombotic disorders. This section includes state-of-the-art chapters on etiology, diagnosis, and pharmacological management of pulmonary embolism and deep venous thrombosis. Part V concludes the book with the remarkable achievements in the interventional laboratory and operating room for patients stricken with extensive and potentially life-threatening venous thromboembolism.

In addition to our role as co-editors, we co-authored 5 of the 20 chapters. In all cases, we ensured that the chapters are filled with summary tables, illustrative figures, and recent references. Our philosophy was to provide each chapter with a critical analysis of the topic along with conclusions based upon global assessment of all available knowledge. *Thrombosis and Thromboembolism* has achieved the balance for which we strived.

We wish to thank some of the individuals who helped make this book possible. Peter Libby, M.D., Chief of the Cardiovascular Division at Brigham and Women's Hospital, provided the personal encouragement, set the standard of excellence, and has served as a role model for us. We appreciate greatly his Foreword. We have also benefited immeasurably from the mentorship of Eugene Braunwald, M.D., and Arthur Sasahara, M.D., both luminaries in the field of thrombosis and thromboembolism. We are grateful to the individual contributors who have taken time from their multiple demands to write and revise their excellent chapters. With regard to the administrative challenge, Ms. Nicole Grimaldi performed exceptionally. A special word of thanks is due to the professional staff of Marcel Dekker, Inc., especially to Ms. Sandra Beberman, Vice President. Finally, we are profoundly appreciative of our families who supported us during the evolution and completion of this book.

Samuel Z. Goldhaber
Paul M. Ridker

Contents

Contents

Contributors

Lishan Aklog, M.D. Associate Surgeon, Cardiac Surgery Division, Brigham and Women's Hospital, and Assistant Professor of Surgery, Harvard Medical School, Boston, Massachusetts

Arman T. Askari, M.D. Fellow in Cardiovascular Medicine, Department of Cardiology, The Cleveland Clinic Foundation, Cleveland, Ohio

Gavin J. Blake, M.B., M.Sc., M.R.C.P., M.R.C.P.I. Cardiology Fellow, Cardiovascular Division, Brigham and Women's Hospital, and Research Fellow in Medicine, Harvard Medical School, Boston, Massachusetts

Henri Bounameaux, M.D. Chief, Division of Angiology and Hemostasis, University Hospital of Geneva, and Associate Professor of Medicine, Geneva School of Medicine, Geneva, Switzerland

Stephen Bravo, M.D. Clinical Instructor, Cardiovascular and Interventional Radiology Service, Brigham and Women's Hospital, Boston, Massachusetts

Christopher P. Cannon, M.D. Cardiovascular Division, Brigham and Women's Hospital, and Assistant Professor of Medicine, Harvard Medical School, Boston, Massachusetts

Mark A. Creager, M.D. Associate Professor of Medicine, Harvard Medical School, and Director, Vascular Center, Brigham and Women's Hospital, Boston, Massachusetts

Mark A. Crowther, M. D. Assistant Professor of Medicine, McMaster University, Hamilton, Ontario, Canada

Andrew C. Eisenhauer, M.D.   Director, Interventional Cardiovascular Medicine Service, Cardiovascular Division, Brigham and Women's Hospital, and Assistant Professor of Medicine and Radiology, Harvard Medical School, Boston, Massachusetts

Jeremy P. Feldman, M.D.   Pulmonary and Critical Care Medicine Fellow, University of California at San Francisco, San Francisco, California

Joseph M. Garasic, M.D.   Director, Peripheral Vascular Intervention, Cardiovascular Division, Massachusetts General Hospital, and Instructor in Medicine, Harvard Medical School, Boston, Massachusetts

Marie Gerhard-Herman, M.D.   Associate Physician, Cardiovascular Division, Brigham and Women's Hospital, and Assistant Professor of Medicine, Harvard Medical School, Boston, Massachusetts

Jeffrey S. Ginsberg, M.D., F.R.C.P.C.   Professor of Medicine, Department of Medicine, and Director, Clinical Thromboembolism Program, Hamilton Civic Hospital Research Centre, McMaster University, Hamilton, Ontario, Canada

Robert P. Giugliano, M.D., S.M.   Associate Physician, Cardiovascular Division, Brigham and Women's Hospital, and Assistant Professor of Medicine, Harvard Medical School, Boston, Massachusetts

Samuel Z. Goldhaber, M.D.   Director, Venous Thromboembolism Research Group; Director, Cardiac Center's Anticoagulation Service; Staff Cardiologist, Cardiovascular Division, Brigham and Women's Hospital; and Associate Professor of Medicine, Department of Medicine, Harvard Medical School, Boston, Massachusetts

Francine Grodstein, D.Sc.   Associate Professor of Medicine, Department of Medicine, Brigham and Women's Hospital and Harvard Medical School, Boston, Massachusetts

Kristen Hallisey, BSN, RN, CVN   Surgical Nurse, Connecticut Surgical Group, Hartford, Connecticut

Gordon Haugland, M.D.   Assistant Professor of Radiology, Division of Vascular and Interventional Radiology, Department of Radiology, SUNY–Downstate Medical Center, Brooklyn, New York

Peter Libby, M.D.   Chief, Cardiovascular Division, Brigham and Women's Hospital, and Mallinckrodt Professor of Medicine, Harvard Medical School, Boston, Massachusetts

Mark W. Mewissen, M.D. Vascular Interventionalist/Vascular Disease Consultant, Vascular Lab, Wisconsin Heart and Vascular Clinics, S.C., and Clinical Associate Professor of Radiology, Medical College of Wisconsin, Milwaukee, Wisconsin

Michael F. Meyerovitz, M.D. Director, Interventional Radiology, St. Vincent's Hospital, Worcester Medical Center, Worcester, Massachusetts

David A. Morrow, M.D. Instructor in Medicine, Cardiovascular Division, Brigham and Women's Hospital and Harvard Medical School, Boston, Massachusetts

Marc A. Pfeffer, M.D., Ph.D. Professor of Medicine, Cardiovascular Division; Medical Director, Partners Research and Education Program (PREP), Brigham and Women's Hospital; and Professor of Medicine, Harvard Medical School, Boston, Massachusetts

Jeffrey J. Popma, M.D., F.A.C.C., F.S.C.A.I. Director, Interventional Cardiology, Brigham and Women's Hospital, and Associate Professor of Medicine, Harvard Medical School, Boston, Massachusetts

Paul M. Ridker, M.D., M.P.H. Director, Center for Cardiovascular Disease Prevention, Brigham and Women's Hospital, and Associate Professor of Medicine, Harvard Medical School, Boston, Massachusetts

Meir J. Stampfer, M.D., D.Sc. Professor of Epidemiology and Nutrition, Department of Medicine, Harvard School of Public Health, Boston, Massachusetts

Kanella V. Tsilimingras, BS Pharm. Assistant Director, Anticoagulation Service, Brigham and Women's Hospital, Boston, Massachusetts

Peter W. F. Wilson, M.D. Professor of Medicine, Department of Endocrinology, Boston University School of Medicine, Boston, Massachusetts

Thrombosis and Thromboembolism

1

Inflammation and Arterial Thrombosis

David A. Morrow and Paul M. Ridker
*Brigham and Women's Hospital and Harvard Medical School,
Boston, Massachusetts*

I. INTRODUCTION

Together, laboratory and clinical data have provided substantial evidence supporting a fundamental role of inflammation in atherothrombosis (1). Laboratory researchers have identified macrophages, T-lymphocytes, and their biochemical messengers as key participants in the initiation, progression, and destabilization of atherosclerotic vascular disease (2). These pathobiological insights have directed the attention of clinical investigators to inflammatory markers as potential novel indicators of underlying atherosclerosis and cardiovascular risk. These efforts have produced a consistent body of epidemiological data demonstrating an association between clinical evidence of inflammation and increased risk of atherothrombosis (3). Moreover, the expansion in our understanding of atherogenesis has prompted reevaluation of the therapeutic mechanisms for several established pharmacological interventions, and pointed in new directions for the prevention and treatment of atherosclerotic vascular disease (2).

II. LABORATORY AND PATHOLOGIC EVIDENCE
A. Inflammation in Atherogenesis

Pathological examination of the mature atheroma demonstrates a core composed of a mixture of inflammatory and smooth muscle cells, lipids, and necrotic cellular debris covered by a protective fibrous cap (4,5). Although the evolution of this advanced lesion is complex and occurs in response to a varied group of endothelial insults, the central processes appear largely stereotyped, involving a number of well-described inflammatory elements (1).

1

The vascular endothelium is a highly functional synthetic organ capable of regulating vasomotor function, oxidizing lipoproteins, and directing cellular recruitment and migration through the production of an array of intercellular messengers (6). This organ may be injured by a number of possible insults, including, but not limited to, oxidative stress (7,8), hemodynamic forces (9), modified lipoproteins (10), infectious agents (11–13), and other cytotoxic substances such as advanced glycosylation products and homocysteine (14). Although initially protective, the responding activation and migration of inflammatory and smooth muscle cells coordinated by the vascular endothelium eventually conspire to promote the development of the atheroma (1).

Endothelial cell dysfunction is marked by upregulation of intercellular adhesion molecules and production of chemokines that mediate increased adhesion and migration of monocyte-derived macrophages and T-lymphocytes. Intercellular adhesion molecules, such as vascular cell adhesion molecule 1 (VCAM-1), E-selectin, and intercellular adhesion molecule 1 (ICAM-1) (15–20) interact with integrins on the surface of leukocytes to facilitate movement of inflammatory cells into the subendothelial space (21,22). Concurrently, multiple chemoattractant substances, including thrombin, connective tissue degradation products, oxidized LDL, and specific molecules secreted by endothelial and smooth muscle cells [monocyte chemotactic protein 1 (MCP-1), interleukin-8 (IL-8), and macrophage colony-stimulating factor (M-CSF)] enhance the recruitment of inflammatory cells to the site of injury (23–27). Directed by these mediators, a cellular inflammatory infiltrate is established within the arterial intima (28–30). With the uptake of LDL by subendothelial macrophages, they are transformed into the lipid-laden foam cells that characterize the fatty streak, the first recognizable progenitor of the advanced atherosclerotic lesion (4,31–33).

As they enter the arterial intima, arriving macrophages and T-lymphocytes generate inflammatory cytokines and growth factors that reinforce the influx of mononuclear leukocytes and the production of foam cells, and that initiates the migration and proliferation of vascular smooth muscle cells, which contribute to the maturation of the fatty streak into the intermediate atherosclerotic lesion. In particular, the elaboration of interleukin-1 (IL-1) (34–36), interleukin-6 (IL-6) (37–39), and tumor necrosis factor alpha (TNF-α) (40,41) augment the expression of adhesion molecules, as well as promote the oxidation and uptake of LDL (18,33). Simultaneously released mitogens, including platelet-derived growth factor, heparin-binding growth factor, and fibroblast growth factor, along with IL-1 and IL-6, stimulate the proliferation of smooth muscle cells that lead to formation of an intermediate plaque composed of layers of monocytes and smooth muscle cells (29,42–49). In addition to promoting cellular infiltration of the maturing atheroma, macrophage-monocytes enhance the transport and oxidation of LDL and produce reactive oxygen species that perpetuate injury to the vascular endothelium (29,50). In this fashion, initial endothelial dysfunction results in a series of interdependent processes that begin as a protective response but may eventuate a self-perpetuating pathological progression toward the complex atheroma (1,51).

In the advanced stages of this progression, a resilient fibrous cap forms over the core of intra- and extracellular lipid, inflammatory monocytes, smooth muscle cells, and necrotic debris (1,51). This protective cap is composed of an extracellular matrix that derives its strength primarily from types I and III collagen as well as elastin synthesized by vascular smooth muscle cells (46,52). The dense fibrous matrix constitutes a barrier between the highly prothrombotic contents of the atheroma core and circulating platelets and coagulation proteins. Vascular smooth muscle cells maintain this barrier in the face of macrophage production of collagenases, elastases, and proteases that may cause areas of focal thinning or erosion (53,54). When these forces determining the integrity of the extracellular matrix become unbalanced toward compromise of the barrier, exposure of the atheroma core promotes arterial thrombosis. In some cases, the thrombus is nonocclusive and may, in the absence of symptoms, become organized and incorporated into the existing advanced atherosclerotic plaque (55–58). As such, repeated episodes of plaque disruption, mural thrombosis, and organization with layering of mural thrombi may contribute to progression of the atherosclerotic lesion (59). In contrast, when the forming thrombus leads to abrupt compromise of distal flow, acute tissue ischemia or infarction may result (56).

B. Inflammation and Acute Atherothrombosis

Until recently, it had appeared self-evident that (nonembolic) arterial thrombosis was the culmination of slow enlargement of the mature atherosclerotic lesion with progressive encroachment into the arterial lumen. This pathobiological construct supported the view that the risk of acute thrombosis was dominated by the severity of arterial stenosis. However, over the past decade, angiographic and pathological data obtained in the coronary arterial bed have challenged this construct. Angiography performed prior to or at the time of acute myocardial infarction has demonstrated that the infarct-related coronary atherosclerotic lesion is frequently not "critical" by standard angiographic criteria (60–63). Similarly, pathological examination of culprit lesions has demonstrated that the majority of acute coronary events occur with the formation of thrombus at the site of plaques obstructing <50% of the arterial lumen (64). Taken together with evidence for the importance of plaque disruption in the development of superimposed thrombus (56,65–69), such data have shifted focus from the degree of luminal stenosis to the morphological and histological characteristics of the atheromatous plaque that determine its propensity to rupture (52,70).

1. The Vulnerable Plaque

Histological evaluation of ruptured atheromatous plaques has pointed to the central role of the fibrous cap in maintaining plaque integrity and suggested the importance of inflammatory constituents of the atheroma in destabilization of this protective barrier (52,70). The advanced atheromatous plaque with a thick fibrous cap, a small lipid core, and a predominance of normal vascular smooth muscle cells is resistant to compromise. In contrast, lesions with caps that are thin and friable are more likely to rupture and extrude procoagulant atheromatous materials from the lipid-rich core (5,56,71). Such "vulnerable" plaques are characterized by a large lipid core and a high density of inflammatory monocytes at the edge of the lesion, or "shoulder" region (72,73), where plaque disruption most frequently occurs (57,65,70,74).

Lending further support to the contribution of inflammatory mechanisms to plaque destabilization, onset of acute thrombosis with or without myocardial necrosis is marked by the production of a number of inflammatory cytokines (75–79). In addition, a series of studies have suggested a link between the elaboration of inflammatory cytokines and impairment of the ability of smooth muscle cells to maintain the integrity of the fibrous cap (52). Interferon-gamma (IFN-γ), a cytokine produced by T-lymphocytes within the atheroma core, decreases the production of collagen by vascular smooth muscle cells (80–82). Smooth muscle cells at the site of plaque rupture or erosion have been found to express high levels of the transplant antigen HLA-DRα, a protein induced only by IFN-γ among a wide spectrum of cytokines evaluated (72,83). Further, matrix metalloproteinases, a group of proteolytic enzymes that degrade collagen as well as elastin, are produced in increased quantities by smooth muscle cells and macrophages under the influence of cell–cell interactions with T-lymphocytes and the inflammatory cytokines, interleukin-1, and tumor necrosis factor (84–88). Histological studies of human atheroma samples using immunostaining techniques have documented the presence of metalloproteinases in macrophages and T-lymphocytes, as well as overlying endothelial cells, with increased enzyme activity found particularly in the "shoulder" region (54,89).

Thus, the "vulnerable" plaque is typified by a large lipid pool and a thin or absent fibrous cap (70,74), as well as the predominance of inflammatory monocytes, the expression of HLA-DR antigens, and a decrease in the number smooth muscle cells (72,90). Each of these features either directly, or through mechanisms outlined above, implicate an inflammatory contribution. While other factors (91), such as shear stress (9,92) and vasospasm (93), may also contribute to plaque destabilization, the participation of inflammation in this process appears central.

2. Platelet Activation, Thrombus Formation, and Vascular Reactivity

Disruption of the fibrous cap or endothelium exposes collagen, lipids, and monocyte-bound tissue factor, all of which are potent stimulants of platelet adhesion and aggregation. In addition, tissue factor has strong procoagulant effects that play an important role in the genesis of thrombus in acute coronary syndromes (94). Activated macrophages within the atheroma core produce large amounts of tissue factor, which upon exposure to circulating coagulation proteins initiate the extrinsic coagulation pathway (95–98). Although the stimuli for tissue factor expression are not fully characterized, T-lymphocytes acting through specific cell surface proteins and cell–cell contact can induce its production (86,98).

Vascular inflammation may also influence arterial vasomotor function through several possible mechanisms. Increased concentrations of thromboxane A2 and its metabolites produced in acute coronary syndromes (99,100) mediate further platelet aggregation as well as arterial vasoconstriction (101). Leukocytes also produce endothelin-1, a potent modulator of vasoconstriction. In addition, certain inflammatory cytokines may increase vascular smooth muscle cell reactivity, as demonstrated in an animal model with IL-1 (102). Finally, inflammatory infiltrates have been documented in the arterial adventitia with vascular nerve involvement and thus have been hypothesized to directly stimulate coronary vasospasm (103).

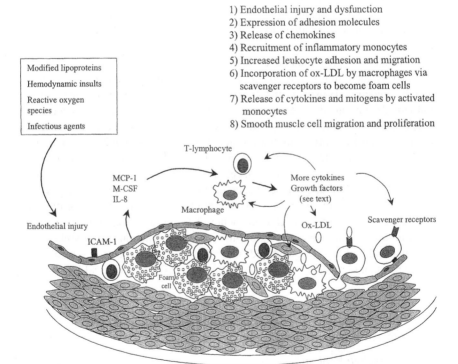

1) Endothelial injury and dysfunction
2) Expression of adhesion molecules
3) Release of chemokines
4) Recruitment of inflammatory monocytes
5) Increased leukocyte adhesion and migration
6) Incorporation of ox-LDL by macrophages via scavenger receptors to become foam cells
7) Release of cytokines and mitogens by activated monocytes
8) Smooth muscle cell migration and proliferation

Modified lipoproteins
Hemodynamic insults
Reactive oxygen species
Infectious agents

T-lymphocyte
MCP-1
M-CSF
IL-8
More cytokines
Growth factors
(see text)
Macrophage
Endothelial injury
Ox-LDL
Scavenger receptors
ICAM-1
Foam cell

Figure 1 Inflammation and formation of the fatty streak. Refer to text for details. ICAM-1, intercellular adhesion molecule 1; MCP-1, monocyte chemotactic protein-1; M-CSF, macrophage colony-stimulating factor; IL, interleukin. (From Ref. 2.)

As such, a substantial body of data implicate the participation of inflammatory cells and/or mediators during every phase of atherogenesis and arterial
thrombosis, including initiation of the fatty streak, progression to an intermediate
atheroma, maturation of the advanced atherosclerotic lesions, thinning and compromise of the fibrous cap, platelet aggregation and thrombosis, and the modulation of coronary vasospasm (Fig. 1).

III. CLINICAL MARKERS OF INFLAMMATION

In spite of continued advancements in the management of acute ischemic heart
disease, morbidity and mortality due to atherosclerotic vascular disease continue
to rise globally (104,105). Thus, the impetus for improving our strategies for the
prevention and management of atherosclerosis has remained strong. In this regard, laboratory and experimental research describing key processes in the initiation, progression, and destabilization of the atheroma have pointed to novel directions for cardiovascular evaluation and management. In particular, recognition
of the role of inflammation in atherothrombosis has directed attention to inflammatory mediators and indicators as potential targets for risk assessment and for
treatment (3).
     Epidemiological data have established a well-characterized set of vascular
risk factors, including advanced age, tobacco use, obesity, diabetes, hypertension,
and dyslipidemia. However, up to one-third of first coronary events occur among
individuals without these traditional risk factors (106). Researchers have thus
sought to identify inflammatory indicators that might add to these clinical factors
for predicting myocardial infarction and stroke (107). Candidate markers have
included several of the cytokines (77,108,109) that promote the recruitment of
monocytes in response to endothelial cell dysfunction; intercellular adhesion molecules (110–112) that mediate the migration of activated monocytes into the
subendothelial space; enzymes (113) that might compromise the integrity of the
protective fibrous cap, as well as the acute-phase proteins that are produced and
released into the systemic circulation in response to inflammatory cytokines. As
an amplified and readily quantified inflammatory signal, the prototypical acute-
phase reactant C-reactive protein (CRP) has been a focus of clinical investigation
to date.

A. High-Sensitivity C-Reactive Protein, Atherosclerosis, and Atherothrombosis

1. C-Reactive Protein

CRP is a pentameric polypeptide initially described as a reactant to the somatic
C-polysaccharide of *Streptococcus pneumonia* (114). This acute-phase protein is

produced exclusively by hepatocytes in response to stimulation by inflammatory cytokines, primarily interleukin-6 (114).

With systemic levels that are dependent on the rate of de novo hepatic production, CRP levels remain stable over long periods of time in the absence of new stimuli (114,115). However, in response to acute tissue injury, infection, or other inflammatory stimuli, CRP levels rise several hundred-fold. As such, CRP and its acute-phase counterpart, serum amyloid A, have been useful in following disease activity in chronic inflammatory conditions such as systemic lupus, inflammatory bowel disease, and rheumatoid arthritis (114,116). Traditional semiquantitative latex agglutination or standard turbidometric methods have been adequate to evaluate such marked elevation of CRP in these disease processes. In contrast, the development of high-sensitivity assays for CRP (hs-CRP) has now enabled detection of CRP within the normal range for healthy individuals (116,117). Further, the introduction of high through-put methods with high analytical sensitivity and reproducibility has provided a simple clinical tool to carefully evaluate the extent of underlying systemic inflammation (116,118).

2. hs-CRP and Prevalent Coronary Heart Disease

Cross-sectional studies have evaluated the association between elevated levels of CRP and the presence and extent of atherosclerotic vascular disease. Elevated levels of CRP have been demonstrated among patients with acute myocardial ischemia (119) and infarction (120), as well as among individuals with stable coronary heart disease (CHD) (121). In a cross-sectional survey of 388 British men aged 50 to 69 recruited from general practice registers, Mendall and colleagues demonstrated a 1.5-fold increase in the prevalence of CHD for each doubling in the levels of hs-CRP (95% CI, 1.25–1.92) (121). Nevertheless, such cross-sectional data cannot exclude the possibility of important confounding, nor do they establish a cause-and-effect relationship (122). For example, blood levels of hs-CRP have been found to increase with age, body-mass index, and tobacco use (121,123), as well as in response to myocardial tissue necrosis. In contrast, prospective studies can control for such confounders and have been important in exploring the independent prognostic information offered by inflammatory markers.

3. hs-CRP and the Risk of Future Cardiovascular Events

Prospective studies have documented a strong and consistent positive correlation between baseline elevation of hs-CRP and the risk of future cardiovascular morbidity and mortality. This predictive capacity of hs-CRP has been demonstrated among apparently healthy individuals free of clinical vascular disease (124–130a) as well as among those with multiple vascular risk factors (131) or recognized coronary artery disease (Fig. 2) (132–135).

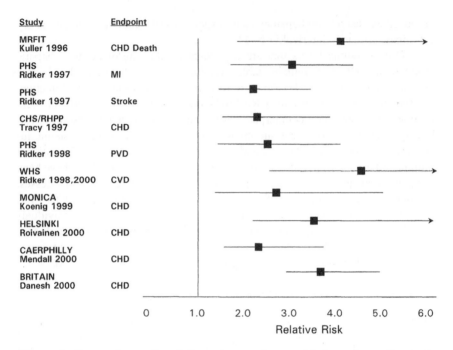

Figure 2 Prospective studies of C-reactive protein as a risk factor for cardiovascular disease among apparently healthy individuals.

Among men with multiple traditional vascular risk factors followed in the MRFIT study, those with the highest baseline levels of hs-CRP were at nearly 3-fold higher risk of CHD mortality (RR 2.8; 95% CI 1.4–5.4) over 17 years of follow-up (131). A similar 2- to 3-fold higher risk of coronary events was evident among elderly men and women with preclinical atherosclerosis and elevated hs-CRP in the Cardiovascular Health Study and Rural Health Promotion Project (127). Further, the prospective European Concerted Action on Thrombosis and Disabilities Study (ECAT) showed that among 2121 patients with angina each standard deviation increase in baseline hs-CRP predicted a 45% increase in the relative risk of nonfatal myocardial infarction (MI) or sudden cardiac death (95% CI; RR 1.15–1.83) through 2 years of follow-up (132). Moreover, in a nested case-control analysis of individuals with stable CHD post-myocardial infarction, hs-CRP predicted a 75% higher relative risk for recurrent nonfatal MI or fatal coronary events in the highest versus lowest hs-CRP quintile (135).

While these data support a prognostic relationship between hs-CRP and future events among persons recognizable as high risk, data from prospective studies of apparently healthy subjects have extended these observations to individuals at seemingly low risk, who may present a particular challenge to clinicians planning strategies for primary CHD prevention (124–126). The Physicians Health Study followed 22,071 apparently healthy men with no clinical vascular disease and low rates of cigarette consumption (136). In this cohort of healthy physicians followed for an average of 8 years, individuals in the highest quartile of hs-CRP had a 2-fold increased risk of future stroke (RR 1.9; 95% CI 1.1–3.3), a 3-fold higher risk of future MI (RR 2.9; 95% CI 1.8–4.6) (124), and a 4-fold higher risk of developing severe peripheral arterial disease (RR 4.1; 95% CI 1.2–6.0) (128,137a,137b). These risk estimates were not modified by smoking status and were independent of other cardiovascular risk factors, including total and HDL cholesterol, triglycerides, lipoprotein(a), and fibrinogen. Moreover, combined determination of hs-CRP and lipid parameters offered a prognostic advantage over measurement of the lipid profile alone, including the total cholesterol to HDL cholesterol ratio (138).

Data from several other prospective studies support these findings (126, 129,130). In the MONICA (Monitoring Trends and Determinants in Cardiovascular Disease) Augsberg Cohort Study of 936 middle-aged healthy European men, a 1 SD increase in log-normalized baseline hs-CRP was associated with a 1.7-fold higher risk of a first major coronary event (95% CI 1.29–2.17) (126). In a nested-case control analysis from a prospective cohort study conducted among general practices from 18 towns in Britain, initially healthy men with hs-CRP levels in the top third had a significantly higher risk of CHD death or nonfatal MI (OR 2.13; 95% CI 1.38–3.28) (129). Similarly, among 482 men followed for an average of 8.5 years in the primary prevention Helsinki Heart Study (PHS), baseline levels of hs-CRP in the highest quartile were associated with a nearly 4-fold higher risk of a first MI or CHD death (OR 3.66; 95% CI 1.97–6.81) (130). Similar to findings in the PHS, the risk relationships observed in these prospective studies were not significantly altered after adjustment for multiple potential confounders, including age and smoking status (126,129,130).

Data from the Women's Health Study (WHS) have corroborated the association between hs-CRP and vascular risk among healthy women. In this prospective study of postmenopausal women, baseline levels of hs-CRP were significantly higher among those who subsequently had a first cardiovascular event compared with those who remained free of vascular disease during 3 years of follow-up (125). Women with hs-CRP in the highest quartile had a 5-fold higher risk of any vascular event (RR 4.8; 95% CI 2.3–10.1), and an 8-fold higher risk of myocardial infarction or stroke (RR 7.7; 95% CI 2.7–19.9) (125). This prognostic association was evident among multiple subgroups of women without traditional risk factors who might otherwise be regarded as low risk. Consistent with findings in men, measurement of hs-CRP added to the predictive value of the lipid profile in determining vascular risk (125,128).

Several prospective analyses have made observations of potential clinical importance regarding levels of hs-CRP among postmenopausal women using hormonal replacement therapy (HRT) (139–141). In the WHS, median levels of hs-CRP were much higher among women using HRT compared with women on no HRT (0.27 vs. 01.4 mg/dL; p = 0.001) (141). As such, while the median level of hs-CRP in WHS (125) was greater than observed in studies consisting only of men, stratification by use of HRT showed that women on no HRT had a distribution of baseline CRP similar to men (141). The association between elevated hs-CRP and HRT was present regardless of the form of HRT used and has been corroborated by data from at least two other studies (139,140). In the Postmenopausal Estrogen/Progestin Interventions Study (139), women allocated to treatment with conjugated equine estrogens had a significant increase in hs-CRP with a mean 85% increase relative to placebo sustained at 3 years (p = 0.0001). Among elderly women treated with unopposed estrogen in the Cardiovascular Health Study, a 59% higher mean hs-CRP level was observed compared to nonusers (140). It has been hypothesized (139) that these data give some mechanistic insight into a transient increase in thrombotic risk associated with initiation of HRT suggested by the higher rate of thrombotic events observed during the first year of active therapy in the Heart and Estrogen/Progestin Replacement Study (HERS) (142). However, further investigation will be important to assess whether these observations supporting the possibility of proinflammatory effects of HRT are clinically relevant (141).

4.   hs-CRP for Risk Assessment in Acute Coronary Syndromes

Data highlighting the importance of the inflammatory constituents of an atheroma in determining the risk of plaque rupture have prompted strong interest in the assessment of inflammatory markers in symptomatic coronary disease (119). CRP level rises in the setting of acute MI (143–145) in close correlation with IL-6 (75,146), and is associated with higher risk of death, pump failure, or myocardial rupture (147). However, the presence and prognostic importance of CRP elevation in acute coronary syndromes without myocardial necrosis remains under investigation with prospective studies among patients with unstable angina showing some heterogeneity in results. Liuzzo and colleagues found that in a group of 31 patients hospitalized with severe unstable angina and no evidence of myocardial necrosis by admission cardiac-specific troponin T, hs-CRP levels exceeding 0.3 mg/dL predicted more frequent recurrent angina and a trend toward higher rates of revascularization, MI, and cardiovascular death prior to hospital discharge (133). These findings with respect to short-term prognosis were corroborated and extended in a study reported by the Thrombolysis in Myocardial Infarction (TIMI) study group (134). In a population of 437 patients presenting with non-ST elevation acute coronary syndromes, a markedly elevated hs-CRP at presentation ($\geq$1.55 mg/dL, 99th percentile of healthy controls) predicted higher mortality by 14 days. Moreover, measurement of hs-CRP added to the prognostic information offered by cardiac-specific troponin T (134). In an additional study using a similar cut-point of 1.5 mg/dL, hs-CRP measured at baseline among 194 patients with unstable angina predicted a higher risk of MI, refractory angina, or death through 90 days (148). In this evaluation, hs-CRP was the strongest independent predictor of coronary events in multivariable analysis, including patient age and ECG findings. Further, analysis of the receiver operating characteristics curves confirmed an optimal threshold of 1.5 mg/dL for the prediction of recurrent coronary events through 90 days (148).

Several other studies have supported the value of baseline hs-CRP determination for assessment of longer term risk in acute coronary syndromes. The FRISC (Fragmin during Instability in Coronary artery disease) study group followed 965 patients for 5 months after initial presentation with a non-ST elevation acute coronary syndrome and found that stratification by tertile of baseline hs-CRP concentration established a gradient of mortality risk (1.6% vs. 4.6% vs. 6.9%, $p = 0.005$) (149). Similarly, among 102 patients with unstable angina followed for 3 months, an hs-CRP level above 0.3 mg/dL (90th percentile of normal controls) at presentation remained an independent predictor of new MI after adjustment for ECG changes and cardiac troponin T (150).

In contrast, two studies have not detected a prognostic relationship between hs-CRP and clinical outcomes in acute ischemic heart disease. In a study of 195 patients with unstable angina followed to hospital discharge, adverse cardiac events occurred with similar frequency in those with or without elevation of baseline hs-CRP (151). A similar evaluation of 140 patients with severe unstable angina found that the risk of suffering a subsequent cardiac event during the initial hospitalization was not statistically different among those with elevated admission CRP (152).

Data from ongoing and future investigation will be necessary to clarify the role of hs-CRP for risk assessment among patients presenting with acute coronary syndromes. In particular, the optimal timing of measurement remains in question. In two studies that included serial measurement of hs-CRP among patients with severe unstable angina, determination of hs-CRP at discharge was a better discriminator of risk of future events than measurement at hospital admission (148,153). However, among patients with myocardial necrosis, it is anticipated that the inflammatory response to tissue injury might confound evidence of systemic inflammation prior to the onset of necrosis, and it remains uncertain as to whether this inflammatory response to MI offers prognostic information beyond other measures of infarct size. In one series of 188 patients treated with thrombolytic therapy, the peak serum CRP concentration was found to correlate with the risk of mortality at 6 months, whereas peak CK and CKMB did not (154). Similar to CK, CRP falls more rapidly and reaches lower peak concentrations in patients with a patent infarct-related artery after reperfusion therapy (155–159). However, the reduction in CRP with early patency of the infarct related artery is greater than that anticipated based on infarct size alone (155,156), raising the possibility that more effective reperfusion reduces inflammation in ST elevation acute coronary syndromes through mechanisms that extend beyond the degree of necrosis (157). In addition, studies that have documented elevated levels of hs-CRP in the absence of elevated cardiac-specific troponins refute a response to myocardial necrosis as the only mechanism for the observed rise (133,134). Such data highlight the need for further careful investigation to expand our understanding of the inflammatory events in acute coronary syndromes. To some extent, this information may come from evaluation of other markers of inflammation.

B. Inflammatory Cytokines

A number of inflammatory indicators other than hs-CRP have been evaluated as potential markers of cardiovascular risk both among individuals presenting with acute ischemic events, as well as among those at risk for atherosclerosis. As the primary stimulant for CRP production, IL-6 levels correlate closely with hs-CRP in noncardiovascular conditions (160). In addition, IL-6 may participate more directly through a broad range of humoral and cellular immune effects (161), as well as procoagulant actions (162,163). Levels of IL-6 are elevated in stable (109) and unstable ischemic heart disease (77). Among patients with unstable angina, increased levels of IL-6 appear to predict higher risk for early adverse outcomes (164). Further, baseline elevation of IL-6 has been associated with increased risk of all-cause mortality among high-functioning elderly men and women from the Iowa 65+ Rural Health Study (108). Data from the Physicians Health Study have shown a 2.3-fold higher risk of MI (95% CI 1.3–4.3; $p = 0.005$) among apparently healthy men with the highest levels of IL-6 (165). Adjustment for baseline differences in total cholesterol, HDL cholesterol, body mass index, blood pressure, smoking status, and diabetes did not substantially alter this risk relationship. Further, the association between IL-6 and future MI persisted even after controlling for levels of hs-CRP (165). In light of these data, it is not surprising that several acute-phase proteins (CRP, serum amyloid A, albumin, and fibrinogen) produced in response to hepatic stimulation by IL-6 have all been associated with increased cardiovascular risk (166).

Several inflammatory cytokines, in addition to IL-6, have been found to correlate with myocardial ischemia (109) and increased risk of recurrent events among those with unstable (164) and stable coronary artery disease (167). For example, TNF-α levels measured in 272 individuals stable for at least 3 months post-MI were significantly higher among those who subsequently suffered a recurrent event compared with age- and gender-matched study participants free from recurrent coronary heart disease events ($p = 0.02$) (167). The risk of experiencing a recurrent cardiac event was 2.7-fold higher ($p = 0.004$) among individuals with TNF-α levels greater than the 95th percentile of the control distribution (167). As such, these data both add to the accumulating evidence that cytokines that play an important role in atherogenesis may be useful in detecting individuals at higher risk for future first or recurrent cardiac events, and lend additional support to the hypothesis that vascular inflammation is a direct contributor to heightened risk of atherothrombosis.

Data demonstrating an association between elevated levels of vascular adhesion molecules and future cardiovascular events further strengthen this evidence for a connection between vascular inflammatory processes and the predictive capacity of inflammatory markers (110,111,128). In contrast to nonspecific markers of systemic inflammation, such as the acute-phase proteins, vascular adhesion molecules are integral to vascular endothelial activation and leukocyte migration, and thus point more directly to the fundamental role of inflammation in mediating cardiovascular risk (111,112).

C. Pathophysiological Correlation

Nevertheless, the pathobiological mechanisms through which elevation of inflammatory markers relate both to increased risk of atherothrombosis, and to higher risk of poor outcomes with acute cardiovascular events remain uncertain. In the setting of acute coronary thrombosis, it is plausible that the increase in circulating markers of inflammation is a manifestation of the intensification of vascular inflammatory processes contributing directly to plaque destabilization. However, this possible explanation has not been conclusively established (168). For example, it has been proposed that repetitive episodes of ischemia and reperfusion may trigger an inflammatory response within the myocardium (79,169–171). Contradicting this hypothesis, Maseri and colleagues have shown that the acute-phase reactants do not rise with recurrent episodes of myocardial ischemia-reperfusion due to coronary vasospasm (172). Nor does activation of the coagulation cascade alone result in increased production of CRP (173).

Alternatively, the possibility of direct contributions from CRP in atherogenesis and acute arterial thrombosis should be considered. CRP has been found within atherosclerotic lesions (174,175) and is known to stimulate the expression of tissue factor (176), influence leukocytes (177), and activate complement (178). Notably, the lack of association between hs-CRP elevation and the burden of coronary atherosclerosis assessed either angiographically (179) or with electron-beam computed tomography (180) support the notion that hs-CRP levels instead reflect pathobiological properties of the atheroma and vascular endothelium (i.e., plaque vulnerability rather than severity). Recent studies demonstrating an association between elevated hs-CRP and endothelial dysfunction determined in studies of human forearm blood flow lend additional credence to this argument (181,182). Further investigation directed at elucidating the precise relationships between the elevation of acute-phase reactants, cytokines, and intercellular adhesion molecules and adverse cardiovascular prognosis will continue to advance our understanding of the pathobiology of atherogenesis and possibly offer new targets for therapeutic intervention.

D. Inflammatory Markers in Clinical Practice

If inflammatory markers such as hs-CRP are to become useful in clinical practice, there must be evidence that they add to the prognostic information offered by traditional cardiovascular risk factors (122). In the case of hs-CRP, baseline elevation of the inflammatory marker remains highly predictive of future events after adjustment for traditional risk factors including age, hypertension, diabetes, body mass, index, and smoking status (124–126). When used in conjunction with lipid measurements in the Women's Health Study and Physicians Health Study, hs-CRP added to the predictive information offered by the total to high-density cholesterol ratio (TC:HDL) (125,183). Moreover, in a prospective evaluation in healthy women that compared traditional (TC and TC:HDL) as well as several "novel" (lipoprotein(a), homocysteine, hs-CRP) markers of cardiovascular risk, the combination of hs-CRP and the TC:HDL ratio was found to be the strongest predictor of first myocardial infarction (Fig. 3) (128). On the basis of these data, high-sensitivity testing for CRP used in conjunction with the TC:HDL ratio has

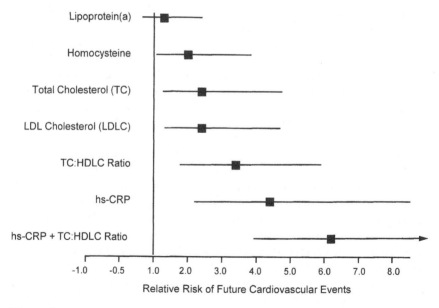

Figure 3   Relative risk of future vascular events associated with base-line elevation (highest quartile) of markers of inflammation and lipids. (From Ref. 128.)

A   1. Determine TC:HDLC Quintile
         2. Determine hs-CRP Quintile
         3. Assess Cardiovascular Relative Risk

B

Quintile	hs-CRP (mg/L)	TC:HDLC (Women)	TC:HDLC (Men)
1	0.1 - 0.7	< 3.4	< 3.4
2	0.7 - 1.1	3.4 - 4.1	3.4 - 4.0
3	1.2 - 1.9	4.1 - 4.7	4.0 - 4.7
4	2.0 - 3.8	4.7 - 5.8	4.7 - 5.5
5	3.9 - 15.0	> 5.8	> 5.5

C

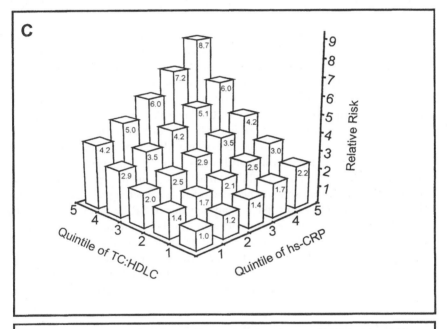

Distribution of hs-CRP derived from ongoing population based surveys. Lipid cutpoints and risk estimates for incident cardiovascular disease derived from N Engl J Med 1997;336:973-979; Circulation 1998;97: 2007-2011; and N Engl J Med 2000;342:836-843.

Figure 4   A proposed cardiovascular risk assessment algorithm using hs-CRP and lipid screening. (From Ref. 184.)

been approved by the Food and Drug Administration for cardiovascular risk stratification among men and women. Algorithms using these data have been proposed (Fig. 4) (184). Clinical algorithms such as this may continue to evolve as new data from large clinical data sets become available.

1. hs-CRP and Therapeutic Interventions: Aspirin

Although the epidemiological data supporting the prognostic utility of hs-CRP are strong and consistent, the inflammatory marker is unlikely to carry significant impact on clinical strategies for management of atherosclerotic vascular disease if the associated risk cannot be modified by available therapies. Thus, data suggesting important interactions between hs-CRP and specific pharmacological therapies are of particular clinical as well as experimental interest.

Aspirin, an agent with both antiplatelet and anti-inflammatory effects, was the first specific pharmacological therapy tested for CRP interaction. In the Physicians Health Study, participants were randomly assigned to low-dose aspirin (325 mg p.o. q.o.d.) or placebo with a 44% reduction in the risk of first MI associated with aspirin use ($p < 0.001$) (136). However, in a nested case control analysis, stratification by quartiles of baseline hs-CRP revealed an increasing gradient of benefit with aspirin, such that those in the highest quartile of hs-CRP realized a 55.7% ($p = 0.002$) reduction in the risk of first MI compared with 13.9% ($p = 0.77$) among those in the lowest quartile of hs-CRP concentration (124). Similar differential effects of aspirin on clinical outcomes in the presence or absence of elevated CRP levels has recently been reported in the setting of unstable angina (124a). Indeed, in this setting, the prognostic value of CRP was found to be quite limited once patients had been treated with aspirin. These data suggest that at least part of the benefit of aspirin may result from an interaction with underlying low-grade vascular inflammation. To date, however, data have been conflicting as to whether aspirin use reduces CRP levels (109,124b). Whether other COX-1 and/or COX-2 inhibitors impact upon CRP levels is currently under investigation.

2. hs-CRP and Therapeutic Interventions: Statins

While data on aspirin are important pathophysiologically, the most provocative data regarding preventive medical therapy interacting with CRP involves the hydroxymethylglutaryl coenzyme A reductase inhibitors, or "statins." In this regard, experimental evidence has for some time supported the idea that, in addition to lowering LDL cholesterol, statins may have relevant anti-inflammatory and thus plaque-stabilizing effects. For example, statins have been shown to reduce macrophage content within atherosclerotic plaques, decrease neointimal inflammation, and suppress matrix metalloproteinase expression, all processes involved in the vulnerability of luminal plaque.

Clinical evidence demonstrating anti-inflammatory and plaque-stabilizing effects of statin drugs has only recently become available (185). The first study to address whether patients with evidence of inflammation benefited from statin therapy was performed within the Cholesterol and Recurrent Events (CARE) trial (135), a secondary-prevention evaluation of pravastatin. Consistent with studies of primary prevention, participants in the CARE trial with elevated CRP levels were found to have higher risks of recurrent coronary events than those with lower levels of CRP. However, a clinically apparent interaction between statin therapy and inflammation was also observed in that the proportion of recurrent events prevented by pravastatin was 54% among those with inflammation compared with 25% among those without inflammation (Fig. 5) (135). Moreover, long-term therapy with pravastatin significantly reduced plasma levels of CRP in a manner that was not related to this agent's effects on LDL cholesterol (186). In fact, in this hypothesis-generating study, there was no relationship between the change in CRP and the change in LDL cholesterol at the end of the 5-year follow-up period. Thus, these initial data provided clinical evidence that statin therapy may well have anti-inflammatory properties.

While the mechanism of this effect is uncertain, the CARE data provide evidence for possible clinical relevance of laboratory observations demonstrating nonlipid effects of the HMG-CoA reductase inhibitors, such as modulation of immune function (187,188), antiproliferative effects on vascular smooth muscle (189,190), and antithrombotic properties (191,192), as well as morphological ef-

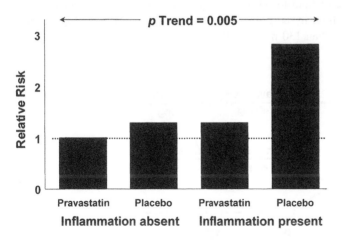

Figure 5 Differential effects of statin therapy in secondary prevention according to the presence or absence of an enhanced inflammatory response: the CARE trial. (From Ref. 135.)

fects on the atherosclerotic plaque (193,194). Indeed, taken together with data from animal studies demonstrating that both dietary and statin-induced lipid lowering result in reduction in metalloproteinase activity (188,195), the data from CARE serve to raise the possibility that statin therapy may achieve a reduction in cardiovascular events through both lipid-dependent and lipid-independent effects on inflammatory cell function and related plaque vulnerability. However, the hypothesis-generating data from CARE—while provocative and initially controversial—require direct evaluation in hypothesis-testing trials.

3. Direct Tests of the Statin/CRP Hypothesis: The PRINCE Trial and the AFCAPS CRP Substudy

Two major studies have now addressed the validity and clinical importance of these observations. The first, the Pravastatin Inflammation/CRP Evaluation (PRINCE) trial, was explicitly designed to address three questions (196). First, can the effects of pravastatin on CRP observed in the CARE trial be confirmed in a direct hypothesis-testing setting? Second, how quickly does any effect of pravastatin on CRP occur and are the effects of pravastatin on CRP truly independent of changes in LDLC? And third, are the effects of pravastatin on CRP observed in CARE (a secondary-prevention study) equally present in primary-prevention populations?

In total, the PRINCE trial evaluated 2884 patients: 1182 in a secondary-prevention cohort who received pravastatin 40 mg daily, and 1702 in a primary-prevention cohort randomly allocated to either pravastatin 40 mg daily or placebo (Fig. 6). Prior use of lipid-lowering therapy within the previous 6 months was not allowed, and those in the primary-prevention arm had to have LDL cholesterol levels greater than 130 mg/dL. Blood samples were collected at baseline,

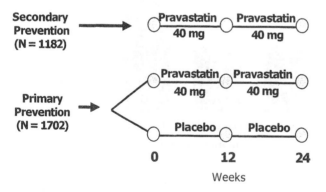

Figure 6 The PRINCE study design. (From Ref. 196.)

12 weeks, and 24 weeks, allowing a direct comparison of the effects of pravastatin on both CRP and lipid levels. Twenty-eight percent of the study participants were taking aspirin, and 9% had a prior history of diabetes.

As ensured by the randomization process, baseline levels of CRP (median 0.20 mg/dL), total cholesterol (231 mg/dL), LDL cholesterol (143 mg/dL), and HDL cholesterol (40 mg/dL) were virtually identical in the two primary-prevention arms of the PRINCE trial. In contrast, compared with those in the primary-prevention cohort, those with a prior history of cardiovascular disease who were enrolled in the secondary-prevention cohort of PRINCE had significantly increased CRP levels (median 0.26 mg/dL). As would be expected, those in the secondary-prevention cohort were also older and more likely to smoke or have diabetes, and the group had a higher proportion of aspirin users than the primary-prevention cohort. During the course of the study, highly significant reductions in total cholesterol, LDL cholesterol, and triglycerides were observed in the pravastatin groups, as was a clinically important increase in HDL cholesterol (all p values <0.001). No change was observed in any of these parameters among those allocated to placebo.

The main analyses of PRINCE were the effects of statin therapy at both 12 and 24 weeks. In the primary-prevention cohort, pravastatin reduced median CRP levels by 16.9% compared with placebo at the end of the 24-week study period ($p < 0.001$). This effect was present at 12 weeks (median reduction in CRP with pravastatin 14.7%; $p < 0.001$). As shown in Figure 7, these effects were observed in all the PRINCE prespecified subgroups, including analyses stratified by age, smoking status, gender, obesity, and lipid levels. As had been hypothesized, virtually no association was observed between CRP and lipid levels either at the study beginning or during follow-up. In fact, in correlational analyses, less than 2% of the variance in the change in CRP could be explained by the change in any lipid parameter. Virtually identical effects were also seen in those in the secondary-prevention cohort of the study.

The PRINCE study thus prospectively confirmed in a large community-based population that statin therapy lowers CRP, and that this effect cannot be predicted by the magnitude of LDL reduction (196). In addition to pravastatin, similar data in smaller studies have also been presented for cerivastatin, simvastatin, and atorvastatin (197,198), although one study failed to show such an effect for fluvastatin (199). Nonetheless, evidence that statins lower CRP does not by itself provide a rationale for broader use of this therapy in primary prevention. However, very recent data from the AFCAPS/TexCAPS CRP substudy suggest that measurement of CRP may provide a novel method to improve the targeting of statin therapy (200).

In the AFCAPS/TexCAPS CRP substudy, CRP levels as well as lipid profiles were measured at study entry and after 1 year in 5742 primary-prevention patients who were then randomly allocated to either lovastatin or placebo. The

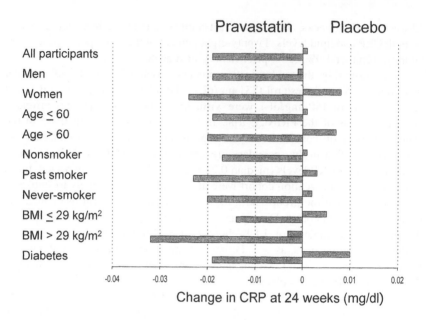

Figure 7 Effects of pravastatin on CRP in PRINCE according to prespecified subgroup analyses. (From Ref. 196.)

AFCAPS/TexCAPS trial had previously shown that lovastatin reduced rates of first acute coronary events by 37%. When the trial data were analyzed in strata based on both CRP and LDL levels, an intriguing pattern was observed (Table 1). Not surprisingly, lovastatin was effective in reducing coronary event rates among those with baseline levels of LDL cholesterol above 150 mg/dL, the me-

Table 1 Event Rates and Number-Needed-to-Treat (NNT) Among Those Allocated to Lovastatin or Placebo in the AFCAPS/TexCAPS Trial, According to Baseline Levels of LDL Cholesterol and CRP

	Statin	Placebo	NNT
Low LDLC/low CRP	0.025	0.022	—
Low LDLC/high CRP	0.029	0.051	48
High LDLC/low CRP	0.020	0.050	33
High LDLC/high CRP	0.038	0.055	58

Median LDLC = 149 mg/dL; median CRP = 0.16 mg/dL.
Source: Ref. 199.

dian LDL value in AFCAPS/TexCAPS; such patients had a number-to-needed-to-treat of 42, a level considered not only cost-effective but cost-saving. However, lovastatin therapy was also effective in reducing the risk of first-ever coronary events among study participants with low levels of LDL cholesterol who had above-average levels of CRP. Specifically, the magnitude of risk reduction associated with statin use for those with above-average CRP levels but normal lipid levels was almost identical to that observed among those with above-median cholesterol levels. Moreover, among such patients who had elevated levels of CRP but normal lipid levels, the event rate was just as high as that observed among those with overt hyperlipidemia. For these individuals, the number-needed-to-treat was also very low (NNT = 48). By contrast, lovastatin appeared to have no effect in participants in AFCAPS/TexCAPS who had below-average LDL levels *and* below-average CRP levels. As might be expected, the absolute event rate was very low in this group, who had normal to low lipid levels and no evidence of inflammation. In this low-risk population defined by both LDL and CRP, the NNT was exceptionally large and statin utility cost-ineffective. Finally, like the PRINCE study, the AFCAPS/TexCAPS CRP substudy showed that lovastatin reduced CRP levels in a lipid-independent manner, this time at 1-year follow-up.

When viewed together, data from the PRINCE study (196) and the AFCAPS/TexCAPS CRP substudy (200) confirm that elevated levels of CRP are a potent independent predictor of heart attack and stroke, and that combining CRP with cholesterol levels provides an improved tool for global risk prediction. Moreover, both of these large studies demonstrate clearly that statin therapy leads to approximately 15% reductions in CRP levels. Last, although hypothesis-generating, the AFCAPS/TexCAPS CRP substudy also suggests that statins may significantly reduce vascular risk even in individuals who do not have overt hyperlipidemia.

IV. SUMMARY

Pathological and experimental data suggest that atherosclerosis is an inflammatory disease. In support of the clinical extension of these observations, prospective epidemiological data provide consistent evidence of an association between sensitive markers of systemic inflammation and the risk of future cardiovascular events. In particular, high-sensitivity testing for CRP identifies apparently healthy individuals who are at higher risk for vascular events at 5 or more years after blood sampling, as well as individuals with stable and unstable coronary disease who are more likely to suffer recurrent atherothrombosis. The predictive capacity of hs-CRP is independent of information offered by traditional vascular risk factors, other novel markers of thrombotic risk, as well as other key participants in the inflammatory cascade. Clinical studies indicate that the risk associated with elevation of inflammatory markers may be modified by established preventive therapies in cardiovascular disease. Experimental data suggest that common therapies such as aspirin and HMG-CoA reductase inhibitors may act in part through modulating inflammatory processes or mediators that may be central to atherothrombosis (109,188). Taken together, these data support the possibility that anti-inflammatory therapies may come to play a role in the prevention and treatment of cardiovascular disease and that inflammatory markers such as hs-CRP may prove clinically useful in targeting therapy to those patients who will derive the greatest benefit.

REFERENCES

1. Ross R. Atherosclerosis—an inflammatory disease. N Engl J Med 1999; 340:115–126.
2. Morrow DA, Ridker PM. Inflammation in cardiovascular disease. In: Topol E, ed. Textbook of Cardiovascular Medicine Updates. Cedar Knolls: Lippincott Williams & Wilkins, 1999:1–12.
3. Morrow DA, Ridker PM. C-reactive protein, inflammation, and coronary risk. Med Clin North Am 2000; 84:149–161.
4. Stary HC. Evolution and progression of atherosclerotic lesions in coronary arteries of children and young adults. Arteriosclerosis 1989; 9:19–32.
5. Davies MJ. A macro and micro view of coronary vascular insult in ischemic heart disease. Circulation 1990; 82:38–46.
6. Gimbrone MA, Jr. Culture of vascular endothelium. Prog Hemost Thromb 1976; 3:1–28.
7. Liao F, et al. Genetic evidence for a common pathway mediating oxidative stress, inflammatory gene induction, and aortic fatty streak formation in mice. J Clin Invest 1994; 94:877–884.
8. Gong KW, et al. Effect of active oxygen species on intimal proliferation in rat aorta after arterial injury. J Vasc Res 1996; 33:42–46.
9. Glagov S, et al. Hemodynamics and atherosclerosis. Insights and perspectives gained from studies of human arteries. Arch Pathol Lab Med 1988; 112:1018–1031.
10. Steinberg D. Antioxidants and atherosclerosis. A current assessment. Circulation 1991; 84:1420–1425.
11. Libby P, Egan D, Skarlatos S. Roles of infectious agents in atherosclerosis and restenosis: an assessment of the evidence and need for future research. Circulation 1997; 96:4095–4103.
12. Benditt EP, Barrett T, McDougall JK. Viruses in the etiology of atherosclerosis. Proc Natl Acad Sci U S A 1983; 80:6386–6389.
13. Lemstrom K, et al. Cytomegalovirus antigen expression, endothelial cell prolifera-

tion, and intimal thickening in rat cardiac allografts after cytomegalovirus infection. Circulation 1995; 92:2594–2604.

14. Harker LA, et al. Homocystine-induced arteriosclerosis. The role of endothelial cell injury and platelet response in its genesis. J Clin Invest 1976; 58:731–741.

15. Quinn MT, et al. Oxidatively modified low density lipoproteins: a potential role in recruitment and retention of monocyte/macrophages during atherogenesis. Proc Natl Acad Sci U S A 1987; 84:2995–2998.

16. Nagel T, et al. Shear stress selectively upregulates intercellular adhesion molecule-1 expression in cultured human vascular endothelial cells. J Clin Invest 1994; 94:885–891.

17. Cybulsky MI, Gimbrone MA, Jr. Endothelial expression of a mononuclear leukocyte adhesion molecule during atherogenesis. Science 1991; 251:788–791.

18. Osborne L, et al. Direct expression cloning of vascular cell adhesion molecule 1, a cytokine-induced protein that binds to lymphocytes. Cell 1989; 59:1203–1211.

19. Poston RN, et al. Expression of intercellular adhesion molecule-1 in atherosclerotic plaques. Am J Pathol 1992; 140:665–673.

20. Nakashima Y, et al. Upregulation of VCAM-1 and ICAM-1 at atherosclerosis-prone siteson the endothelium in the ApoE-deficient mouse. Arterioscler Thromb Vasc Biol 1998; 18:842–851.

21. Osborne L. Leukocyte adhesion to endothelium in inflammation. Cell 1990; 62:3–6.

22. Navab M, et al. Monocyte adhesion and transmigration in atherosclerosis. Coronary Artery Dis 1994; 5:198–204.

23. Valente AJ, et al. Mechanisms in intimal monocyte-macrophage recruitment. A special role for monocyte chemotactic protein-1. Circulation 1992; 86:20–25.

24. Nelken NA, et al. Monocyte chemoattractant protein-1 in human atheromatous plaques. J Clin Invest 1991; 88:1121–1127.

25. Wang JM, et al. Expression of monocyte chemotactic protein and interleukin-8 by cytokine-activated human vascular smooth muscle cells. Arterioscler Thromb 1991; 11:1166–1174.

26. Cushing SD, et al. Minimally modified low density lipoprotein induces monocyte chemotactic protein 1 in human endothelial cells and smooth muscle cells. Proc Natl Acad Sci U S A 1990; 87:5134–5138.

27. Rajavashisth TB, et al. Induction of endothelial cell expression of granulocyte and macrophage colony-stimulating factors by modified low-density lipoproteins. Nature 1990; 344:254–257.

28. Jonasson L, et al. Regional accumulations of T cells, macrophages, and smooth muscle cells in the human atherosclerotic plaque. Arteriosclerosis 1986; 6:131–138.

29. Mitchinson MJ, Ball RY. Macrophages and atherogenesis. Lancet 1987; 2:146–148.

30. Yla-Herttuala S, et al. Expression of monocyte chemoattractant protein 1 in macrophage-rich areas of human and rabbit atherosclerotic lesions. Proc Natl Acad Sci U S A 1991; 88:5252–5256.

31. Aqel NM, et al. Monocytic origin of foam cells in human atherosclerotic plaques. Atherosclerosis 1984; 53:265–271.

32. Yla-Herttuala S, et al. Evidence for the presence of oxidatively modified low density lipoprotein in atherosclerotic lesions of rabbit and man. J Clin Invest 1989; 84:1086–1095.

33. Steinberg D, et al. Beyond cholesterol. Modifications of low-density lipoprotein that increase its atherogenicity. N Engl J Med 1989; 320:915–924.

34. Mantovani A, Bussolino F, Dejana E. Cytokine regulation of endothelial cell function. FASEB J 1992; 6:2591–2599.

35. Raines EW, Dower SK, Ross R. Interleukin-1 mitogenic activity for fibroblasts and smooth muscle cells is due to PDGF-AA. Science 1989; 243:393–396.

36. Libby P, Friedman GB, Salomon RN. Cytokines as modulators of cell proliferation in fibrotic diseases. Am Rev Respir Dis 1989; 140:1114–1117.

37. Seino Y, et al. Interleukin 6 gene transcripts are expressed in human atherosclerotic lesions. Cytokine 1994; 6:87–91.

38. Rus HG, Vlaicu R, Niculescu F. Interleukin-6 and interleukin-8 protein and gene expression in human arterial atherosclerotic wall. Atherosclerosis 1996; 127:263–271.

39. Sukovich DA, et al. Expression of interleukin-6 in atherosclerotic lesions of male ApoE-knockout mice: inhibition by 17beta-estradiol. Arterioscler Thromb Vasc Biol 1998; 18:1498–1505.

40. Old LJ. Tumor necrosis factor (TNF). Science 1985; 230:630–632.

41. Libby P, et al. Endotoxin and tumor necrosis factor induce interleukin-1 gene expression in adult human vascular endothelial cells. Am J Pathol 1986; 124:179–185.

42. Schwartz SM, Reidy MA. Common mechanisms of proliferation of smooth muscle in atherosclerosis and hypertension. Hum Pathol 1987; 18:240–247.

43. Libby P, Warner SJ, Friedman GB. Interleukin 1: a mitogen for human vascular smooth muscle cells that induces the release of growth-inhibitory prostanoids. J Clin Invest 1988; 81:487–498.

44. Winkles JA, et al. Human vascular smooth muscle cells both express and respond to heparin-binding growth factor I (endothelial cell growth factor). Proc Natl Acad Sci U S A 1987; 84:7124–7128.

45. Libby P, et al. Production of platelet-derived growth factor-like mitogen by smooth-muscle cells from human atheroma. N Engl J Med 1988; 318:1493–1498.

46. Ip JH, et al. Syndromes of accelerated atherosclerosis: role of vascular injury and smooth muscle cell proliferation. J Am Coll Cardiol 1990; 15:1667–1687.

47. Ikeda U, et al. Interleukin 6 stimulates growth of vascular smooth muscle cells in a PDGF-dependent manner. Am J Physiol 1991; 260:H1713–1717.

48. Ross R, et al. Localization of PDGF-B protein in macrophages in all phases of atherogenesis. Science 1990; 248:1009–1012.

49. Shimokado K, et al. A significant part of macrophage-derived growth factor consists of at least two forms of PDGF. Cell 1985; 43:277–286.

50. Meier B, et al. Human fibroblasts release reactive oxygen species in response to interleukin-1 or tumour necrosis factor-alpha. Biochem J 1989; 263:539–545.

51. Rosenfeld ME, Ross R. Macrophage and smooth muscle cell proliferation in atherosclerotic lesions of WHHL and comparably hypercholesterolemic fat-fed rabbits. Arteriosclerosis 1990; 10:680–687.

52. Libby P. Molecular bases of the acute coronary syndromes. Circulation 1995; 91: 2844–2850.
53. Lendon CL, et al. Atherosclerotic plaque caps are locally weakened when macrophages density is increased. Atherosclerosis 1991; 87:87–90.
54. Henney AM, et al. Localization of stromelysin gene expression in atherosclerotic plaques by in situ hybridization. Proc Natl Acad Sci U S A 1991; 88:8154–8158.
55. Bini A, et al. Identification and distribution of fibrinogen, fibrin, and fibrin(ogen) degradation products in atherosclerosis. Use of monoclonal antibodies. Arteriosclerosis 1989; 9:109–121.
56. Davies MJ, Thomas AC. Plaque fissuring—the cause of acute myocardial infarction, sudden ischaemic death, and crescendo angina. Br Heart J 1985; 53:363–373.
57. Davies M. Thrombosis and coronary atherosclerosis. In: Julian D, Kublen W, Norris R, Swan H, Collen D, Verstraete M, eds. Thrombolysis in Cardiovascular Disease. New York: Marcel Dekker; 1989:25–43.
58. Roberts WC, Buja LM. The frequency and significance of coronary arterial thrombi and other observations in fatal acute myocardial infarction: a study of 107 necropsy patients. Am J Med 1972; 52:425–443.
59. Fuster V, et al. Atherosclerotic plaque rupture and thrombosis. Evolving concepts. Circulation 1990; 82:47–59.
60. Serruys PW, et al. Is transluminal coronary angioplasty mandatory after successful thrombolysis? Quantitative coronary angiographic study. Br Heart J 1983; 50:257–265.
61. Hackett D, Davies G, Maseri A. Pre-existing coronary stenoses in patients with first myocardial infarction are not necessarily severe. Eur Heart J 1988; 9:1317–1323.
62. Ambrose JA, et al. Angiographic progression of coronary artery disease and the development of myocardial infarction. J Am Coll Cardiol 1988; 12:56–62.
63. Little WC, et al. Can coronary angiography predict the site of a subsequent myocardial infarction in patients with mild-to-moderate coronary artery disease? Circulation 1988; 78:1157–1166.
64. Falk E, Shah PK, Fuster V. Coronary plaque disruption. Circulation 1995; 92:657–671.
65. Constantinides P. Plaque fissuring in human coronary thrombosis. J Atheroscler Res 1966; 6:1–17.
66. Falk E. Plaque rupture with severe pre-existing stenosis precipitating coronary thrombosis. Characteristics of coronary atherosclerotic plaques underlying fatal occlusive thrombi. Br Heart J 1983; 50:127–134.
67. Ambrose JA, et al. Coronary angiographic morphology in myocardial infarction: a link between the pathogenesis of unstable angina and myocardial infarction. J Am Coll Cardiol 1985; 6:1233–1238.
68. Fuster V. Lewis A. Conner Memorial Lecture. Mechanisms leading to myocardial infarction: insights from studies of vascular biology. Circulation 1994; 90:2126–2146.
69. Lee RT, et al. Mechanical deformation promotes secretion of IL-1 alpha and IL-1 receptor antagonist. J Immunol 1997; 159:5084–5088.

70. Falk E. Why do plaques rupture? Circulation 1992; 86:30–42.
71. Loree HM, et al. Effects of fibrous cap thickness on peak circumferential stress in model atherosclerotic vessels. Circ Res 1992; 71:850–858.
72. van der Wal AC, et al. Site of intimal rupture or erosion of thrombosed coronary atherosclerotic plaques is characterized by an inflammatory process irrespective of the dominant plaque morphology. Circulation 1994; 89:36–44.
73. Moreno PR, et al. Macrophage infiltration in acute coronary syndromes. Implications for plaque rupture. Circulation 1994; 90:775–778.
74. Richardson PD, Davies MJ, Born GV. Influence of plaque configuration and stress distribution on fissuring of coronary atherosclerotic plaques. Lancet 1989; 2:941–944.
75. Miyao Y, et al. Elevated plasma interleukin-6 levels in patients with acute myocardial infarction. Am Heart J 1993; 126:1299–1304.
76. Pannitteri G, et al. Interleukins 6 and 8 as mediators of acute phase response in acute myocardial infarction. Am J Cardiol 1997; 80:622–625.
77. Biasucci LM, et al. Elevated levels of interleukin-6 in unstable angina. Circulation 1996; 94:874–877.
78. Marx N, et al. Induction of cytokine expression in leukocytes in acute myocardial infarction. J Am Coll Cardiol 1997; 30:165–170.
79. Neumann FJ, et al. Cardiac release of cytokines and inflammatory responses in acute myocardial infarction. Circulation 1995; 92:748–755.
80. Amento EP, et al. Cytokines and growth factors positively and negatively regulate interstitial collagen gene expression in human vascular smooth muscle cells. Arterioscler Thromb 1991; 11:1223–1230.
81. Hansson GK, et al. Immune mechanisms in atherosclerosis. Arteriosclerosis 1989; 9:567–578.
82. Rekhter MD, et al. Type I collagen gene expression in human atherosclerosis. Localization to specific plaque regions. Am J Pathol 1993; 143:1634–1648.
83. Warner SJ, Friedman GB, Libby P. Regulation of major histocompatibility gene expression in human vascular smooth muscle cells. Arteriosclerosis 1989; 9:279–288.
84. Galis ZS, et al. Cytokine-stimulated human vascular smooth muscle cells synthesize a complement of enzymes required for extracellular matrix digestion. Circ Res 1994; 75:181–189.
85. Saren P, Welgus HG, Kovanen PT. TNF-alpha and IL-1beta selectively induce expression of 92-kDa gelatinase by human macrophages. J Immunol 1996; 157:4159–4165.
86. Mach F, et al. Activation of monocyte/macrophage functions related to acute atheroma complication by ligation of CD40: induction of collagenase, stromelysin, and tissue factor. Circulation 1997; 96:396–399.
87. Rajavashisth TB, et al. Membrane type 1 matrix metalloproteinase expression in human atherosclerotic plaques: evidence for activation by proinflammatory mediators. Circulation 1999; 99:3103–3109.
88. Moreau M, et al. Interleukin-8 mediates downregulation of tissue inhibitor of metalloproteinase-1 expression in cholesterol-loaded human macrophages: relevance to stability of atherosclerotic plaque. Circulation 1999; 99:420–426.

89. Galis ZS, et al. Increased expression of matrix metalloproteinases and matrix degrading activity in vulnerable regions of human atherosclerotic plaques. J Clin Invest 1994; 94:2493–2503.

90. van der Wal AC, Becker AE. Atherosclerotic plaque rupture—pathologic basis of plaque stability and instability. Cardiovasc Res 1999; 41:334–344.

91. Fuster V, et al. Insights into the pathogenesis of acute ischemic syndromes. Circulation 1988; 77:1213–1220.

92. Lee RT, et al. Structure-dependent dynamic mechanical behavior of fibrous caps from human atherosclerotic plaques. Circulation 1991; 83:1764–1770.

93. Lin CS, et al. Morphodynamic interpretation of acute coronary thrombosis, with special reference to volcano-like eruption of atheromatous plaque caused by coronary artery spasm. Angiology 1988; 39:535–547.

94. Annex BH, et al. Differential expression of tissue factor protein in directional atherectomy specimens from patients with stable and unstable coronary syndromes. Circulation 1995; 91:619–622.

95. Moreno PR, et al. Macrophages, smooth muscle cells, and tissue factor in unstable angina. Implications for cell-mediated thrombogenicity in acute coronary syndromes. Circulation 1996; 94:3090–3097.

96. Wilcox JN, et al. Localization of tissue factor in the normal vessel wall and in the atherosclerotic plaque. Proc Natl Acad Sci U S A 1989; 86:2839–2843.

97. Neri Serneri G, et al. Transient intermittent lymphocyte activation is responsible for the instability of angina. Circulation 1992; 86:790–797.

98. Camerer E, et al. Cell biology of tissue factor, the principal initiator of blood coagulation. Thromb Res 1996; 81:1–41.

99. Hirsh PD, et al. Release of prostaglandins and thromboxane into the coronary circulation in patients with ischemic heart disease. N Engl J Med 1981; 304:685–691.

100. Fitzgerald DJ, et al. Platelet activation in unstable coronary disease. N Engl J Med 1986; 315:983–989.

101. Willerson JT, et al. Specific platelet mediators and unstable coronary artery lesions. Experimental evidence and potential clinical implications. Circulation 1989; 80: 198–205.

102. Shimokawa H, et al. Chronic treatment with interleukin-1 beta induces coronary intimal lesions and vasospastic responses in pigs in vivo. The role of platelet-derived growth factor. J Clin Invest 1996; 97:769–776.

103. Kohchi K, et al. Significance of adventitial inflammation of the coronary artery in patients with unstable angina: results at autopsy. Circulation 1985; 71:709–716.

104. Braunwald E. Shattuck Lecture—cardiovascular medicine at the turn of the millennium: triumphs, concerns, and opportunities. N Engl J Med 1997; 337:1360–1369.

105. Manson JE, et al. Primary Prevention of Myocardial Infarction. New York: Oxford University Press, 1997.

106. Ridker PM, Haughie P. Prospective studies of C-reactive protein as a risk factor for cardiovascular disease. J Invest Med 1998; 46:391–395.

107. Ridker P. Fibrinolytic and inflammatory markers for arterial occlusion: the evolving epidemiology of thrombosis and hemostasis. Thromb Haemost 1997; 78:53–59.

108. Harris TB, et al. Associations of elevated interleukin-6 and C-reactive protein levels with mortality in the elderly. Am J Med 1999; 106:506–512.

109. Ikonomidis I, et al. Increased proinflammatory cytokines in patients with chronic stable angina and their reduction by aspirin. Circulation 1999; 100:793–798.

110. Hwang SJ, et al. Circulating adhesion molecules VCAM-1, ICAM-1, and E-selectin in carotid atherosclerosis and incident coronary heart disease cases: the Atherosclerosis Risk In Communities (ARIC) study. Circulation 1997; 96:4219–4225.

111. Ridker PM, et al. Plasma concentration of soluble intercellular adhesion molecule 1 and risks of future myocardial infarction in apparently healthy men. Lancet 1998; 351:88–92.

112. Aukrust P, et al. Enhanced levels of soluble and membrane-bound CD40 ligand in patients with unstable angina. Possible reflection of T lymphocyte and platelet involvement in the pathogenesis of acute coronary syndromes. Circulation 1999; 100:614–620.

113. Kai H, et al. Peripheral blood levels of matrix metalloproteases-2 and -9 are elevated in patients with acute coronary syndromes. J Am Coll Cardiol 1998; 32:368–372.

114. Pepys MB, Baltz ML. Acute phase proteins with special reference to C-reactive protein and related proteins (pentaxins) and serum amyloid A protein. Adv Immunol 1983; 34:141–212.

115. Macy E, Hayes T, Tracy R. Variability in the measurement of C-reactive protein in healthy subjects: implications for reference interval and epidemiologic applications. Clin Chem 1997; 43:52–58.

116. Ledue TB, et al. Analytical evaluation of particle-enhanced immunonephelometric assays for C-reactive protein, serum amyloid A and mannose-binding protein in human serum. Ann Clin Biochem 1998; 35:745–753.

117. Wilkins J, et al. Rapid automated high sensitivity enzyme immunoassay of C-reactive protein. Clin Chem 1998; 44:1358–1361.

118. Rifai N, Tracy RP, Ridker PM. Clinical efficacy of an automated high-sensitivity C-reactive protein assay. Clin Chem 1999; 45:2136–2141.

119. Berk BC, Weintraub WS, Alexander RW. Elevation of C-reactive protein in "active" coronary artery disease. Am J Cardiol 1990; 65:168–172.

120. Pietila K, et al. C-reactive protein in subendocardial and transmural myocardial infarcts. Clin Chem 1986; 32:1596–1597.

121. Mendall MA, et al. C reactive protein and its relation to cardiovascular risk factors: a population based cross sectional study. Br Med J 1996; 312:1061–1065.

122. Ridker PM. Evaluating novel cardiovascular risk factors: can we better predict heart attacks? Ann Intern Med 1999; 130:933–937.

123. Tracy RP, et al. Lifetime smoking exposure affects the association of C-reactive protein with cardiovascular disease risk factors and subclinical disease in healthy elderly subjects. Arterioscler Thromb Vasc Biol 1997; 17:2167–2176.

124a. Kennon S, et al. The effect of aspirin on C-reactive protein as a marker of risk in unstable angina. J Am Coll Cardiol 2001; 37:1266–1270.

124b. Feldman M, et al. Effects of low-dose aspirin on serum C-reactive protein and thromboxane B2 concentrations: A placebo controlled study using a highly sensitive C-reactive protein assay. J Am Coll Cardiol 2001; 37:2036–2041.

125. Ridker PM, et al. Prospective study of C-reactive protein and the risk of future

cardiovascular events among apparently healthy women. Circulation 1998; 98: 731–733.

126. Koenig W, et al. C-reactive protein, a sensitive marker of inflammation, predicts future risk of coronary heart disease in initially healthy middle-aged men: Results from the MONICA (Monitoring trends and determinants in cardiovascular disease) Augsberg Cohort Study, 1984 to 1992. Circulation 1999; 99:237–242.

127. Tracy RP, et al. Relationship of C-reactive protein to risk of cardiovascular disease in the elderly. Results from the Cardiovascular Health Study and the Rural Health Promotion Project. Arterioscler Thromb Vasc Biol 1997; 17:1121–1127.

128. Ridker PM, et al. C-reactive protein and other markers of inflammation in the prediction of cardiovascular disease in women. N Engl J Med 2000; 342:836–843.

129. Danesh J, et al. Low grade inflammation and coronary heart disease: prospective study and updated meta-analyses. Br Med J 2000; 321:199–204.

130. Roivainen M, et al. Infections, inflammation, and the risk of coronary heart disease. Circulation 2000; 101:252–257.

130a. Ridker PM. High-sensitivity C-reactive protein: potential adjunct for global risk assessment in the primary prevention cardiovascular disease. Circulation 2001; 103:1813–1818.

131. Kuller LH, et al. Relation of C-reactive protein and coronary heart disease in the MRFIT nested case-control study. Multiple Risk Factor Intervention Trial. Am J Epidemiol 1996; 144:537–547.

132. Haverkate F, et al. Production of C-reactive protein and risk of coronary events in stable and unstable angina. European Concerted Action on Thrombosis and Disabilities Angina Pectoris Study Group. Lancet 1997; 349:462–466.

133. Liuzzo G, et al. The prognostic value of C-reactive protein and serum amyloid a protein in severe unstable angina. N Engl J Med 1994; 331:417–424.

134. Morrow DA, et al. C-Reactive protein is a potent predictor of mortality independently and in combination with troponin T in acute coronary syndromes. J Am Coll Cardiol 1998; 31:1460–1465.

135. Ridker PM, et al. Inflammation, pravastatin, and the risk of coronary events after myocardial infarction in patients with average cholesterol levels. Cholesterol and Recurrent Events (CARE) Investigators. Circulation 1998; 98:839–844.

136. Steering Committee of the Physicians' Health Study Research G. Final report on the aspirin component of the ongoing Physicians' Health Study. N Engl J Med 1989; 321:129–135.

137a. Ridker PM, et al. Plasma concentration of C-reactive protein and risk of developing peripheral vascular disease. Circulation 1998; 97:425–428.

137b. Ridker PM, et al. Novel risk factors for systemic atherosclerosis. A comparison of C-reactive protein, fibrinogen, homocysteine, lipoprotein(a), and standard cholesterol screening as predictors of peripheral arterial disease. JAMA 2001; 285: 2481–2485.

138. Ridker P, Glynn R, Hennekens C. C-reactive protein adds to the predictive value of total and HDL cholesterol in determining risk of first myocardial infarction. Circulation 1998; 97:2007–2011.

139. Cushman M, et al. Effect of postmenopausal hormones on inflammation-sensitive

proteins: the Postmenopausal Estrogen/Progestin Interventions (PEPI) Study. Circulation 1999; 100:717–722.

140. Cushman M, et al. Hormone replacement therapy, inflammation, and hemostasis in elderly women. Arterioscler Thromb Vasc Biol 1999; 19:893–899.

141. Ridker PM, et al. Hormone replacement therapy and increased plasma concentration of C-reactive protein. Circulation 1999; 100:713–716.

142. Hulley S, et al. Randomized trial of estrogen plus progestin for secondary prevention of coronary heart disease in postmenopausal women. Heart and Estrogen/Progestin Replacement Study (HERS) Research Group. JAMA 1998; 280:605–613.

143. Kushner I, Broder ML, Karp D. Control of the acute phase response. Serum C-reactive protein kinetics after acute myocardial infarction. J Clin Invest 1978; 61: 235–242.

144. de Beer FC, et al. Measurement of serum C-reactive protein concentration in myocardial ischaemia and infarction. Br Heart J 1982; 47:239–243.

145. Voulgari F, et al. Serum levels of acute phase and cardiac proteins after myocardial infarction, surgery, and infection. Br Heart J 1982; 48:352–356.

146. Ikeda U, et al. Serum interleukin 6 levels become elevated in acute myocardial infarction. J Mol Cell Cardiol 1992; 24:579–584.

147. Anzai T, et al. C-reactive protein as a predictor of infarct expansion and cardiac rupture after a first Q-wave acute myocardial infarction. Circulation 1997; 96:778–784.

148. Ferreiros ER, et al. Independent prognostic value of elevated C-reactive protein in unstable angina. Circulation 1999; 100:1958–1963.

149. Toss H, et al. Prognostic influence of increased fibrinogen and C-reactive protein levels in unstable coronary artery disease. FRISC Study Group. Fragmin during Instability in Coronary Artery Disease. Circulation 1997; 96:4204–4210.

150. Rebuzzi A, et al. Incremental prognostic value of serum levels of troponin T and C-reactive protein on admission in patients with unstable angina pectoris. Am J Cardiol 1998; 82:715–719.

151. Benamer H, et al. Comparison of the prognostic value of C-reactive protein and troponin I in patients with unstable angina pectoris. Am J Cardiol 1998; 82:845–850.

152. Oltrona L, et al. C-reactive protein elevation and early outcome in patients with unstable angina pectoris. Am J Cardiol 1997; 80:1002–1006.

153. Biasucci L, et al. Elevated levels of C-reactive protein at discharge in patients with unstable angina predict recurrent instability. Circulation 1999; 99:855–860.

154. Pietila KO, et al. Serum C-reactive protein concentration in acute myocardial infarction and its relationship to mortality during 24 months of follow-up in patients under thrombolytic treatment. Eur Heart J 1996; 17:1345–1349.

155. Pietila K, et al. Intravenous streptokinase treatment and serum C-reactive protein in patients with acute myocardial infarction. Br Heart J 1987; 58:225–229.

156. Pietila K, et al. Serum C-reactive protein and infarct size in myocardial infarct patients with a closed versus an open infarct-related coronary artery after thrombolytic therapy. Eur Heart J 1993; 14:915–919.

157. Pietila K, et al. Comparison of peak serum C-reactive protein and hydroxybutyrate dehydrogenase levels in patients with acute myocardial infarction treated with alteplase and streptokinase. Am J Cardiol 1997; 80:1075–1077.

158. Pudil R, et al. The effect of reperfusion on plasma tumor necrosis factor alpha and C reactive protein levels in the course of acute myocardial infarction. Acta Medica 1996; 39:149–153.

159. Andreotti F, et al. Early coronary reperfusion blunts the procoagulant response of plasminogen activator inhibitor-1 and von Willebrand factor in acute myocardial infarction. J Am Coll Cardiol 1990; 16:1553–1560.

160. Bataille R, Klein B. C-reactive protein levels as a direct indicator of interleukin-6 levels in humans in vivo. Arthr Rheum 1992; 35:982–984.

161. Van Snick J. Interleukin-6: an overview. Ann Rev Immunol 1990; 8:253–278.

162. Mestries JC, et al. In vivo modulation of coagulation and fibrinolysis by recombinant glycosylated human interleukin-6 in baboons. Euro Cyto Netw 1994; 5:275–281.

163. Stouthard JM, et al. Interleukin-6 stimulates coagulation, not fibrinolysis, in humans. Thromb Haemost 1996; 76:738–742.

164. Biasucci LM, et al. Increasing levels of interleukin (IL)-1Ra and IL-6 during the first 2 days of hospitalization in unstable angina are associated with increased risk of in-hospital coronary events. Circulation 1999; 99:2079–2084.

165. Ridker PM, et al. Plasma concentration of interleukin-6 and the risk of future myocardial infarction among apparently healthy men. Circulation 2000; 101:1767–1772.

166. Danesh J, et al. Association of fibrinogen, C-reactive protein, albumin, or leukocyte count with coronary heart disease: meta-analyses of prospective studies. JAMA 1998; 279:1477–1482.

167. Ridker PM, et al. Elevation of tumor necrosis factor—alpha and increased risk of recurrent coronary events following myocardial infarction. Circulation 2000; 101:2149–2153.

168. Crea F, et al. Role of inflammation in the pathogenesis of unstable coronary artery disease. Am J Cardiol 1997; 80:10E–16E.

169. Kukielka GL, et al. Induction of interleukin-6 synthesis in the myocardium. Potential role in postreperfusion inflammatory injury. Circulation 1995; 92:1866–1875.

170. Hawkins HK, et al. Acute inflammatory reaction after myocardial ischemic injury and reperfusion. Development and use of a neutrophil-specific antibody. Am J Pathol 1996; 148:1957–1969.

171. Gwechenberger M, et al. Cardiac Myocytes Produce Interleukin-6 in Culture and in Viable Border Zone of Reperfused Infarctions. Circulation 1999; 99:546–551.

172. Liuzzo G, et al. Plasma protein acute-phase response in unstable angina is not induced by ischemic injury. Circulation 1996; 94:2373–2380.

173. Biasucci LM, et al. Episodic activation of the coagulation system in unstable angina does not elicit an acute phase reaction. Am J Cardiol 1996; 77:85–87.

174. Reynolds GD, Vance RP. C-reactive protein immunohistochemical localization in normal and atherosclerotic human aortas. Arch Pathol Lab Med 1987; 111:265–269.

175. Torzewski J, et al. C-reactive protein frequently colocalizes with the terminal complement complex in the intima of early atherosclerotic lesions of human coronary arteries. Arterioscler Thromb Vasc Biol 1998; 18:1386–1392.

176. Cermak J, et al. C-reactive protein induces human peripheral blood monocytes to synthesize tissue factor. Blood 1993; 82:513–520.

177. Zouki C, et al. Prevention of in vitro neutrophil adhesion to endothelial cells through shedding of L-selectin by C-reactive protein and peptides derived from C-reactive protein. J Clin Invest 1997; 100:522–529.

178. Wolbink GJ, et al. CRP-mediated activation of complement in vivo: assessment by measuring circulating complement-C-reactive protein complexes. J Immunol 1996; 157:473–479.

179. Azar RR, et al. Relation of C-reactive protein to extent and severity of coronary narrowing in patients with stable angina pectoris or abnormal exercise tests. Am J Cardiol 2000; 86:205–206.

180. Redberg RF, et al. Lack of association of C-reactive protein and coronary calcium by electron beam computed tomography in postmenopausal women: implications for coronary artery disease screening. J Am Coll Cardiol 2000; 36:39–43.

181. Sinisalo J, et al. Relation of inflammation to vascular function in patients with coronary heart disease. Atherosclerosis 2000; 149:403–411.

182. Fichtlscherer S, et al. Elevated C-reactive protein levels and impaired endothelial vasoreactivity in patients with coronary artery disease. Circulation 2000; 102: 1000–1006.

183. Ridker PM, Glynn RJ, Hennekens CH. C-reactive protein adds to the predictive value of total and HDL cholesterol in determining risk of first myocardial infarction. Circulation 1998; 97:2007–2011.

184. Rifai N, Ridker P. A Proposed cardiovascular risk assessment algorithm employing high-sensitivity C-reactive protein and lipid screening. Clin Chem 2001; 47:28–30.

185. Vaughan CJ, Murphy MB, Buckley BM. Statins do more than just lower cholesterol. Lancet 1996; 348:1079–1082.

186. Ridker PM, et al. Long-term effects of pravastatin on plasma concentration of C-reactive protein. Circulation 1999; 100:230–235.

187. Kurakata S, et al. Effects of different inhibitors of 3-hydroxy-3-methylglutaryl coenzyme A (HMG-CoA) reductase, pravastatin sodium and simvastatin, on sterol synthesis and immunological functions in human lymphocytes in vitro. Immunopharmacology 1996; 34:51–61.

188. Aikawa M, et al. An HMG-CoA reductase inhibitor (cervistatin) suppresses accumulation of macrophages expressing matrix metalloproteinases and tissue factor in atheroma of WHHL rabbits. Circulation 1998; 98:47.

189. Munro E, et al. Inhibition of human vascular smooth muscle cell proliferation by lovastatin: the role of isoprenoid intermediates of cholesterol synthesis. Eur J Clin Invest 1994; 24:766–772.

190. Rogler G, Lackner KJ, Schmitz G. Effects of fluvastatin on growth of porcine and human vascular smooth muscle cells in vitro. Am J Cardiol 1995; 76:114A–116A.

191. Rosenson RS, Tangney CC. Antiatherothrombotic properties of statins: implications for cardiovascular event reduction. JAMA 1998; 279:1643–1650.

192. Corsini A, et al. Non-lipid-related effects of 3-hydroxy-3-methylglutaryl coenzyme A reductase inhibitors. Cardiology 1996; 87:458–468.

193. Shiomi M, et al. Reduction of serum cholesterol levels alters lesional composition of atherosclerotic plaques. Effect of pravastatin sodium on atherosclerosis in mature WHHL rabbits. Arterioscler Thromb Vasc Biol 1995; 15:1938–1944.

194. Williams JK, et al. Pravastatin has cholesterol-lowering independent effects on the artery wall of atherosclerotic monkeys. J Am Coll Cardiol 1998; 31:684–691.

195. Aikawa M, et al. Lipid lowering by diet reduces matrix metalloproteinase activity and increases collagen content of rabbit atheroma: a potential mechanism of lesion stabilization. Circulation 1998; 97:2433–2444.

196. Albert MA, et al. for the PRINCE investigators. Effect of statin therapy on C-reactive protein levels. The Pravastatin Inflammation/CRP Evaluation (PRINCE): A randomized trial and cohort study. JAMA 2001; 286:64–70.

197. Ridker PM, et al. Rapid reduction in C-reactive protein with cerivastatin among 785 patients with primary hypercholesterolemia. Circulation 2001; 103:1191–1193.

198. Jialal I, et al. Effect of hydroxymethyl glutaryl coenzyme A reductase inhibitor therapy on high sensitive C-reactive protein levels. Circulation 2001; 103:1933–1935.

199. Cortellaro M, et al. Effects of fluvastatin and bezafibrate combination on plasma fibrinogen, t-plasminogen activator inhibitor and C-reactive protein levels in coronary artery disease patients with mixed hyperlipidemia (FACT study). Thromb Hemost 2000; 83:549–553.

200. Ridker PM, et al. Measurement of C-reactive protein for the targeting of statin therapy in the primary prevention of acute coronary events. N Engl J Med 2001; 344:1959–1965.

2

Homocysteine and Vascular Disease Risk

Peter W. F. Wilson
Boston University School of Medicine, Boston, Massachusetts

I. METABOLISM

Several decades ago, homocystinuria, a rare pediatric condition, was noted to be associated with musculoskeletal abnormalities and the development of venous thromboembolism and arterial disease in adolescence. The underlying metabolic defect for this condition was shown to be decreased enzymatic activity of cystathionine beta-synthase (1). This deficiency was associated with increased levels of methionine and homocysteine and a decrease in blood levels of cysteine. Later investigations of a patient with elevated homocysteine levels and similar clinical findings, but with a low concentration of methionine in the plasma and evidence of abnormal vitamin B_{12} metabolism, led to the conclusion that another defect could account for elevated homocysteine levels and vascular disease (2,3).

The metabolism for homocysteine has become more clear over time and it is now evident that there is a methionine cycle, a folate cycle, and a transsulfuration pathway (Fig. 1). Defects in transsulfuration, especially congenital deficiency of cystathionine beta-synthase, may account for some of the persons with elevated homocysteine concentrations, and other pathways were important for the recycling of homocysteine to methionine. Vitamins in the B group often acted as cofactors for reactions at several of the key branching points in the pathways.

Assays for homocysteine improved and researchers reported that mildly increased homocysteine levels were associated with premature vascular disease, and those affected had no obvious genetic defects (3). Furthermore, mild eleva-

35

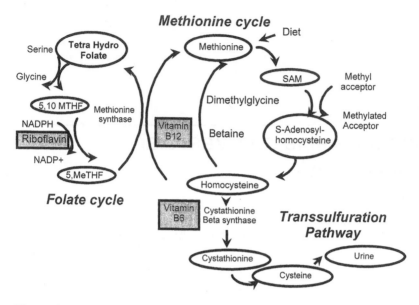

Figure 1 Metabolic pathways for homocysteine.

tions in homocysteine levels were relatively common (4). This brief review will focus on the determinants of homocysteine and the consequences of elevated levels in the population setting, emphasizing some of the most recent vascular disease studies.

II. POPULATION LEVELS AND DETERMINANTS

A large variety of factors have been associated with increased levels of homocysteine, and only the key topics in healthy outpatients will be considered here (Table 1) (5). Fasting blood homocysteine concentrations are typically greater in the elderly compared with middle-aged adults, and higher in men than in women. Analyses of the Framingham Heart Study and the National Health and Nutrition Examination Survey data have shown that the prevalence of elevated homocysteine (>14 μmol/L) increases with age in both sexes, and plasma homocysteine levels are inversely correlated with vitamin intake (Fig. 2) (6,7). Vitamins B_1, B_2, B_6, B_{12}, folate, niacin, retinol, vitamin C, and vitamin E have all been studied, but the greatest interest has been shown for vitamins B_6, B_{12}, and folate, as these nutrients act as cofactors for several homocysteine metabolic pathways. The two lowest deciles of folate, the lowest decile of vitamin B_{12}, and the lowest decile

Table 1 Factors Associated with
Elevated Homocysteine Levels

Enzyme deficiencies and mutations
Cystathionine beta-synthase
Methionine synthase
Methylenetetrahydrofolate reductase
Cobalamin mutations
Vitamin deficiencies
Folate
Vitamin B_6
Vitamin B_{12}
Increased methionine consumption
Demographics
Increasing age
Male sex
Postmenopausal status
Medical disorders
Renal insufficiency
Hypothyroidism
Drugs
Antifolate medications (methotrexate)
Vitamin B_{12} antagonists (nitrous oxide)
Bile acid resins
Thiazide diuretics
Cyclosporine

Source: Ref. 5.

of pyridoxal phosphate were significantly associated with higher mean levels of homocysteine in the older Framingham Heart Study participants (6). Similarly, homocysteine concentrations were elevated among participants in the Health Professionals Study, who consumed <280 μg/day of folate. Data from the early 1990s in Framingham showed that suboptimal vitamin B_6 (pyridoxine), vitamin B_{12}, or folate were relatively common, and approximately 25 to 30% of adults were affected (6). Moderately elevated homocysteine levels frequently accompanied these subclinical deficiencies. Recently published homocysteine and B vitamin data from the National Health and Nutrition Examination Survey generally corroborate the patterns above: homocysteine levels typically were greater in men than women; positively associated with age; and inversely associated with vitamin B_{12} and folate. Reference ranges were developed for American adults, and, as an example, the 95th percentile of homocysteine range was 12.9 μmol/L in men and 10.2 μmol/L in women 40 to 59 years of age (8).

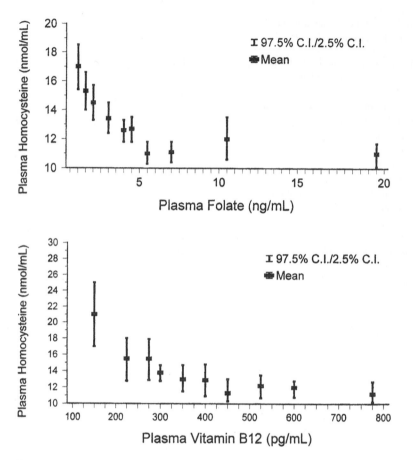

Figure 2 Relations between homocysteine levels and plasma levels of vitamin B$_{12}$ and folate. (From Ref. 6.)

Naturally occurring sources of folate in the diet include orange juice and green, leafy vegetables. Cold breakfast cereals are often fortified with folate and recently this food item has become an increasingly important source of dietary folate. There are strong positive associations between cereal consumption and plasma folate levels, but the relation plateaus near five to six servings per week of cereal (9). Approximately one-quarter of the adult population in the United States consumes vitamin supplements that contain folate (and often vitamins B$_6$ and B$_{12}$) and these persons tend to have lower homocysteine levels (10).

Low vitamin B$_{12}$ status can also account for elevated homocysteine levels, as this vitamin is a necessary cofactor in several homocysteine metabolic steps. Inadequate production of intrinsic factor in the stomach can result in a severe vitamin B$_{12}$ deficiency, with substantially elevated homocysteine concentrations, but this etiology is an infrequent cause of low vitamin B$_{12}$ status. Hypochlorhydria and achlorhydria are more common than inadequate intrinsic factor deficiency, especially in older individuals, and can lead to impaired absorption of vitamin B$_{12}$ because low pH is needed to dissociate B$_{12}$ from food.

Studies of birth defects showed that inadequate folate intake in the early stages of pregnancy was associated with fetal abnormalities such as spina bifida and anencephaly (11,12). Increased folate in the diet showed promise in preventing the occurrence of these birth defects, and in 1996 the Food and Drug Administration mandated fortification of American flour and cereal products made on or before January 1, 1998. Framingham analyses estimated that the fraction of persons with a dietary folate intake <200 µg/day would decline from 18 to 8% and that the prevalence of homocysteine levels >14 µmol/L would decrease from 26 to 22% of the population (Fig. 3) (9). In fact, nutritional and biochemical data from the Framingham Offspring subjects who were not taking folate supplements demonstrated a reduction in the prevalence of folate deficiency and a dramatic decline in the prevalence of elevated homocysteine levels (>13 µmol/L) from 18.7% before fortification to 9.8% after fortification (Table 2) (13).

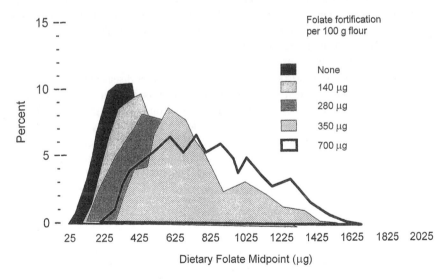

Figure 3 Estimated effects of folate fortification on a population basis, taken from Framingham experience. (From Ref. 9.)

Table 2 Plasma Folate and Homocysteine Concentrations Before and After Folic Acid Fortification (Framingham Offspring Study Participants not Taking Vitamin B Supplements)

Characteristic	Study group[a] (n = 248)	Control group (n = 553)
Plasma folate < 3 ng/mL (%)		
Baseline	22.0 (17.3–26.7)[b]	25.3 (22.1–28.4)
Follow-up	1.7 (0.0–5.4)	20.7 (18.3–23.2)
Fasting total homocysteine > 13 μmol/L (%)		
Baseline	18.7 (14.5–22.9)	17.6 (14.8–20.4)
Follow-up	9.8 (5.6–14.0)	21.0 (18.2–23.8)

[a] Study group was examined before exposure to foods fortified with folic acid (baseline) and approximately 3 years later, after exposure to fortification (follow-up). The control group was examined before fortification on two occasions separated by approximately 3 years.
[b] Numbers in parentheses are the 95% confidence intervals for the estimates.
Source: Ref. 7.

III. GENETICS

There are many genetic causes of elevated homocysteine levels. Enzymatic defects and variants have been associated with cystathionine beta-synthetase, methylene tetrahydrofolate reductase (MTHFR), thermolabile and nonthermolabile variants, and methionine synthetase, to name a few. The MTHFR variant 677-C → T has gotten the most attention, as it is relatively common and affects 10 to 15% of North Americans and 5 to 25% of Europeans. This MTHFR variant has also been studied for associations with cardiovascular disease (14), and homozygosity has generally been associated with an increased occurrence of disease; however, several studies demonstrated no association between the MTHFR and vascular outcomes. A meta-analysis concluded that a modest association with increased risk for cardiovascular disease was present (15). The inconsistent association between MTHFR variants and vascular disease may be partially explained by population dietary data. Persons homozygous for MTHFR 677-C → T and who had suboptimal folate status were especially likely to have elevated homocysteine levels (16).

Variants of methionine synthase, one of the enzymes responsible for remethylation of homocysteine to methionine, are also being studied for associations with vascular disease. This enzyme is dependent upon B$_{12}$ nutrition and metabolism, and deficiencies of this enzyme are associated with elevated homocysteine, low methionine, and neurological disorders. Studies of potential associations between methionine synthase variants and vascular disease are underway (17).

IV. CARDIOVASCULAR DISEASE RISK

Increased homocysteine levels are more common in persons who develop athero-sclerotic vascular disease (18), and evidence has been derived from observational studies of coronary heart disease. Positive associations between elevated homo-cysteine levels and carotid stenosis, stroke, and peripheral vascular disease have all been reported. A meta-analysis concerning homocysteine levels and athero-sclerotic disease has also been undertaken and reached the conclusion that a 5 μmol/L increment in homocysteine levels was associated with a 1.6-fold risk for coronary artery disease in men and a 1.8-fold risk in women. The authors con-cluded that 10% of coronary artery disease risk could be attributed to homocyste-ine elevations (Fig. 4) (19).

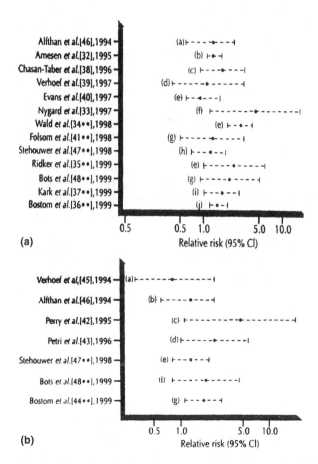

Figure 4   Odds ratio for coronary artery disease associated with a 5 μmol/L difference in homocysteine in group of observational studies. (From Ref. 18.)

More recent population reports generally show a positive association between higher homocysteine levels and lower vitamin B intake and coronary artery disease. As an example, the European Concerted Action Project (COMAC), involving 750 European men and women with vascular disease and a similar number of controls, showed that a homocysteine level >12 μmol/L (the top 20% of the homocysteine distribution for controls), was associated with significantly elevated odds ratios for all vascular disease, coronary heart disease, cerebrovascular disease, and peripheral vascular disease (19).

Other studies have not always corroborated these results. In some instances, the associations with adverse outcomes were demonstrated for nutrient status, but not for homocysteine levels. For instance, higher homocysteine levels were not associated with greater risk in a MRFIT-nested case-control analysis (20); the ARIC study demonstrated higher folate and B_6 intake to be associated with lower CVD risk but associations with higher homocysteine were not significant (21); and the Nurses' Health Study investigators found that higher folate and B_6 intake was associated with lower cardiovascular risk (22). Elevated homocysteine concentrations in the plasma may potentiate thrombin generation and may have relevance in the setting of acute coronary syndromes. A study of approximately 100 persons with acute coronary syndromes was found to have positive associations with F1 + 2 and Factor VIIa levels (23). It has been proposed that hyperhomocysteinemia potentiates a procoagulant state that may adversely affect the endothelium and enhance tissue factor activity (24).

Large-scale interventional data that reduce homocysteine levels and demonstrate favorable effects on cardiovascular risk are lacking, but vitamin supplements are being included in a variety of ongoing studies and the results should be forthcoming (5). The minimal daily dose of folic acid that appears to have maximal efficacy to decrease plasma homocysteine is estimated as 0.4 μg/day, with higher doses not generally being more effective. It is recommended that vitamin B_{12} deficiency be ruled out prior to initiating folic acid therapy. Alternatively, persons on folic acid therapy can be supplemented with a dose of 400 to 1000 μg/day of vitamin B_{12}. The dose of vitamin B_6 recommended was 25 to 50 mg/day and there is little risk of developing complications such as sensory neuropathy at this supplement level (5).

V. ELDERLY AND MORTALITY RISK

Data from elderly subjects have shown associations between homocysteine levels and a variety of vascular outcomes (25–27). A cross-sectional study demonstrated an association between elevated homocysteine levels and moderate degrees of carotid stenosis (25), and more recent prospective investigations have been undertaken. A 10-year follow-up study from Framingham showed that persons with homocysteine >14 μmol/L have 1.5 times greater odds of total mortality and cardiovascular mortality than persons with levels below that threshold. This relation was evident even after adjustment for the usual cardiovascular risk factors of age, gender, diabetes, smoking, systolic blood pressure, total cholesterol, and HDL cholesterol (27). Homocysteine was also found to be associated with an increased risk for incident stroke among Framingham participants. In proportional hazards models that adjusted for age, sex, systolic blood pressure, diabetes, smoking, and history of atrial fibrillation and prevalent coronary heart disease, the odds ratio for stroke was 1.82 (95% CI 1.14–2.91) for persons in the top quartile of homocysteine (26). An increased risk of death has also been reported in middle-aged and elderly men and women from Jerusalem. This investigation included more than 11 years of follow-up for approximately 1800 persons >50 years of age at baseline, and showed an increasing risk of death for greater quintiles of homocysteine, and the hazard ratios were 1.0, 1.4, 1.3, 1.5, and 2.0 ($p < 0.001$ for trend) (28).

Although the pathogenic mechanisms are not definite, current models favor direct angiotoxicity involving endothelial and vascular smooth muscle cells, as well as impaired thrombolysis. Testing for homocysteine has not been recommended as a component of population screening for cardiovascular disease risk factors. The American Heart Association Nutrition Committee recommended measuring homocysteine levels in "high-risk patients with a strong family history for premature atherosclerosis or with arterial occlusive diseases, particularly in the absence of other risk factors, as well as in members of their families" (29).

VI. DIABETES AND RENAL DISEASE

Interest in homocysteine levels among diabetics has grown over the past few years. Elevated homocysteine levels do not appear to be more common in type 1 diabetics (30), but a different situation may hold when renal impairment is present. Elevated levels are common in diabetes and are particularly associated with mild increases in serum creatinine and urinary excretion of albumin in type 1 diabetes (31). Young diabetics who smoke have been reported to have higher homocysteine levels than diabetic nonsmokers (32). Similarly, the Hoorn Study in the Netherlands demonstrated very strong associations between elevated homocysteine and death and disease in a nested case-control study that included approximately 800 subjects. In this study, the relative odds for mortality was similar for elevated homocysteine (>14 μmol/L), hypertension, current smoking, and elevated cholesterol (>200 mg/dL). The authors report emphasized that the homocysteine associations were stronger in diabetic than in nondiabetic participants (33).

An intriguing new research area is the role of homocysteine levels and atherosclerotic disease among persons with renal disease, as it is appreciated that heart disease, particularly atherosclerotic disease, is an important cause of debility and death in dialysis patients. While mean levels of homocysteine are approximately 10 μmol/L in healthy adults and 14 to 15 μmol/L in coronary disease cases, higher levels are commonly observed in persons with end-stage renal disease, where levels are typically in the 20 to 30 μmol/L range (34–36). These elevations are often present despite regular use of folate supplementation and demonstration of normal folate levels in the plasma. Recent cross-sectional data from Rhode Island dialysis patients suggest that elevated homocysteine levels are present even after folate fortification was instituted, and clinical trials of high-dose folate supplementation for renal patients have been suggested as a tactic to prevent atherosclerotic disease in this high-risk patient group (36).

VII. INCORPORATION OF NEW RISK FACTORS INTO PREDICTION OF CORONARY HEART DISEASE

New factors associated with increased risk for coronary heart disease arouse great interest and enthusiasm, kindling the hope that we may enhance identification of individuals at risk for CHD. Important concerns are that such metabolic factors be biologically plausible, measurable, repeatable, strong, graded, and treatable (37–39). Measurement issues include accuracy and precision for the factor in the laboratory and evidence of low or modest variability in the clinical setting. If the laboratory or biological variability is very large, the utility of the measurement for predictive purposes is seriously reduced. Many years of experience and standardization of measurements are available for some vascular risk factors, and less experience is available for homocysteine. New risk factors may provide clues to pathogenesis and in some instances may improve our ability to predict disease. The ability to predict new vascular disease events should be demonstrated after consideration of the core set of factors that are currently available, including age, sex, blood pressure, cholesterol or LDL cholesterol, HDL cholesterol, smoking, and diabetes mellitus. This criterion is often not met in new investigations and considerable experience and relatively large data sets and follow-up may be necessary to assure that new factors, such as homocysteine, prove useful in predicting vascular disease risk.

VIII. SUMMARY

Higher homocysteine levels have been associated with a greater risk of coronary artery disease, carotid stenosis, stroke, and cardiovascular disease in general (25–27). A meta-analysis demonstrated the results are consistent across a variety of population groups (18). Elevated homocysteine levels may be accompanied by decreased blood levels and intake of folate, vitamin B_6, or vitamin B_{12} (6). These vitamins are important cofactors in the metabolism of homocysteine, and borderline deficiencies are relatively common, affecting approximately 30% of the elderly participants in the Framingham Heart Study (6). Greater intake of these vitamins in the diet, with supplements in the form of multivitamins, or through fortification of foods, has led to less vitamin deficiency and a decrease in the prevalence of elevated homocysteine levels (6,9). Fortification of the food supply in the United States with folate was announced in early 1996 with a mandated enactment date of January 1, 1998. Analyses of homocysteine and folate levels before and after fortification have been undertaken in Framingham Heart Study participants and showed a dramatic decline in the prevalence of low folate levels, a reduction in the prevalence of elevated homocysteine from approximately 20 to 10%, and a modest decrease in mean homocysteine levels from approximately 10 to 9 μmol/L (13).

REFERENCES

1. Mudd SH, Finkelstein IF, Laster L. Homocystinuria: An enzymatic defect. Science 1964; 143:1443.
2. Mudd SH, Levy HL, Abeles RH, Jennedy JP Jr. A derangement in B_{12} metabolism leading to homocystinemia, cystathioninemia and methylmalonic aciduria. Biochem Biophys Res Commun 1969; 35:121.
3. McCully KS. Vascular pathology of homocysteinemia: implications for the pathogenesis of arteriosclerosis. Am J Pathol 1969; 56:111.
4. Lee TH, Juarez G, Cook EF, Weisberg MC, Rouan GW, Brand DA, Goldman L. Ruling out acute myocardial infarction: a prospective multicenter validation of a 12-hour strategy for patients at low risk. N Engl J Med 1991; 324:1239.
5. Eikelboom JW, Lonn E, Genest J Jr, Hankey G, Yusuf S. Homocyst(e)ine and cardiovascular disease: a critical review of the epidemiologic evidence. Ann Intern Med 1999; 131:363.
6. Selhub J, Jacques PF, Wilson PWF, Rush D, Rosenberg IH. Vitamin status and intake as primary determinants of homocysteinemia in the elderly. JAMA 1993; 270:2693.
7. Jacques PF, Rosenberg IH, Rogers G, Selhub J, Bowman BA, Gunter EW, Wright JD, Johnson CL. Serum total homocysteine concentrations in adolescent and adult Americans: results from the third National Health and Nutrition Examination Survey. Am J Clin Nutr 1999; 69:482.
8. Selhub J, Jacques PF, Rosenberg IH, Rogers G, Bowman BA, Gunter EW, Wright JD, Johnson CL. Serum total homocysteine concentrations in the third National Health and Nutrition Examination Survey (1991–1994): population reference ranges and contribution of vitamin status to high serum concentrations. Ann Intern Med 1999; 131:331.

9. Tucker KL, Mahnken B, Wilson PW, Jacques P, Selhub J. Folic acid fortification of the food supply. Potential benefits and risks for the elderly population. JAMA 1996; 276:1879.

10. Jacques PF, Rosenberg IH, Rogers G, Selhub J, Bowman BA, Gunter EW, Wright JD, Johnson CL. Serum total homocysteine concentrations in adolescent and adult Americans: results from the third National Health and Nutrition Examination Survey (NHANES III). Am J Clin Nutr 1998; 67:722.

11. Botto LD, Moore CA, Khoury MJ, Erickson JD. Neural-tube defects. N Engl J Med 1999; 341:1509.

12. Berry RJ, Li Z, Erickson JD, Li S, Moore CA, Wang H, Mulinare J, Zhao P, Wong LY, Gindler J, Hong SX, Correa A. Prevention of neural-tube defects with folic acid in China. China-U.S. Collaborative Project for Neural Tube Defect Prevention. N Engl J Med 1999; 341:1485.

13. Jacques PF, Selhub J, Bostom AG, Wilson PW, Rosenberg IH. The effect of folic acid fortification on plasma folate and total homocysteine concentrations. N Engl J Med 1999; 340:1449.

14. Gallagher PM, Meleady R, Shields DC, Tan KS, McMaster D, Rozen R, Evans A, Graham IM, Whitehead AS. Homocysteine and risk of premature coronary heart disease. Evidence for a common gene mutation. Circulation 1996; 94: 2154.

15. Kluijtmans LA, Kastelein JJ, Lindemans J, Boers GH, Heil SG, Bruschke AV, Jukema JW, van den Heuvel LP, Trijbels FJ, Boerma GJ, Verheugt FW, Willems F, Blom HJ. Thermolabile methylenetetrahydrofolate reductase in coronary artery disease. Circulation 1997; 96:2573.

16. Jacques PF, Bostom AG, Williams RR, Ellison RC, Eckfeldt JH, Rosenberg IH, Selhub J, Rozen R. Relation between folate status, a common mutation in methylenetetrahydrofolate reductase, and plasma homocysteine concentrations. Circulation 1996; 93:7.

17. van der Put NM, van der Molen EF, Kluijtmans LA, Heil SG, Trijbels JM, Eskes TK, Oppenraaij-Emmerzaal D, Banerjee R, Blom HJ. Sequence analysis of the coding region of human methionine synthase: relevance to hyperhomocysteinaemia in neural-tube defects and vascular disease. Q J Med 1997; 90:511.

18. Boushey CJ, Beresford SAS, Omenn GS, Motulsky AG. A quantitative assessment of plasma homocysteine as a risk factor for vascular disease: Probable benefits of increasing folic acid intakes. JAMA 1995; 274:1049.

19. Graham IM, Daly LE, Refsum HM, Robinson K, Brattstrom LE, Ueland PM, Palma-Reis RJ, Boers GH, Sheahan RG, Israelsson B, Uiterwaal CS, Meleady R, McMaster D, Verhoef P, Witteman J, Rubba P, Bellet H, Wautrecht JC, de Valk HW, Sales Luis AC, Parrot-Rouland FM, Tan KS, Higgins I, Garcon D, Andria G, et al. Plasma homocysteine as a risk factor for vascular disease. The European Concerted Action Project. JAMA 1997; 277:1775.

20. Evans RW, Shaten BJ, Hempel JD, Cutler JA, Kuller LH. Homocyst(e)ine and risk of cardiovascular disease in the Multiple Risk Factor Intervention Trial. Arterioscler Thromb Vasc Biol 1997; 17:1947.

21. Folsom AR, Nieto FJ, McGovern PG, Tsai MY, Malinow MR, Eckfeldt JH, Hess DL, Davis CE. Prospective study of coronary heart disease incidence in relation

to fasting total homocysteine, related genetic polymorphisms, and B vitamins: the Atherosclerosis Risk in Communities (ARIC) study. Circulation 1998; 98:204.

22. Rimm EB, Willett WC, Hu FB, Sampson L, Colditz GA, Manson JE, Hennekens C, Stampfer MJ. Folate and vitamin B_6 from diet and supplements in relation to risk of coronary heart disease among women. JAMA 1998; 279:359.

23. Al Obaidi MK, Philippou H, Stubbs PJ, Adami A, Amersey R, Noble MM, Lane DA. Relationships between homocysteine, factor VIIa, and thrombin generation in acute coronary syndromes. Circulation 2000; 101:372.

24. Fryer RH, Wilson BD, Gubler DB, Fitzgerald LA, Rodgers GM. Homocysteine, a risk factor for premature vascular disease and thrombosis, induces tissue factor activity in endothelial cells. Arterioscler Thromb 1993; 13:1327.

25. Selhub J, Jacques PF, Bostom AG, D'Agostino RB, Wilson PWF, Belanger AJ, O'Leary DH, Wolf PA, Schaefer EJ, Rosenberg IH. Association between plasma homocysteine and extracranial carotid stenosis. N Engl J Med 1995; 332:286.

26. Bostom AG, Rosenberg IH, Silbershatz H, Jacques PF, Selhub J, D'Agostino RB, Wilson PW, Wolf PA. Nonfasting plasma total homocysteine levels and stroke incidence in elderly persons: the Framingham Study. Ann Intern Med 1999; 131:352.

27. Bostom AG, Silbershatz H, Rosenberg IH, Selhub J, D'Agostino RB, Wolf PA, Jacques PF, Wilson PW. Nonfasting plasma total homocysteine levels and all-cause and cardiovascular disease mortality in elderly Framingham men and women. Arch Intern Med 1999; 159:1077.

28. Kark JD, Selhub J, Adler B, Gofin J, Abramson JH, Friedman G, Rosenberg IH. Nonfasting plasma total homocysteine level and mortality in middle-aged and elderly men and women in Jerusalem. Ann Intern Med 1999; 131:321.

29. Malinow MR, Bostom AG, Krauss RM. Homocyst(e)ine, diet, and cardiovascular diseases: a statement for healthcare professionals from the Nutrition Committee, American Heart Association. Circulation 1999; 99:178.

30. Pavia C, Ferrer I, Valls C, Artuch R, Colome C, Vilaseca MA. Total homocysteine in patients with type 1 diabetes [In Process Citation]. Diabetes Care 2000; 23:84.

31. Hofmann MA, Kohl B, Zumbach MS, Borcea V, Bierhaus A, Henkels M, Amiral J, Fiehn W, Ziegler R, Wahl P, Nawroth PP. Hyperhomocyst(e)inemia and endothelial dysfunction in IDDM. Diabetes Care 1997; 20:1880.

32. Targher G, Bertolini L, Zenari L, Cacciatori V, Muggeo M, Faccini G, Zoppini G. Cigarette smoking and plasma total homocysteine levels in young adults with type 1 diabetes [In Process Citation]. Diabetes Care 2000; 23:524.

33. Hoogeveen EK, Kostense PJ, Jakobs C, Dekker JM, Nijpels G, Heine RJ, Bouter LM, Stehouwer CD. Hyperhomocysteinemia increases risk of death, especially in type 2 diabetes: 5-year follow-up of the Hoorn Study. Circulation 2000; 101:1506.

34. Bostom AG, Shemin D, Lapane KL, Sutherland P, Nadeau MR, Wilson PW, Yoburn D, Bausserman L, Tofler G, Jacques PF, Selhub J, Rosenberg IH. Hyperhomocysteinemia, hyperfibrinogenemia, and lipoprotein (a) excess in maintenance dialysis patients: a matched case-control study. Atherosclerosis 1996; 125:91.

35. Bostom AG, Shemin D, Lapane KL, Hume AL, Yoburn D, Nadeau MR, Bendich A, Selhub J, Rosenberg IH. High dose-B-vitamin treatment of hyperhomocysteinemia in dialysis patients. Kidney Int 1996; 49:147.

36. Bostom AG, Gohh RY, Tsai MY, Hopkins-Garcia BJ, Nadeau MR, Bianchi LA,

Jacques PF, Rosenberg IH, Selhub J. Excess prevalence of fasting and postmethio-nine-loading hyperhomocysteinemia in stable renal transplant recipients. Arterioscler Thromb Vasc Biol 1997; 17:1894.

37. Ridker PM. Evaluating novel cardiovascular risk factors: can we better predict heart attacks? Ann Intern Med 1999; 130:933.

38. Wilson PW. Metabolic risk factors for coronary heart disease: current and future prospects. Curr Opin Cardiol 1999; 14:176.

39. Harjai KJ. Potential new cardiovascular risk factors: left ventricular hypertrophy, homocysteine, lipoprotein(a), triglycerides, oxidative stress, and fibrinogen. Ann Intern Med 1999; 131:376.

3

Antiphospholipid Antibody Syndrome

Mark A. Crowther and Jeffrey S. Ginsberg
McMaster University, Hamilton, Ontario, Canada

I. LABORATORY CHARACTERISTICS

A. Definition

Antiphospholipid antibodies (APLA) are a heterogeneous group of autoantibodies associated with both arterial and venous thrombosis, recurrent pregnancy loss, and thrombocytopenia. They can occur either in association with other autoimmune conditions, most frequently systemic lupus erythematosus (SLE), or in isolation, a condition known as the primary antiphospholipid antibody syndrome. In the research laboratory, many antiphospholipid antibodies (with varying epitope specificity) can be identified. However, in clinical practice, the antiphospholipid antibodies are divided into two large groups, the lupus anticoagulants and the anticardiolipin antibodies.

Lupus anticoagulants or nonspecific inhibitors interfere with the assembly of procoagulant complexes. In vitro, these antibodies are associated with the prolongation of phospholipid-dependent blood-clotting times. Characteristically, clotting times return to normal with the addition of exogenous phospholipid. Lupus anticoagulants may demonstrate specificity for blood-clotting proteins, in particular prothrombin. However, the mechanism by which they promote thrombosis is unknown. Lupus anticoagulants are likely associated with a high risk of first and recurrent thrombosis as well as recurrent pregnancy loss.

Anticardiolipin antibodies (ACA) were historically detected using VDRL testing but are now detected with specific enzyme-linked immunosorbent assays (ELISA) and, unlike the lupus anticoagulants, the ACA levels can be quantified. In vivo, ACA frequently demonstrate specificity for beta-2 glycoprotein-1, a circulating plasma glycoprotein. Anticardiolipin antibodies are likely associated with titer-dependent increases in the risk of thrombosis and recurrent pregnancy loss.

ACA, and to a lesser extent lupus anticoagulants, may demonstrate specificity for certain anionic phospholipids, in particular phosphatidylserine, phosphatidylinositol, and phosphatidylcholine. The clinical importance of this epitope specificity is controversial.

B. Prevalence in the General and Selected Populations

APLA are found in about 20% of patients presenting with venous thromboembolism (1,2), in about 10% of patients presenting with first ischemic stroke (3), and in approximately 5 to 10% of young people presenting with first myocardial infarction (4). Their prevalence in the unselected population is unknown; reported rates vary widely with the test system used and the population being studied. About 30% of individuals with systemic lupus erythematosus have an APLA (5). Low-titer anticardiolipin antibodies are frequently detected in otherwise well individuals; repeat testing reveals a high rate of spontaneous resolution.

C. Laboratory Characteristics

Many ACA are specific for beta-2 glycoprotein-1 in concert with cell-surface anionic phospholipid (6) and are detected and quantified using accurate ELISA (7,8). The levels of IgG, IgA, and IgM antiphospholipid antibodies can be quantified and are usually reported in phospholipid antibody units (PL units). The isotype and subgroup specificity of ACA appears to be important. For example, high-titer IgG ACA is associated with a high risk of clinical complications, while the clinical significance of IgM or IgA ACA, even when present in high titer, is less clear. Anticardiolipin antibody testing is notoriously inaccurate; both within- and between-center reliability is poor.

LAC are a heterogeneous group of autoantibodies, which prolong the clotting time in a variety of assays (9,10) and may demonstrate specificity for beta-2 glycoprotein-1 (11). LAC do not prolong clotting times in assays in which phospholipid is present in excess. This suggests that LAC inhibit in vitro coagulation by interfering with the assembly of procoagulant complexes on phospholipid surfaces. This observation also forms the basis for the test for LAC—a prolonged clotting time, in a phospholipid-limited assay system, that normalizes with the addition of excess phospholipid confirms the presence of LAC. Anecdotal experience suggests that lupus anticoagulants are much less common than anticardiolipin antibodies, that they are infrequently transient, and that they are associated with a high risk of complications, although none of these observations has been adequately studied. Furthermore, laboratory assays for lupus anticoagulants, particularly potent lupus anticoagulants, are much more reliable than available tests for anticardiolipin antibodies (11).

II. CLINICAL COMPLICATIONS

A. Arterial and Venous Thromboembolism

1. Background and Historical Aspects

ACA are associated with both first and recurrent thromboembolism. Finazzi et al. (12) followed 360 patients with APLA for a mean of 3.9 years and demonstrated that ACA of IgG isotype with a titer greater than 40 GPL (anti-IgG antiphospholipid antibody) units were strongly associated with the development of thromboembolism. Others have shown that ACA are associated with first stroke [odds ratio (OR) 2.31; 95% CI 1.09 to 4.90] (3) and with thromboembolism in patients with SLE (13). The best evidence that ACA are associated with recurrent thromboembolism comes from a large prospective study performed by Schulman et al. (14). This study followed 412 patients with a first episode of venous thromboembolism, and demonstrated the risk of recurrence was 29% in patients with ACA antibodies and 14% in those without antibodies ($p = 0.0013$).

LAC are associated with thromboembolism either in the presence (OR 2.7; 95% CI 0.97 to 7.70) (13) or absence (OR 9.4 to 10.7) of SLE (1,15).

After a first episode of arterial or venous thromboembolism, the risk of recurrence is higher in patients with APLA than in those without APLA (14, 16,17), and in patients with an ACA, the risk of thromboembolism is higher in those with a previous history of thromboembolism than in those without such a history (12). This increased risk of recurrent thromboembolism has also been reported in patients with stroke (18–20), with venous thromboembolism (14), and with other types of thromboembolism (16,17).

In summary, patients with APLA, particularly those with a LAC, those with higher titer ACA, and those with a history of previous thrombosis are at increased risk of both first and recurrent thrombosis in either the arterial or venous circulation.

2. Evidence-Based Treatment Recommendations

Warfarin reduces the risk of recurrent TE by competitively inhibiting two hepatic vitamin K–dependent enzymes (21). These enzymes are required for gamma-carboxylation of coagulation factors II, VII, IX, and X. Coagulation factors lacking gamma-carboxyl residues have reduced functional activity and do not participate normally in the coagulation cascade (22,23). Warfarin is a very effective antithrombotic. Kearon et al. (17) demonstrated that warfarin, administered to achieve an INR of 2.0 to 3.0, reduced the risk of recurrent venous thromboembolism compared with placebo by 95% (hazard ratio 0.05; 95% CI, 0.01 to 0.37). Similarly, Hull et al. (24) demonstrated that in patients with acute venous thromboembolism, warfarin reduced the risk of recurrence to 3% (compared with 26% with low-dose heparin [$p = 0.014$; relative risk reduction (RRR) 90%]). The risk of arterial thromboembolism is also reduced by warfarin. A pooled analysis of seven well-designed trials found that warfarin reduces the risk of embolic stroke in patients with nonvalvular atrial fibrillation from 8.8 to 3.4%, RRR 61%; $p < 0.0001$ (25). In a comprehensive overview of the effectiveness of warfarin in patients with coronary artery disease involving 10,056 patients in 16 trials, Anand and Yusuf (26) demonstrated that oral anticoagulants reduced the risk of mortality [odds reduction (ORed) 22%; 95% CI, 0.13 to 0.31], myocardial infarction (ORed 42%; 95% CI, 0.34 to 0.48), and thromboembolic complications including stroke (ORed 63%; 95% CI, 0.53 to 0.71).

For the prevention of thromboembolism, high-intensity warfarin (target INR > 2.8) has been evaluated in five settings: (1) patients with tissue heart valves (27); (2) patients with acute deep vein thrombosis (28); (3) patients with APLA (16,29,30); (4) patients with previous stroke (31); and (5) patients with coronary artery disease (26). High-intensity warfarin was not more effective than standard-intensity warfarin in the first two studies: these results contrast with those reported in patients with coronary artery disease in whom high-intensity warfarin was associated with a reduced risk of death, myocardial infarction, and stroke at a cost of an increased risk of hemorrhage. In patients with previous stroke (31), the SPIRIT study demonstrated that, compared with aspirin (80 mg/ day), warfarin administered with a target intensity of 3.0 to 4.5 resulted in a significant increase in the risk of hemorrhage (hazard ratio 2.3; 95% CI, 1.6 to 3.5). The incidence of bleeding increased by a factor of 1.43 (95% CI, 0.96 to 2.13) for each 0.5-unit increase of the achieved INR. A similar increase in the risk of hemorrhage was reported in the other investigations of warfarin administered with a target intensity of more than 3.0 (16,27–30).

Anticoagulant therapy reduces the risk of recurrent thromboembolism in a variety of patient populations, including those with APLA. Thus, Schulman et al. (14) treated patients with acute venous thromboembolism (VTE) with warfarin for 6 months. In the 68 patients with an ACA, no cases of recurrent thromboembolism occurred while on anticoagulant therapy. Similarly, Kearon et al. (17) demonstrated that although APLA were associated with an increased risk of recurrent VTE, recurrent thromboembolism was only observed in patients with APLA after warfarin discontinuation.

Despite the evidence of the effectiveness of warfarin for the prevention of recurrent thromboembolism in patients with an APLA and a history of thromboembolism, there is evidence that these patients might be resistant to the usual intensities of warfarin. Three studies (16,29,30) suggest that patients with APLA and thromboembolism have an increased risk of recurrent thromboembolism, despite therapeutic anticoagulation with warfarin (administered to achieve an INR of ≤3.0). Data derived from these studies suggest that the risk of recurrent thromboembolism is highest in patients who do not receive anticoagulants (0.21 events/patient/year), and lowest in those who receive warfarin with a target INR of >3.0 (0.02 events/patient/year). The annual rate of major bleeding in the three studies varied from 3 to 7%. Table 1 presents a summary of evidence from the available literature, estimating the risk of recurrent thromboembolism.

The annual risk of fatal, major, and minor bleeding in patients receiving warfarin with a target INR of 2.0 to 3.0 is 0.4% to 1.0%, 1.3% to 6.6%, and 8% to 22%, respectively, rates approximately 5 times those seen in patients not receiving warfarin (17,26,32–34). The risk of hemorrhage varies with the duration of anticoagulant therapy, with the greatest risk in the first year of therapy (32,33). In addition, the major bleeding rate increases in proportion to the INR (31–33). Based on many prospective studies, the annual risk of major hemorrhage in a patient treated with long-term warfarin with a target INR of 2.0 to 3.0 is likely to be 3% or less (32,35). The risk increases as the INR target range is increased beyond 3.0. Based on a comprehensive review of the literature, Landefeld estimated that the risk of hemorrhage increases threefold when the target INR is increased from 2.5 to 3.5 (32), a figure also reported by the SPIRIT investigators (31). This potential for warfarin resistance explains why most ongoing trials evaluating long-term, low-dose warfarin regimens (INR 1.5–2.0) have excluded patients with known ACA syndromes.

Table 1 Recurrent TE in Patients with APLA

Intervention	Pt yrs of follow-up	Number of recurrences	Rate (events/pt/yr)
No anticoagulants (all studies)	740.2	155	0.21
Retrospective studies	532.6	131	0.25
Prospective studies	207.6	24	0.12
ASA alone[a]	50.8	16	0.31
Warfarin target INR < 3.0			
All studies	312	52	0.17
Retrospective studies	278	52	0.19
Prospective studies	36	0	0.00
Warfarin target INR > 3.0	332	5	0.015
INR > 3.0 + ASA	44.8	0	0

[a] ASA dose varied between 80 and 325 mg/day.
Source: Modified from Refs. 14, 16, 17, 29, 30.

3. Diagnostic Pathway

A congenital or acquired hypercoagulable state should be suspected in all patients presenting with unusual forms of thrombosis or in whom thrombosis occurs at a young age in the absence of identifiable risk factors. Hypercoagulable states associated with venous thrombosis include activated protein C resistance (with or without factor V Leiden), the prothrombin gene 20210A mutation, and deficiencies of protein C, protein S, or antithrombin. Hyperhomocysteinemia can be either congenital or acquired and is associated with both arterial and venous thrombosis, as are the antiphospholipid antibodies. Unexpected arterial thrombosis in otherwise well patients can be associated with hyperhomocysteinemia or antiphospholipid antibodies.

All patients with unexplained venous thrombosis, in particular those with thrombosis in unusual sites (such as the cerebral veins or mesenteric veins), should be screened for an antiphospholipid antibody. Both a lupus and an anticardiolipin antibody should be sought. Testing should be carried out in accordance with the recommendations of the International Society of Thrombosis and Hemostasis, with appropriate confirmatory assays for suspected lupus anticoagulants.

Patients with arterial thrombosis should also be screened for a hypercoagulable state if their thrombosis has occurred at a young age, or in an unusual location in the absence of other risk factors such as valvular heart disease. Testing of cholesterol and triglyceride levels, homocysteine levels, preferably in the fasting state, and antiphospholipid antibodies may reveal a treatable cause for their episode of arterial thrombosis.

4. Unanswered Questions

Many questions remain unanswered in patients with antiphospholipid antibodies. First, many patients, particularly those with systemic lupus erythematosus, are screened for the presence of an antiphospholipid antibody despite their never having had an episode of thrombosis. When detected, the clinical importance of the antibody is unknown. As a result, some such patients (who are suspected to have a high risk of first thrombosis) are treated with warfarin with varying INR target ranges, while others are treated with aspirin or other antiplatelet agents, and many receive no antithrombotic prophylaxis. To address the need for routine antithrombotic prophylaxis in this problematic patient population, a large, randomized clinical trial is currently being carried out. Within this study, adults and children, with both an antiphospholipid antibody and systemic lupus erythematosus, are allocated to long-term warfarin with a target INR of 2.0, or no therapy. The primary outcome measure of the study is the rate of objectively confirmed arterial and venous thrombosis.

A second frequently encountered clinical problem is determining the optimal intensity of warfarin anticoagulation in patients with an APLA and a history of previous thrombosis. Evidence-based treatment recommendations are not available, and there is a large variation in practice habits for patients with this problem. Two large, multicenter trials are currently under way which will address this issue. In both, patients with a persistently positive APLA and a history of arterial or venous thrombosis are allocated to receive warfarin with a target INR that exceeds 3.0 versus lower intensity anticoagulation. These studies will provide (1) guidance for the optimal intensity of warfarin therapy and (2) reliable estimates of the risk of recurrent thrombosis in patients treated with warfarin with a target intensity of less than 3.0.

B. Recurrent Pregnancy Loss

1. Background and Historical Aspects

There is a large body of evidence that patients with antiphospholipid antibodies have an increased risk of pregnancy complications, including pregnancy loss (36–38). The pathophysiology of recurrent pregnancy loss in such patients is not completely understood, and current theories revolve around placental pathology leading to fetal hypoxia. These theories invoke either placental vascular thrombosis leading to placental infarction; abnormal uteroplacental vascular conversion, as in spiral artery vasculopathy; or a combination of the two (39–41). In particular, recent interest has focused on changes in cell-surface annexin V in response to antiphospholipid antibodies. Reductions in the levels of annexin V might be associated with the development of a procoagulant state in the uterus (42).

In an effort to improve the rate of successful pregnancy outcomes, a variety of interventions, including low-dose aspirin (ASA), heparin, prednisone, intravenous immunoglobulins, and combinations of these therapies, have been used (43–59). It is plausible that antithrombotic therapy (heparin and aspirin) might reduce the risk of pregnancy loss, if this loss is due to placental vascular thrombosis. Prednisone has anti-inflammatory and immunosuppressive properties, which might reduce the risk of fetal loss either by reducing the production of APLA or by reducing placental vascular changes that promote a prothrombotic state (49,52,58,60). Intravenous immunoglobulin is believed to improve the likelihood of successful pregnancy outcomes in patients with APS by either blocking the activity of autoantibodies (mediated by passively transferred anti-idiotypic antibodies) or by immune modulation (up-regulation of suppressor T-cell function) (61); both antibody blockade and immune modulation could theoretically prevent placental thrombosis by reducing the levels of APLA.

2. Clinical Presentation and Characteristics

In a large tertiary care referral center, as many as 45% of patients presenting with recurrent pregnancy loss will have a positive antiphospholipid antibody as the only detectable cause of pregnancy loss. Recent publications suggest that other congenital or acquired hypercoagulable states may be associated with recurrent pregnancy loss.

3. Diagnostic Pathway

Before a prothrombotic state is sought in patients with recurrent pregnancy loss, structural, cytogenetic, and endocrinological abnormalities should be ruled out. If no other cause for the pregnancy loss can be discerned, an antiphospholipid antibody should be sought. It remains controversial whether other causes of a prothrombotic condition should be investigated such as the factor V Leiden mutation, the prothrombin gene mutation, or hyperhomocysteinemia.

4. Evidence-Based Treatment Recommendations

There are many published reports of strategies used for the prevention of fetal loss in patients with APS. However, only a few present data derived from well-designed and executed clinical trials. To provide the most rigorous possible conclusions, we have limited this review to treatment recommendations derived from studies in which all patients had a persistently positive antiphospholipid antibody and two or more first-trimester pregnancy losses or one or more second- or third-trimester losses. We excluded studies including patients with secondary APLA, such as those with SLE, to eliminate confounding effects of the underlying disease on the likelihood of successful pregnancy outcome, and we excluded nonrandomized studies with less than 10 patients because of the potential for bias in these small case series.

There are four randomized controlled trials that satisfied the inclusion criteria for this review (44,49,55,58). In addition, there are two controlled trials in which treatment allocation was not randomized (47,48); one nonrandomized controlled trial (46); three case series (57,62,63); and one prospective cohort study (64). The studies by Kutteh and colleagues (47,48) were considered to be "quasi-randomized," because treatment was assigned in an alternate (47) or consecutive (48) manner. In addition, the "high-dose" heparin arm was reported in both of these trials. Of the 150 patients reported in the case series by Backos et al. (62), 45 had been previously reported in the randomized trial of Rai et al. (55).

The live birth rate reported in these studies demonstrates both the diverse treatment regimens as well as varying successful pregnancy rates that have been reported to date. The rate varies from 42% with ASA alone (55) to 100% with

ASA alone (58), ASA in combination with prednisone (57,58), or with heparin (56). Only two (47,55) of the six randomized controlled trials or quasirandomized controlled trials had equivalent treatment arms (aspirin alone compared with aspirin and heparin). Combining the results of these studies using the Mantel–Haenszel weighted odds ratio for two categorical independent variables revealed an odds ratio of 3.86 (95% CI, 1.78–8.47), and the weighted relative risk of 1.73 (95% CI, 1.28–2.35), in favor of treatment with heparin and aspirin, compared with aspirin alone. These results suggest that treatment with heparin in addition to ASA is 1.7 times as likely to result in a live birth than treatment with ASA alone.

The remaining randomized controlled trials and quasirandomized controlled trials do not have similar treatment arms and thus cannot be combined to produce an odds ratio as an estimate of their effectiveness. However, the frequency of live births from each treatment arm of the randomized controlled trials was extracted and a weighted mean frequency was calculated. Either heparin or prednisone in addition to ASA resulted in live birth frequencies of 0.75 and 0.70, respectively. Treatments with ASA alone or with placebo led to calculated live birth rates of 0.56 and 0.52, respectively.

One recently reported study is relevant to this review, but is not included in the analysis because it did not satisfy the inclusion criteria. The randomized controlled trial published by the Pregnancy Loss Study Group (59) enrolled 16 patients, 9 of whom received heparin and ASA, and 7 of whom received heparin, ASA, and IVIG administered in a dose of 2 g/kg monthly from documentation of pregnancy until 36 weeks gestation. All 16 patients enrolled in this study delivered successfully. However, it was not clear whether the antiphospholipid antibody titer was confirmed on at least two occasions.

We also attempted to evaluate the maternal and fetal toxicities of therapy. Treatment with prednisone in women with APS has been reported to be associated with preterm birth (44,49,57,58), premature rupture of membranes (44,49,58), maternal hypertension, preeclampsia (44,49,57,58), cataracts (44,49), and gestational diabetes mellitus (44,49,58). In these studies, treatment with ASA plus prednisone resulted in an obstetric weighted mean frequency of obstetric events 0.33 compared to 0.12 for ASA plus heparin treatment. The weighted maternal event frequency for ASA plus heparin was 0.043 compared to 0.375 for ASA plus prednisone. Thus, for both obstetric and maternal events, the regimen of prednisone plus ASA resulted in a substantial increase in the risk of an adverse maternal event. The frequency of adverse outcomes in patients treated with heparin was low. In the randomized controlled trial that evaluated heparin (55), there were no reported instances of major bleeding, thrombocytopenia, or osteoporotic fractures. Although heparin is considered to be safe for the fetus (65), its long-term use can lead to maternal adverse effects including osteoporosis (66), thrombocytopenia (67), and bleeding (68,69). One study (55) measured the bone density of women taking heparin plus ASA before and after therapy. There was a decrease in lumbar spine bone density in these women; however, no comparison group was evaluated. Other reported toxicities of heparin were few. A recently completed study of heparin plus aspirin found a frequency of gestational diabetes of 2.7% (62), which compares favorably to the reported incidence of 2 to 3.5% in the general population (70,71).

Low-molecular-weight heparins are an attractive alternative to standard heparin for many indications because, in animal models, they produce less osteoporosis than standard heparin (72), yet they appear to be at least as effective as standard heparin (73,74). This suggests that low-molecular-weight heparins would be an excellent choice for anticoagulation during pregnancy. However, until good-quality evidence exists for the effectiveness of the low-molecular-weight heparins in patients with an antiphospholipid antibody and recurrent pregnancy loss, their routine use cannot be recommended.

In summary, based on currently available literature, it appears that the treatment of choice for the prevention of pregnancy loss in women with APS is low-dose heparin and aspirin. Although we cannot confidently exclude the possibility that prednisone plus ASA therapy is as, or more, effective than heparin plus aspirin therapy, prednisone-containing regimens are associated with a higher risk of maternal and obstetric toxicity. In addition, based on our analysis, we conclude that rigorous clinical trials designed to determine the optimal type and duration of treatment to enhance the likelihood of live birth are urgently needed.

5. Unanswered Questions

As with all other areas in this field, there remain many unanswered questions. Although one small study suggests that low-dose unfractionated heparin increases the likelihood of successful pregnancy outcome, there are no independent, randomized studies to support this conclusion. Low-molecular-weight heparins have replaced unfractionated heparin in many clinical circumstances; whether low-molecular-weight heparin can replace unfractionated heparin in this patient population has never been tested in a randomized clinical trial. Aspirin therapy is widely accepted in this patient population, yet its efficacy has never been proven in a methodologically rigorous study. Finally, the role of anticoagulants or immunosuppressant therapy has never been tested in women who are unable to concieve, or those with pregnancy loss at less than 8 weeks gestation.

C. Thrombocytopenia

Thrombocytopenia is a commonly observed clinical finding in patients with antiphospholipid antibodies. Cuadrado et al. (75) reported a prevalence of 23.4% in 171 patients with antiphospholipid antibody syndrome. Thrombocytopenia occurs in patients with both primary and secondary antiphospholipid antibody syndrome (76). Although the cause of thrombocytopenia in these patients is unknown, the similarities between immune thrombocytopenia purpura and antiphospholipid antibody–associated thrombocytopenia suggest that immune-mediated platelet destruction underlies both disorders. Furthermore, the response of patients with antiphospholipid antibody–associated thrombocytopenia to immunomodulatory therapy supports the hypothesis that the thrombocytopenia is due to immune platelet destruction. No large prospective studies of therapy for antiphospholipid antibody–associated thrombocytopenia have been reported. However, based on anecdotal experience, therapy with corticosteroids, intravenous immunoglobulin, immunosuppressive agents, and, ultimately, splenectomy for patients with severe, refractory thrombocytopenia may be effective. Galindo and colleagues (77) reported their experience with 11 patients who underwent splenectomy for severe, refractory thrombocytopenia. Nine patients had a good clinical response, as defined by platelet counts in excess of 100×10^9/L without pharmacological therapy. Many patients with immune platelet destruction will have markedly low platelet counts (30 to 50×10^9) yet be asymptomatic; such patients are best treated with careful monitoring, rather than potentially toxic interventions. If therapy for thrombocytopenia is required, platelet counts can usually be temporarily increased with corticosteroids or intravenous immunoglobulin.

III. CLINICAL SCENARIOS AND SUGGESTED MANAGEMENT

Treatment recommendations are based on anecdotal clinical experience and the published literature, where available. These are treatment recommendations that should be interpreted in the face of each patient's unique clinical presentation.

> **Case 1** A 36-year-old mother of two presents with acute arterial ischemia of the right leg. Angiography reveals thrombotic occlusion of the femoral artery. All laboratory tests are normal, with the exception of a positive lupus anticoagulant. Thrombolytic therapy is successful at recanalizing the artery. She is treated with warfarin (target INR 2.0 to 3.0), and has a repeat lupus anticoagulant assay at 3 months. This is positive. She presents for advice about therapy.

Many experts would recommend that this woman be treated with a higher target INR (3.0 to 4.0), and others would consider adding aspirin therapy, given that her initial event was arterial. Our recommendations are to treat with warfarin to achieve a target INR of 2.0 to 3.0, pending the results of ongoing studies. Aspirin therapy will increase the risk of hemorrhage; whether it will reduce the risk of recurrent thrombosis is unknown. Although we cannot exclude the possibility that high-intensity warfarin therapy might be more effective than standard-intensity therapy, it is clearly associated with an increased risk of hemorrhage. Most experts would recommend, pending the results of ongoing studies, that she be treated with warfarin for an indefinite duration.

> **Case 2** A 45-year-old construction worker presents with transient ischemic attacks. He is otherwise well but is discovered to have an anticardiolipin antibody titer of 19 (normal to 10) GPL units. This is repeated and confirmed 3 months after the initial test. Carotid Doppler ultrasound, 24-h cardiac monitor, cerebral CT scan, and transesophageal ultrasound are all normal. He is started on aspirin by his family physician. You are consulted to provide guidance on optimal anticoagulant therapy.

This patient presents with a common and problematic clinical situation. No studies have examined optimal therapy for such a patient. Extrapolating from other clinical situations associated with a high risk of arterial thromboembolism, long-term aspirin therapy is likely associated with a reduced risk of thrombosis, with only marginal toxicity. However, its effectiveness in this clinical situation is unknown. Warfarin is likely to be associated with an annual risk of major hemorrhage of 2 to 5%, and an annual risk of fatal hemorrhage of 0.5%. Given that the benefit of warfarin in this setting is unknown, it does not seem prudent to recommend warfarin.

> **Case 3** A 58-year-old male presents after an acute myocardial infarction. His cholesterol and triglycerides are normal, and angiography demonstrates occlusion of the right coronary system at the ostium. Lupus anticoagulant is repeatedly positive; homocysteine levels are within the normal range. He is placed on warfarin and sent for assessment.

Several studies (outlined in Table 1) suggest that patients with a lupus anticoagulant are at increased risk of recurrent thrombosis. Therefore, this man is likely to be at high risk of recurrent arterial or venous thrombosis, events that might occur despite therapeutic anticoagulation with warfarin. Some experts would recommend that this patient be maintained on long-term warfarin administered with a target intensity of at least 2.0 to 3.0. Because his thrombotic event was arterial—an acute myocardial infarction—some cardiologists would recommend that he receive aspirin in addition to warfarin. On the other hand, this regimen is likely to be associated with increased long-term risk of hemorrhage, and thus aspirin alone might also be considered.

> **Case 4** A 42-year-old woman with a known lupus anticoagulant and systemic lupus erythematosus is seen in clinic because of a new pulmonary embolism, which has occurred despite warfarin administered with a target INR of 3.0 to 4.0. She is otherwise well, except for lupus nephritis for which she receives monthly cyclophosphamide.

Recurrent thrombosis despite therapeutic anticoagulation is well described in patients with a lupus anticoagulant. Most experts would recommend that this patient receive therapeutic-dose heparin, either unfractionated or low-molecular-weight, for secondary prevention of thrombosis. Whether warfarin therapy can be reinstituted after a prolonged course of heparin is unknown.

REFERENCES

1. Ginsberg JS, Wells PS, Brill-Edwards P, Donovan D, Moffatt K, Johnston M, Stevens P, Hirsh Antiphospholipid antibodies and venous thromboembolism. Blood 1995; 86:3685–3691.
2. Doig RG, O'Malley CJ, Dauer R, McGrath KM. An evaluation of 200 consecutive patients with spontaneous or recurrent thrombosis for primary hypercoagulable states. Am J Clin Pathol 1994; 102:797–801.
3. Anonymous. Anticardiolipin antibodies are an independent risk factor for first ischemic stroke. The Antiphospholipid Antibodies in Stroke Study (APASS) Group. Neurology 1993; 43:2069–2073.
4. Adler Y, Finkelstein Y, Zandeman-Goddard G, Blank M, Lorber M, Lorber A, Faden D, Shoenfeld Y. The presence of antiphospholipid antibodies in acute myocardial infarction. Lupus 1995; 4:309–313.
5. Love PE, Santoro SA. Antiphospholipid antibodies: anticardiolipin and the lupus anticoagulant in systemic lupus erythematosus (SLE) and in non-SLE disorders. Prevalence and clinical significance. Ann Intern Med 1990; 112:682–698.
6. Wang MX, Kandiah DA, Ichikawa K, Khamashta M, Hughes G, Koike T, Roubey R, Krilis SA. Epitope specificity of monoclonal anti-beta 2-glycoprotein I antibodies derived from patients with the antiphospholipid syndrome. J Immunol 1995; 155: 1629–1636.
7. Brandt JT, Triplett DA, Alving B, Scharrer I. Criteria for the diagnosis of lupus anticoagulants: an update. On behalf of the Subcommittee on Lupus Anticoagulant/ Antiphospholipid Antibody of the Scientific and Standardisation Committee of the ISTH. Thromb Haemost 1995; 74:1185–1190.
8. Triplett DA. Antiphospholipid-protein antibodies: laboratory detection and clinical relevance. Thromb Res 1995; 78:1–31.
9. Martin BA, Branch DW, Rodgers GM. Sensitivity of the activated partial thromboplastin time, the dilute Russell's viper venom time, and the kaolin clotting time for the detection of the lupus anticoagulant: a direct comparison using plasma dilutions. Blood Coag Fibrinolysis 1996; 7:31–38.
10. Pengo V, Thiagarajan P, Shapiro SS, Heine MJ. Immunological specificity and mechanism of action of IgG lupus anticoagulants. Blood 1987; 70:69–76.
11. Arnout J, Meijer P, Vermylen J. Lupus anticoagulant testing in Europe: an analysis of results from the first European Concerted Action on Thrombophilia (ECAT) survey using plasmas spiked with monoclonal antibodies against human beta 2-glycoprotein I. Thromb Haemost 1999; 81(6):929–934.

12. Finazzi G, Brancaccio V, Moia M, Ciaverella N, Mazzucconi MG, Schinco PC, Ruggeri M, Pogliani EM, Gamba G, Rossi E, et al. Natural history and risk factors for thrombosis in 360 patients with antiphospholipid antibodies: a four-year prospective study from the Italian Registry. Am J Med 1996; 100:530–536.

13. Long AA, Ginsberg JS, Brill-Edwards P, Johnston M, Turner C, Denburg JA, Bensen WG, Cividino A, Andrew M, Hirsh J. The relationship of antiphospholipid antibodies to thromboembolic disease in systemic lupus erythematosus: a cross-sectional study. Thrombos Haemost 1991; 66:520–524.

14. Schulman S, Svenungsson E, Granqvist S. Anticardiolipin antibodies predict early recurrence of thromboembolism and death among patients with venous thromboembolism following anticoagulant therapy. Duration of Anticoagulation Study Group. Am J Med 1998; 104(4):332–338.

15. Simioni P, Prandoni P, Zanon E, Saracino MA, Scudeller A, Villalta S, Scarano L, Girolami B, Benedetti L, Girolami A. Deep venous thrombosis and lupus anticoagulant. A case-control study. Thromb Haemost 1996; 76(2):187–189.

16. Khamashta MA, Cuadrado MJ, Mujic F, Taub NA, Hunt BJ, Hughes GR. The management of thrombosis in the antiphospholipid-antibody syndrome. N Engl J Med 1995; 332:993–997.

17. Kearon C, Gent M, Hirsh J, Weitz JI, Kovacs MJ, Anderson D, Turpie AG, Green D, Ginsberg JS, Wells PS, et al. A comparison of three months of anticoagulation with extended anticoagulation for a first episode of idiopathic venous thromboembolism. N Engl J Med 1999; 340(12):901–907.

18. Levine SR, Brey RL, Joseph CL, Havstad S. Risk of recurrent thromboembolic events in patients with focal cerebral ischemia and antiphospholipid antibodies. The Antiphospholipid Antibodies in Stroke Study Group. Stroke 1992; 23:129–132.

19. Levine SR, Brey RL, Sawaya KL, Salowich-Palm L, Kokkinos J, Kostrzema B, Perry M, Havstad S, Carey J. Recurrent stroke and thrombo-occlusive events in the antiphospholipid syndrome. Ann Neurol 1995; 38:119–124.

20. Nencini P, Baruffi MC, Abbate R, Massai G, Amaducci L, Inzitari D. Lupus anticoagulant and anticardiolipin antibodies in young adults with cerebral ischemia. Stroke 1992; 23:189–193.

21. Furie B, Bouchard BA, Furie BC. Vitamin K-dependent biosynthesis of gamma-carboxyglutamic acid. Blood 1999; 93(6):1798–1808.

22. Malhotra OP, Nesheim ME, Mann KG. The kinetics of activation of normal and gamma-carboxyglutamic acid-deficient prothrombins. J Biol Chem 1985; 260:279–287.

23. Malhotra OP. Dicoumarol-induced prothrombins containing 6, 7, and 8 gamma-carboxyglutamic acid residues: isolation and characterization. Biochem Cell Biol 1989; 67(8):411–421.

24. Hull R, Delmore T, Genton E, Hirsh J, Gent M, Sackett D, McLoughlin D, Armstrong P. Warfarin sodium versus low-dose heparin in the long-term treatment of venous thrombosis. N Engl J Med 1979; 301:855–858.

25. Cleland J, Cowburn PJ, Falk RH. Should all patients with atrial fibrillation receive warfarin? Eur Heart J 1996; 17:674–681.

26. Anand SS, Yusuf S. Oral anticoagulant therapy in patients with coronary artery disease: a meta-analysis. JAMA 1999; 282(21):2058–2067.

27. Turpie AG, Gunstensen J, Hirsh J, Nelson H, Gent M. Randomised comparison of two intensities of oral anticoagulant therapy after tissue heart valve replacement. Lancet 1988; 1:1242–1245.

28. Hull R, Hirsh J, Jay R, Carter C, England C, Gent M, Turpie AG, McLoughlin D, McBride JA, Dodd P, et al. Different intensities of oral anticoagulant therapy in the treatment of proximal-vein thrombosis. N Engl J Med 1982; 307:1676–1681.

29. Rosove MH, Brewer PM. Antiphospholipid thrombosis: clinical course after the first thrombotic event in 70 patients. Ann Intern Med 1992; 117:303–308.

30. Rousseau A, Berube C. Prevention of thrombotic recurrences after an initial thrombotic event in antiphospholipid syndrome: a retrospective study. Lupus 1996; 5(5): 557.

31. The SPIRIT study group. A randomized trial of anticoagulants versus aspirin after cerebral ischemia of presumed arterial origin. The Stroke Prevention in Reversible Ischemia Trial (SPIRIT) Study Group. Ann Neurol 1997; 42(6):857–865.

32. Landefeld CS, Beyth RJ. Anticoagulant-related bleeding: clinical epidemiology, prediction, and prevention. Am J Med 1993; 95:315–328.

33. Fihn SD, McDonell M, Martin D, Henikoff J, Vermes D, Kent D, White RH. Risk factors for complications of chronic anticoagulation. A multicenter study. Warfarin Optimized Outpatient Follow-up Study Group. Ann Intern Med 1993; 118:511–520.

34. Turpie AG, Gent M, Laupacis A, Latour Y, Gunstensen J, Basile FKM, Hirsh J. A comparison of aspirin with placebo in patients treated with warfarin after heart-valve replacement. N Engl J Med 1993; 329:524–529.

35. Anonymous. Adjusted-dose warfarin versus low-intensity, fixed-dose warfarin plus aspirin for high-risk patients with atrial fibrillation: Stroke Prevention in Atrial Fibrillation III randomized trial. Lancet 1996; 348:633–638.

36. Branch DW. Antiphospholipid antibodies and reproductive outcome: the current state of affairs. J Reprod Immunol 1998; 38(1):75–87.

37. Hewell SW, Hammer RH. Antiphospholipid antibodies: a threat throughout pregnancy. J Obstet Gynecol Neonat Nurs 1997; 26(2):162–168.

38. Faden D, Tincani A, Tanzi P, Spatola L, Lojacono A, Tarantini M, Balestrieri G. Anti-beta2 glycoprotein I antibodies in a general obstetric population: preliminary results on the prevalence and correlation with pregnancy outcome. Anti-beta2 glycoprotein I antibodies are associated with some obstetrical complications, mainly preeclampsia-eclampsia. Eur J Obst Gynecol Reprod Biol 1997; 73(1):37–42.

39. Shapiro SS. The lupus anticoagulant/antiphospholipid syndrome. Ann Rev Med 1996; 47:533–553.

40. Salafia CM, Parke AL. Placental pathology in systemic lupus erythematosus and phospholipid antibody syndrome. Rheum Dis Clin North Am 1997; 23(1):85–97.

41. Welsch S, Branch DW. Antiphospholipid syndrome in pregnancy. Obstetric concerns and treatment. Rheum Dis Clin North Am 1997; 23(1):71–84.

42. Rand JH, Wu XX, Andree HA, Lockwood CJ, Guller S, Scher J, Harpel PC. Pregnancy loss in the antiphospholipid-antibody syndrome—a possible thrombogenic mechanism. N Engl J Med 1997; 337(3):154–160.

43. Branch DW, Silver RM, Blackwell JL, Reading JC, Scott JR. Outcome of treated pregnancies in women with antiphospholipid syndrome: an update of the Utah experience. Obstet Gynecol 1992; 80(4):614–620.

44. Cowchock FS, Reece EA, Balaban D, Branch DW, Plouffe L. Repeated fetal losses associated with antiphospholipid antibodies: a collaborative randomized trial comparing prednisone with low-dose heparin treatment. Am J Obstet Gynecol 1992; 166:1318–1323.

45. Christiansen OB, Mathiesen O, Husth M, Rasmussen KL, Ingerslev HJ, Lauritsen JG, Grunnet N. Placebo-controlled trial of treatment of unexplained secondary recurrent spontaneous abortions and recurrent late spontaneous abortions with i.v. immunoglobulin. Hum Reprod 1995; 10(10):2690–2695.

46. Hasegawa I, Takakuwa K, Goto S, Yamada K, Sekizuka N, Kanazawa K, Tanaka K. Effectiveness of prednisolone/aspirin therapy for recurrent aborters with antiphospholipid antibody. Hum Reprod 1992; 7(2):203–207.

47. Kutteh WH. Antiphospholipid antibody-associated recurrent pregnancy loss: treatment with heparin and low-dose aspirin is superior to low-dose aspirin alone. Am J Obstet Gynecol 1996; 174(5):1584–1589.

48. Kutteh WH, Ermel LD. A clinical trial for the treatment of antiphospholipid antibody-associated recurrent pregnancy loss with lower dose heparin and aspirin. Am J Reprod Immunol 1996; 35(4):402–407.

49. Laskin CA, Bombardier C, Hannah ME, Mandel FP, Knox-Ritchie JW, Farewell V, Farine D, Spitzer K, Fielding L, Soloninka CA, et al. Prednisone and aspirin in women with autoantibodies and unexplained recurrent fetal loss. New Engl J Med 1997; 337:148–153.

50. Lima F, Khamashta MA, Buchanan NM, Kerslake S, Hunt BJ, Hughes GR. A study of sixty pregnancies in patients with the antiphospholipid syndrome. Clin Exp Rheumatol 1996; 14(2):131–136.

51. Lockshin MD, Druzin ML, Qamar T. Prednisone does not prevent recurrent fetal death in women with antiphospholipid antibody. Am J Obstet Gynecol 1989; 160: 439–443.

52. Lubbe WF, Butler WS, Palmer SJ, Liggins GC. Fetal survival after prednisone suppression of maternal lupus-anticoagulant. Lancet 1983; 1:1361–1363.

53. Marzusch K, Dietl J, Klein R, Hornung D, Neuer A, Berg PA. Recurrent first trimester spontaneous abortion associated with antiphospholipid antibodies: a pilot study of treatment with intravenous immunoglobulin. Acta Obstet Gynecol Scand 1996; 75(10):922–926.

54. Passaleva A, Massai G, D'Elios MM, Livi C, Abbate R. Prevention of miscarriage in antiphospholipid syndrome. Autoimmunity 1992; 14:121–125.

55. Rai R, Cohen H, Dave M, Regan L. Randomised controlled trial of aspirin and aspirin plus heparin in pregnant women with recurrent miscarriage associated with phospholipid antibodies (or antiphospholipid antibodies). Br Med J 1997; 314(7076): 253–257.

56. Ruffatti A, Orsini A, Di LL, Nardelli GB, Patrassi GM, Truscia D, Brigato G, Grella P, Todesco S. A prospective study of fifty-three consecutive calcium heparin treated pregnancies in patients with antiphospholipid antibody-related fetal loss. Clin Exp Rheumatol 1997; 15(5):499–505.

57. Silveira LH, Hubble CL, Jara LJ, Saway S, Martinez-Osuna P, Seleznick MJ, Angel J, O'Brien W, Espinoza LR. Prevention of anticardiolipin antibody-related pregnancy losses with prednisone and aspirin. Am J Med 1992; 93:403–411.

58. Silver RK, MacGregor SN, Sholl JS, Hobart JM, Neerhof MG, Ragin A. Comparative trial of prednisone plus aspirin versus aspirin alone in the treatment of anticardiolipin antibody-positive obstetric patients. Am J Obstet Gynecol 1993; 169:1411–1417.

59. Branch DW, Peaceman AM, Druzin M, Silver RK, El-Sayed Y, Silver RM, Esplin MS, Spinnato J, Harger J. A multicenter, placebo-controlled pilot study of intravenous immune globulin treatment of antiphospholipid syndrome during pregnancy. The Pregnancy Loss Study Group. Am J Obstet Gynecol 2000; 182(1 Pt 1):122–127.

60. Lubbe WF, Butler WS, Palmer SJ, Liggins GC. Lupus anticoagulant in pregnancy. Br J Obstet Gynaecol 1984; 91:357–363.

61. Orvieto R, Achiron A, Ben-Rafael Z, Achiron R. Intravenous immunoglobulin treatment for recurrent abortions caused by antiphospholipid antibodies. Fertility Sterility 1991; 56:1013–1020.

62. Backos M, Rai R, Baxter N, Chilcott IT, Cohen H, Regan L. Pregnancy complications in women with recurrent miscarriage associated with antiphospholipid antibodies treated with low dose aspirin and heparin. Br J Obstet Gynaecol 1999; 106(2):102–107.

63. Ruffatti A, Orsini A, Di LL, Nardelli GB, Patrassi GM, Truscia D, Brigato G, Grella P, Todesco S. A prospective study of fifty-three consecutive calcium heparin treated pregnancies in patients with antiphospholipid antibody-related fetal loss. Clin Exp Rheumatol 1997; 15(5):499–505.

64. Rai RS, Clifford K, Cohen H, Regan L. High prospective fetal loss rate in untreated pregnancies of women with recurrent miscarriage and antiphospholipid antibodies. Hum Reprod 1995; 10(12):3301–3304.

65. Bates SM, Ginsberg JS. Anticoagulants in pregnancy: fetal effects. Baillieres Clin Obstet Gynaecol 1997; 11(3):479–488.

66. Douketis JD, Ginsberg JS, Burrows RF, Duku EK, Webber CE, Brill-Edwards P. The effects of long-term heparin therapy during pregnancy on bone density. A prospective matched cohort study. Thromb Haemost 1996; 75(2):254–257.

67. Warkentin TE, Kelton JG. Heparin-induced thrombocytopenia. Progr Hemost Thromb 1991; 10:1–34.

68. Ginsberg JS, Hirsh J. Use of antithrombotic agents during pregnancy. Chest 1998; 114(suppl 5):524S–30S.

69. Levine MN, Raskob G, Landefeld S, Kearon C. Hemorrhagic complications of anticoagulant treatment. Chest 1998; 114(suppl 5):511S–523S.

70. Koukkou E, Taub N, Jackson P, Metcalfe G, Cameron M, Lowy C. Difference in prevalence of gestational diabetes and perinatal outcome in an innercity multiethnic London population. Eur J Obstet Gynecol Reprod Biol 1995; 59(2):153–157.

71. Engelgau MM, Herman WH, Smith PJ, German RR, Aubert RE. The epidemiology of diabetes and pregnancy in the U.S,. 1988. Diabetes Care 1995; 18(7):1029–1033.

72. Shaughnessy SG, Young E, Deschamps P, Hirsh J. The effects of low molecular weight and standard heparin on calcium loss from fetal rat calvaria. Blood 1995; 86:1368–1373.

73. Levine MN, Gent M, Hirsh J, Leclerc J, Anderson D, Weitz J, Ginsberg J, Turpie AG, Demers C, Kovacs M, et al. A comparison of low-molecular-weight heparin

administered primarily at home with unfractionated heparin administered in the hospital for proximal deep-vein thrombosis. N Engl J Med 1996; 334(11):677–681.

74. Cohen M, Demers C, Gurfinkel EP, Turpie AG, Fromell GJ, Goodman S, Langer A, Califf RM, Fox KA, Premmereur J, et al. Low-molecular-weight heparins in non-ST-segment elevation ischemia: the ESSENCE trial. Efficacy and Safety of Subcutaneous Enoxaparin versus intravenous unfractionated heparin, in non-Q-wave Coronary Events. Am J Cardiol 1998; 82(5B):19L–24L.

75. Cuadrado MJ, Mujic F, Munoz E, Khamashta MA, Hughes GR. Thrombocytopenia in the antiphospholipid syndrome. Ann Rheum Dis 1997; 56(3):194–196.

76. Vianna JL, Khamashta MA, Ordi-Ros J, Font J, Cervera R, Lopez-Soto ATC, Franz J, Selva A, Ingelmo M, et al. Comparison of the primary and secondary antiphospholipid syndrome: a European Multicenter Study of 114 patients. Am J Med 1994; 96: 3–9.

77. Galindo M, Khamashta MA, Hughes GR. Splenectomy for refractory thrombocytopenia in the antiphospholipid syndrome. Rheumatology (Oxford) 1999; 38(9):848–853.

4

The Epidemiology of Postmenopausal Hormone Therapy and Cardiovascular Disease

Francine Grodstein
Brigham and Women's Hospital and Harvard Medical School, Boston, Massachusetts

Meir J. Stampfer
Harvard School of Public Health, Boston, Massachusetts

I. INTRODUCTION

Considerable evidence supports a relation between postmenopausal hormone therapy and cardiovascular disease. Specifically, long-term use of hormone therapy is associated with substantial protection against heart disease. This protection, observed largely in observational epidemiological studies, may be due, in part, to self-selection bias. Women who take hormones may not be completely comparable to those who do not; women on hormone therapy see a physician regularly and may lead generally healthier lifestyles. However, adjustment for known cardiac risk factors in many of the large studies of homogeneous populations had little impact on their results, implying an equivalent risk status for users and nonusers. To date, however, no randomized trial data in primary prevention have been presented. The effect of progestin added to estrogen therapy has not been adequately assessed, but initial evidence suggests that most of the coronary benefit is probably retained. Considerable controversy exists regarding the effect of hormones in women with established coronary disease, although, like the studies of primary prevention, existing data suggest long-term benefits. On the other hand, the only randomized trial in secondary prevention, the HERS study, failed to show the expected benefits of this approach over a 4-year period of observation.

It is becoming increasingly clear that hormone therapy is not related to risk of stroke, and that rates of venous thromboembolism are higher in women who take hormone therapy than those who do not. Importantly, sparse evidence also suggests that there may be short-term higher risks of cardiovascular disease when women initiate hormone use. An increase in breast cancer is also a concern. In promoting healthy aging in women, alternatives to hormone therapy should be considered; estimates suggest that 82% of coronary disease could be eliminated through adherence to basic guidelines involving moderate exercise, a good diet, and abstinence from smoking.

Cardiovascular diseases (CVD) remain the leading cause of death in women. The role of hormone therapy in CVD remains a controversial topic, despite clear evidence from randomized clinical trials that hormone use improves the lipid profile, enhances blood flow, and has numerous other beneficial effects on intermediate endpoints. This chapter summarizes the epidemiological investigations regarding the association between postmenopausal hormone therapy and cardiovascular disease, including primary and secondary prevention of coronary heart disease, stroke, and pulmonary embolism. For coronary heart disease, substantial evidence on primary prevention has accumulated from numerous observational studies. Less consistent information is available on the relationship between stroke and hormone therapy. Finally, few studies have examined the relation of hormone use to second coronary events or to pulmonary embolism, but the only completed large-scale clinical trial of hormone therapy addresses these issues.

II. CORONARY HEART DISEASE

A. Primary Prevention

Overwhelming evidence from epidemiological studies indicates an inverse relation between hormone use and heart disease in healthy women. Several observational study designs have been used to examine this association: hospital and community-based case-control studies; cross-sectional studies; and prospective studies; virtually all report a lower risk of heart disease for women who take hormones than those who do not. In addition, results from all the studies have been combined in several meta-analyses (1,2), with summary relative risk estimates in all these indicating approximately a 35% lower rate of coronary heart disease (CHD) for hormone users than nonusers (Fig. 1). However, many studies suggest that current hormone users enjoy greater protection against heart disease than past users. Thus, combining investigations of current, past, and ever use in a summary estimate is misleading because the results will be directly affected by the proportion of past and current use in the studies included. As expected, summary estimates based on analyses of current use are lower than those derived by combining studies of any hormone use (Fig. 1). For all studies of current use,

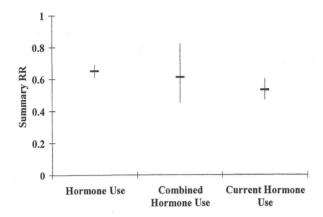

Figure 1 Summary relative risks from meta-analyses of observational studies of post-menopausal hormone therapy and primary prevention of coronary heart disease.

the summary RR is 0.53 (95% CI, 0.47–0.60), and for prospective studies, the summary estimate was 0.60 (95% CI, 0.50–0.72). While the prospective studies are generally considered to be the least biased of the observational study designs, one potential limitation of most prospective studies is that hormone use is often assessed only at the start of the study. With subsequent long-term follow-up, there can be substantial misclassification of hormone use, since many women will stop or start taking hormones after the baseline assessment; this would lead to an underestimate of the benefit of postmenopausal hormone therapy.

Of the studies included in the meta-analyses, the Nurses' Health Study (3) is the largest prospective cohort to investigate hormone use and heart disease. The study was established in 1976 when 121,700 married female registered nurses aged 30 to 55 years completed a mailed questionnaire. Information on coronary risk factors and hormone use was updated with follow-up questionnaires sent every 2 years. Reports of coronary disease are confirmed by medical record review, and data on hormones and other possible risk factors are likely to be reliable since all subjects are registered nurses, with a demonstrated interest in medical research. In the analysis of hormones and heart disease, a total of 70,543 postmenopausal women without prior coronary heart disease were followed for up to 20 years; 945 nonfatal myocardial infarctions and 186 confirmed coronary deaths were documented.

Substantial coronary benefits were observed for current hormone users, who had a 40% lower risk of heart disease compared to women who had never taken hormones (RR = 0.60; 95% CI, 0.52–0.70), after adjustment for a wide array of CHD risk factors. The relation was substantially attenuated among past hormone users (RR = 0.82; 95% CI, 0.72–0.94). Interestingly, the dose of oral conjugated estrogen did not appear to affect these results; women taking 0.325 mg of estrogen had a similarly reduced risk of CHD as those taking 0.625 mg (RR = 0.53; 95% CI, 0.43–0.67 for 0.625 mg; and RR = 0.58; 95% CI, 0.37–0.92 for 0.325 mg).

The Nurses' Health Study cohort includes predominantly young postmenopausal women, and data for women of older ages are sparse. Ettinger et al. (4) studied 454 women with an average age of 77 years at the end of follow-up, and reported a relative risk of 0.40 (95% CI, 0.16–1.02) for coronary death among long-term hormone users. In the Leisure World cohort (5), estrogen status and other cardiovascular risk factors were ascertained in 8807 women aged 40 through 101 living in a retirement community in 1981 (median age = 73); 203 deaths due to MI were identified over 7.5 years of follow-up. The rate of fatal myocardial infarction was substantially reduced among estrogen users (RR = 0.60; $p < 0.001$).

1. Duration of Hormone Use

Preliminary data released from the Women's Health Initiative, an ongoing, large randomized clinical trial of hormone therapy and cardiovascular disease in healthy women, suggested that there may be a slight rise in the risk of heart disease, stroke, and venous thrombosis during the initial 1 to 2 years of hormone use, followed by a decrease in risk with continued use. Unfortunately, there is very little additional evidence available on this issue; most of the observational studies mentioned above primarily consist of long-term hormone users, and very few investigations have specifically examined the short-term effects of hormone therapy on CVD. In the Leisure World Study (5), a large prospective observational cohort, the relative risk of CHD was 0.73 (95% CI, 0.46–1.16) for recent hormone users of 3 or fewer years duration compared to nonusers; although this estimate of duration was based on a single assessment of hormone use at baseline. In the Nurses' Health Study (3), current hormone users of less than 2 years had a relative risk of CHD of 0.53 (95% CI, 0.31–0.93); but, since information is collected biennially, the actual duration of use would be underestimated. In a small prospective study, Avila et al. (6) found little relation between less than 1 year of current hormone use (RR = 0.9; 95% CI, 0.4–1.9) and MI. In case-control studies, Sidney et al. (7) observed no association between current hormone use of less than 1 year and MI (RR = 0.95; 95% CI, 0.37–2.45), and Heckbert et al. (8) also reported that current hormone use of less than 1.8 years was not related to myocardial infarction (RR = 0.91; 95% CI, 0.60–1.38). In the latter study, there was a trend of decreasing risk of MI with increasing duration of hormone use (RR = 0.55; 9% CI, 0.34–0.88 for 8.2 years or more), similar to that reported in the information released by the Women's Health Initiative. Clearly additional data are necessary.

2. Combined Hormone Therapy

Currently, progestins are prescribed along with estrogen in women with a uterus to reduce or eliminate the excess risk of endometrial cancer due to unopposed estrogen. However, progestin use was quite uncommon during the period that most of the epidemiological studies were conducted. Hence, most of the data are related directly to use of estrogen alone. In studies of intermediate endpoints, randomized clinical trials report significant decreases in LDL and increases in HDL for women assigned to estrogen combined with progestin, but for HDL, the elevation among users of estrogen with medroxyprogesterone acetate (the most commonly used progestin in the U.S.) is significantly less than that for users of estrogen alone. In addition, while estrogen therapy improves blood flow, limited studies suggest that this benefit may be diminished with the addition of progestin. Thus, progestin might be hypothesized to detract from the overall beneficial effects of estrogen on heart disease.

Nonetheless, in the few observational epidemiological studies of primary prevention which separately examine combined hormone therapy, virtually all strongly suggest a similar impact of estrogen combined with progestin and estrogen alone (Fig. 1). In a follow-up study in Uppsala, Sweden (9), the relative risk of MI was 0.64 (95% CI, 0.45–0.90) for women taking estrogen with progestin. In the Nurses' Health Study, the relation of hormone use to CHD was similar for users of estrogen alone (RR = 0.56; 95% CI, 0.46–0.68) and estrogen combined with progestin (RR = 0.66; 95% CI, 0.49–0.87), after adjusting for an array of coronary risk factors.

3. Secondary Prevention

Although limited data are available regarding hormone therapy and secondary prevention of CHD, the only published, large-scale randomized clinical trial on hormones and CVD included only women with established CHD. The Heart and Estrogen/progestin Replacement Study (HERS) (10) randomized 2763 women with coronary disease to 0.625 mg of oral conjugated estrogen combined with 2.5 mg of continuous medroxyprogesterone acetate ($n = 1380$) or placebo ($n = 1383$). Surprisingly, there was no overall protection against second coronary events for women assigned to treatment, compared to those given placebo (RR = 0.99; 95% CI, 0.80–1.22). However, as also suggested by the preliminary results released from the Women's Health Initiative, there was a strong trend of decreasing risk of heart disease with increasing duration of hormone use (p-trend = 0.009). In the first year of the trial, the risk of major coronary disease increased 52% among treated women; in the second year, there was no relation between treatment and disease (RR = 1.00), and in the third year the relative risk was 0.87. By the fourth to fifth years of the trial, rates of coronary events were 33% lower in women assigned to hormone therapy; this decrease is virtually identical to the 40% lower risk of MI in the long-term prospective observational studies of primary prevention. Furthermore, the average duration of treatment in the HERS trial was 4.1 years, and 25% of women assigned to treatment had discontinued use at the end of 3 years; thus, in an intention-to-treat analysis, the decreased risk observed during years 4 to 5 is likely an underestimate of the long-term benefits of hormone therapy.

Recent data from the Nurses' Health Study (11) report similar results to the HERS trial. Among 2489 postmenopausal participants with previous coronary disease, we identified 213 cases of recurrent nonfatal myocardial infarctions or coronary deaths. We also observed a trend of decreasing risk of recurrent events with increasing time since initiation of current hormone use (p-trend = 0.002). For users of less than 1 year, the multivariate-adjusted relative risk of major CHD was 1.25 (95% CI, 0.78–2.00), compared to never users. After 2 or more years since beginning hormone use, we found a significantly lower rate of CHD events in current hormone users than in never users (RR = 0.38; 95% CI, 0.22–0.66). Overall, with up to 20 years of follow-up, the relative risk of a second event for current hormone users was 0.65 (95% CI, 0.45–0.95); one can only speculate whether the HERS results may also have indicated overall protection had the follow-up been extended for a longer period of time.

Additional support for the long-term benefits of hormone therapy for secondary prevention of CHD comes from the prior observational studies of women with prior CHD; these have largely included hormone users of relatively long duration and all have reported lower risks of second cardiovascular events or death among the hormone users. For example, O'Keefe et al. (12) reported better survival over 7 years among women with coronary angioplasty who continued taking estrogen.

In the Nurses' Health Study analyses, the data suggested that the short-term increase in risk appeared to be concentrated in women who first began therapy after their initial coronary disease, whereas women who had been long-term users prior to their initial disease seemed to benefit from continued hormone use; thus, perhaps new hormone use after a coronary event may not be advisable, but continued use could contribute to a decrease in the risk of second events. Unfortunately, it is unlikely that many studies will have adequate data to address this issue.

4. Combined Hormone Therapy

It has been suggested that the unexpected HERS results of no overall benefits of hormone therapy on recurrent heart disease may have been due to the combined therapy regimen used in that trial. However, as discussed previously, the observational data from studies of healthy women provide no evidence of a difference between combined therapy or estrogen alone on risk of clinical events. In addition, in our study of hormone therapy in women with established coronary disease, we also found the suggestion of a similar impact of estrogen alone and with progestin on recurrent coronary events in the Nurses' Health Study. Furthermore, in preliminary data from the ERA study, a 3-year randomized clinical trial of atherosclerosis progression in women with heart disease, neither estrogen alone nor estrogen with progestin resulted in a decrease of plaque area, compared to placebo.

5. Association of Hormones with Lower Risk of CHD: Cause and Effect or Selection?

The findings from the observational studies that hormone users are at generally lower risk from coronary disease do not necessarily imply cause and effect. Women and their physicians decide on estrogen therapy. Often the health status of the woman will have an important influence on this decision and on the results of studies that examine these women. Thus, some have argued that hormone use is merely a marker rather than a cause of good health.

Most of the observational studies reviewed here have provided some information bearing on this critical point. The Nurses' Health Study tried to evaluate whether increased medical care of women using postmenopausal hormones might be responsible for the benefit observed. In an analysis limited to women who reported regular physician visits (50% of the cohort), results were similar to those found in the larger population of all subjects: the relative risk for major coronary heart disease was 0.52 (95% CI, 0.37–0.74) for current hormone use.

Another approach is to examine the risk profile of estrogen users and nonusers to determine whether the differences, if any, are sufficient to explain the large decrease in risk among estrogen users. Barrett-Connor (13) observed that, in a cohort of postmenopausal women, those taking estrogens reported more intensive health-care behavior, including frequent screening tests such as blood cholesterol measurement and mammograms. An examination of determinants of estrogen therapy in 9704 women participating in a large, multicenter study of osteoporotic fractures found that hormone users tended to be better educated, less obese, and drank alcohol and participated in sports more often than nonusers. Similarly, in a prospective study of randomly selected premenopausal women, Matthews et al. (14) observed a better cardiovascular risk factor profile prior to hormone use among the women who subsequently took hormones at menopause than among women who did not.

However, many of the large studies reviewed here are based upon homogeneous groups, chosen because of their common profession or community. In the Nurses' Health Study, all women are registered nurses with access to health care and medical knowledge, and the distribution of established coronary risk factors was similar among current and never users of hormone therapy (Table 1). In the Leisure World Study of women in a retirement community, multivariate control for risk factors had only modest impact on the relative risk estimates; the age-

Table 1 Distribution of Characteristics of Participants in the Nurses' Health Study

	Hormone use	
	Never	Current
Parental MI before the age of 60 (%)	29.6	21.8
Hypertension (%)	32.9	35.6
Diabetes mellitus (%)	5.8	3.8
High serum cholesterol level (%)	9.4	5.5
Vitamin E use (%)	9.5	17.4
Aspirin use (%)	33.6	46.9
Mean body mass index	26.3	25.1
Mean alcohol consumption (g/day)	4.7	6.4
Mean consumption of saturated fat (g/day)	31.2	41.9

adjusted relative risk of all-cause mortality was 0.80 (95% CI, 0.70–0.87) for hormone users compared to nonusers and, after further adjustment for high blood pressure, history of angina, MI, or stroke, alcohol use, smoking, body mass index, and age at menopause, the relative risk was virtually the same (RR = 0.79; 95% CI, 0.71–0.88), implying an equivalent risk status for users and nonusers. In addition, to further examine this issue, the Nurses' Health Study conducted an analysis limited to a subgroup of low-risk women (i.e., those with no diagnosis of hypertension, diabetes, or high serum cholesterol who were nonsmokers and had a Quetelet's Index below 32 kg/m²). Even with such restrictions, the relative risk for coronary disease was almost 40% lower for current hormone users. In summary, to explain the overall benefit of hormone therapy as a result of confounding by health status, one would have to presume unknown risk factors which are extremely strong predictors of CHD and very closely associated with estrogen use.

III. CEREBROVASCULAR DISEASE

Fewer investigations of stroke than of heart disease have been conducted; however, there is little evidence that hormone use is inversely related to stroke. In the largest study (15), based on 1422 cases from the Danish National Patient Register and 3171 controls, the association between nonfatal stroke and hormone use was examined by the type of stroke. Current unopposed estrogen use was not related to thromboembolic infarction (RR = 1.16; 95% CI, 0.86–1.58), although there were decreased risks of subarachnoid and intracerebral hemorrhages (RR = 0.52; 95% CI, 0.23–1.22 and RR = 0.15; 95% CI, 0.02–1.09, respectively); however, the numbers of cases of hemorrhagic stroke were somewhat small and the relative risk estimates were not statistically significant. In a recent prospective study, 9236 women in Uppsala, Sweden (9) were followed for 8 years and 289 strokes were identified; the relative risk of stroke for recent compared to never hormone users was 0.88 (95% CI, 0.65–1.19) and the relative risks were similar for ischemic and hemorrhagic strokes. In the most recent data from the Nurses' Health Study (3), with 714 stroke cases, current hormone therapy was not associated with the incidence of stroke; for all strokes, the relative risk was 1.13 (95% CI, 0.94–1.24). For ischemic strokes, this risk was 1.27 (95% CI, 1.00–1.61) and for hemorrhagic strokes, 0.96 (95% CI, 0.65–1.40). Furthermore, there was a strong trend of increasing risk of stroke with increasing dose of estrogen used; for women taking 0.625 mg or more of oral conjugated estrogen, there was a significantly higher risk of stroke compared to women who had never taken hormones (RR = 1.38; 95% CI, 1.11–1.73 for 0.625 mg; RR = 1.57; 95% CI, 1.12–2.20 for 1.25 mg; and RR = 0.57; 95% CI, 0.29–1.11 for 0.3 mg). Since 0.625 mg of estrogen was used in the Women's Health Initiative trial, this may be consistent with the slightly increased risk of stroke reported by those investigators.

A. Combined Hormone Therapy

Even fewer studies have examined the effect of added progestin on stroke risk, but most report similarly null results for both regimens. For example, in one of the largest studies, Pedersen et al. (15) reported an odds ratio of 1.16 (95% CI, 0.86–1.58) for current use of estrogen alone and 1.17 (95% CI, 0.92–1.47) for estrogen combined with progestin. Interestingly, for hemorrhagic strokes (n = 160), current use of estrogen was associated with an odds ratio of 0.52 (95% CI, 0.23–1.22) and with added progestin it was 1.22 (95% CI, 0.79–1.89); but the confidence intervals around both estimates were wide. In another case-control study of fatal and nonfatal ischemic stroke, Petitti et al. (16) found an odds ratio of 1.04 (95% CI, 0.60–1.10) for estrogen alone and 0.60 (95% CI, 0.31–1.16) for estrogen with progestin. In the Nurses' Health Study (3), for women currently taking estrogen alone, the risk of stroke was 1.17 (95% CI, 0.94–1.46) compared to women who had never taken hormones, and for women taking combined therapy, this relative risk was 1.44 (95% CI, 1.08–1.92). Again, additional information is clearly necessary, but it is certainly unlikely that either estrogen alone or combined with progestin has any cerebrovascular benefits.

IV. VENOUS THROMBOSIS

All the recent studies of postmenopausal hormone therapy and venous thrombosis have consistently reported elevated rates of disease in current hormone users. In observational studies (17,18), there is approximately a two- to threefold higher rate of venous thrombosis among current hormone users compared to never users, and in results from the HERS trial, the relative risk was 2.89 (95% CI, 1.50–5.58). Few data are available regarding the effect of different estrogen doses, durations of use, and types of regimens. However, most evidence suggests that the risk diminishes with hormone cessation. In addition, since pulmonary embolism is not a common disease, the absolute impact of an increased risk may be limited; based on data from the Nurses' Health Study, one would expect to find five extra cases of PE for every 100,000 women given hormone therapy for 1 year.

V. SUMMARY

The preponderance of evidence from the epidemiological studies strongly supports the view that long-term use of postmenopausal hormone therapy can reduce the risk for coronary heart disease in healthy women, and possibly in women with prior heart disease as well. However, there appears to be an increased risk of venous thromboembolism, and the data on stroke are inconclusive. The only completed large-scale clinical trial of hormone use indicates that combined therapy in women with established coronary disease leads to a short-term increase in the risk of second events, and this increase may exist in women without coronary disease. In addition, abundant evidence from observational studies indicates that hormone use increases the risk of breast cancer. Thus, alternatives to hormone therapy deserve consideration.

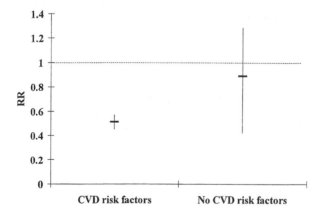

Figure 2   Risk of total mortality for current postmenopausal hormone users compared to women who never used hormones, according to risk factor groups.

Table 2 Coronary Risk Reduction Through Lifestyle Factors in the Nurses' Health Study

	RR	PAR%
Healthy diet[a]	0.17 (0.07–0.41)	82% (58–93)
Nonsmoking		
Moderate exercise 30^+ min/day[a]		
BMI <25 kg/m^2		
Alcohol $>1/2$ glass/day		

[a] Dietary components include high cereal fiber, high n-3 fatty acids, high folate, high ratio of polyunsaturated to saturated fat, low trans fat, and low glycemic load. Moderate exercise may include brisk walking.
RR = relative risk; PAR% = population attributable risk percent.

In assessing the overall risks and benefits of hormone therapy, we found that among women with CVD risk factors, mortality rates were substantially lower for those who used hormone therapy, but among women without any major CVD risk factors, mortality rates were similar for current and never hormone users (Fig. 2); this suggests that lifestyle modification could supersede hormone therapy. In particular, many known lifestyle factors appear to substantially decrease the risk of cardiovascular disease in both healthy women and those with established disease. In conclusion, in a recent study of 84,000 women (19), the investigators estimated that 82% of heart disease could be eliminated if the population adhered to basic guidelines (Table 2) involving moderate exercise, a good diet, and abstinence from smoking. Thus, if the only reason for considering hormone replacement therapy in a given woman is for cardiovascular risk reduction, many physicians would first encourage use of lipid-lowering agents such as statins where randomized trial data demonstrate clear efficacy.

REFERENCES

1. Grodstein F, Stampfer MJ. The epidemiology of coronary heart disease and estrogen replacement in postmenopausal women. Prog Cardiovasc Dis 1995; 38:199–210.
2. Grady D, Rubin SM, Petitti DB, Fox CS, Black D, Ettinger B, Ernster VL, Cummings SR. Hormone therapy to prevent disease and prolong life in postmenopausal women. Ann Intern Med 1992; 117:1016–1037.
3. Grodstein F, Manson JE, Colditz GA, Willett WC, Speizer FE, Stampfer MJ. A prospective observational study of postmenopausal hormone therapy and primary prevention of cardiovascular disease. Ann Intern Med 2000; 133:933–941.
4. Ettinger B, Friedman GD, Bush T, Quesenberry CP. Reduced mortality associated with long-term postmenopausal estrogen therapy. Obstet Gynecol 1996; 87:6–12.

5. Henderson BE, Paganini-Hill A, Ross RK. Decreased mortality in users of estrogen replacement therapy. Arch Intern Med 1991; 151:75–78.
6. Avila MH, Walker AM, Jick H. Use of replacement estrogens and the risk of myocardial infarction. Epidemiology 1990; 1:128–133.
7. Sidney S, Petitti DB, Quesenberry CP. Myocardial infarction and the use of estrogen and estrogen-progestogen in postmenopausal women. Ann Intern Med 1997; 127: 501–508.
8. Heckbert SR, Weiss NS, Koepsell TD, Lemaitre RN, Smith NL, Siscovick DS, Lin D, Psaty BM. Duration of estrogen replacement therapy in relation to the risk of incident myocardial infarction in postmenopausal women. Arch Intern Med 1997; 157:1330–1336.
9. Grodstein F, Stampfer MJ, Fulkeborn M, Naessen T, Persson I. Postmenopausal hormone therapy and risk of cardiovascular disease and hip fracture in a cohort of Swedish women. Epidemiology 1999; 5:476–480.
10. Hulley S, Grady D, Bush T, Friberg C, Harrington D, Riggs B, Vittinghoff E. Randomized trial of estrogen plus progestin for secondary prevention of coronary heart disease in post menopausal women: The Heart and Estrogen/progestin Replacement Study (HERS). JAMA 1998; 280:605–613.
11. Grodstein F, Manson JE, Stampfer MJ. Postmenopausal hormone use and secondary prevention of coronary events in the Nurses' Health Study: A prospective, observational study. Ann Intern Med 2001; 135:1–8.
12. O'Keefe JH, Kim SC, Hall RR, Cochran VC, Lawhorn SL, McCallister BD. Estrogen replacement therapy after coronary angioplasty in women. J Am Coll Cardiol 1997; 29:1–5.
13. Barrett-Connor E. Postmenopausal estrogen and prevention bias. Ann Intern Med 1991; 115:455–456.
14. Matthews KA, Kuller LH, Wing RR, Meilahn EN, Plantinga P. Prior to estrogen replacement therapy, are users healthier than nonusers? Am J Epidemiol 1996; 143: 971–978.
15. Pedersen AT, Lidegaard O, Kreiner S, Ottesen B. Hormone replacement therapy and risk of non-fatal stroke. Lancet 1997; 350:1277–1283.
16. Petitti DB, Sidney S, Quesenberry CP, Bernstein A. Ischemic stroke and use of estrogen and estrogen/progestogen as hormone replacement therapy. Stroke 1998; 29:23–28.
17. Grodstein F, Stampfer MJ, Goldhaber SZ, Manson JE, Colditz GA, Speizer FE, Willett WC, Hennekens CH. Prospective study of exogenous hormones and risk of pulmonary embolism in women. Lancet 1996; 348:983–987.
18. Daly E, Vessey MP, Hawkins MM, Carson JL, Gough P, Marsh S. Risk of venous thromboembolism in users of hormone replacement therapy. Lancet 1996; 348:977–988.
19. Stampfer MJ, Hu FB, Manson JE, Rimm EB, Willett WC. Primary prevention of coronary heart disease in women through diet and lifestyle. N Engl J Med 2000; 343:16–22.

5

Low-Molecular-Weight Heparins and Direct Thrombin Inhibitors in Acute Coronary Syndromes

Robert P. Giugliano
*Brigham and Women's Hospital and Harvard Medical School,
Boston, Massachusetts*

I. INTRODUCTION

Acute coronary syndromes are defined as unstable angina or non-Q-wave myocardial infarction. The goals of antithrombotic therapy in the treatment of acute coronary syndromes are threefold: (1) to prevent progression of intracoronary thrombus (Fig. 1); (2) to promote stabilization of the atherosclerotic plaque; and (3) to reduce the risk of subsequent ischemic events (1,2). An overview (3) of antiplatelet therapy in patients with arterial disease clearly established the benefit of aspirin; however, rates of (re)infarction or death remain elevated in the short-term even with aspirin therapy. One such strategy to prevent recurrent ischemic events has been the concomitant administration of antithrombotic therapy.

Unfractionated heparin (UFH), until recently the antithrombin of choice in acute coronary syndromes, became entrenched in clinical practice *prior* to the modern era of clinical trials. Thus, convincing data in large numbers of patients are lacking. In patients without ST elevation, the addition of UFH to aspirin has been studied in several moderate-sized trials (4–9). Overviews (9,10) of these studies suggest that UFH reduces the rate of death or (recurrent) myocardial infarction (MI) by one-third to one-half.

In patients receiving fibrinolytic therapy, the benefit of adding UFH to aspirin is less clear (improved mid- and late-term infarct artery patency) (11–13), and may depend on the particular fibrinolytic agent (14) and route of administra-

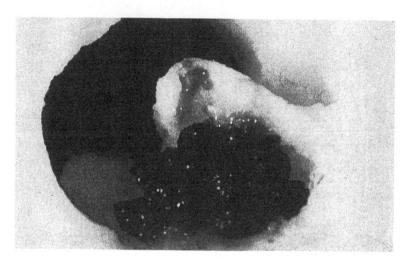

Figure 1 Intracoronary thrombus following plaque rupture in a patient with an acute coronary syndrome. (Courtesy of Davies MJ, Heart 2000; 83:261, with permission.)

tion (15). Moreover, large trials (GISSI-2, ISIS-3, and GUSTO-1) (16–18) have not shown a consistent reduction in clinical events.

In addition, UFH has several limitations, including an unpredictable dose response, low bioavailability, dose-dependent clearance with a prolonged half-life at higher dosages, need for frequent monitoring and dose adjustment, and risk of thrombocytopenia with or without thrombosis (19). Thus, several new classes of antithrombotic agents have been developed and systematically studied. This chapter will focus on the emerging data with two of these new antithrombotic drugs—low-molecular-weight heparins (LMWH) and direct thrombin inhibitors—and their role in the management of acute coronary syndromes (unstable angina/non-ST-elevation MI and ST-elevation MI).

II. LOW-MOLECULAR-WEIGHT HEPARINS

A. Pharmacology

Heparin refers not to a single structure but instead to a family of mucopolysaccharide chains of alternating residues of D-glucosamine and uronic acid (20). These chains are of varying length and composition. LMWHs have a lower mean molecular weight, 4000–5000 daltons (range 1000–10,000 daltons) compared to UFH (mean 15,000 daltons; range 1000–30,000 daltons).

LMWHs, like UFH, bind a cofactor called antithrombin to produce their predominant anticoagulant effect. Binding is mediated through a unique pentasaccharide sequence of the mucopolysaccharide that increases by 1000-fold both the interaction between antithrombin and thrombin (factor II_a), and the interaction between antithrombin and factor Xa (21). However, a minimum chain length of 15 to 18 saccharides (corresponding to a molecular weight of $\geq$ 5400 daltons) is required to inactivate thrombin (22). In contrast, inhibition of factor Xa can occur with short polysaccharide chains. Thus, one potentially important distinction between UFH and LMWH, and among LMWHs themselves, is the varying ratio of factor Xa to factor IIa. The factor Xa:IIa activity for UFH is approximately 1.2, while ratios for the various LMWH preparations vary from 2 to 4. Table 1 lists LMWHs in order of anti Xa:IIa ratio.

Agents with a high anti–factor Xa activity were designed specifically with the hope that inhibition of earlier steps in the blood coagulation system would be associated with a more potent antithrombotic effect than inhibition of subsequent steps (Fig. 2). Because of the amplification process of the coagulation cascade, a single factor Xa molecule can lead to the generation of hundreds of thrombin molecules; hence "upstream" inhibition of factor Xa can lead to dramatic reductions in thrombin generation further "downstream."

Clinical advantages of LMWHs include simpler (subcutaneous) administration, no need to monitor anticoagulant effect, weight-based dosing not requiring daily adjustment, uninterrupted therapy, and facilitation of outpatient use if needed (Table 2). Furthermore, the overall cost to the health-care system may be lower (23), despite higher drug costs, due to infrequent need for laboratory testing.

B. Use in Unstable Angina and Non-ST-Elevation MI

Six large phase III randomized controlled trials (FRISC, FRIC, ESSENCE, TIMI-11B, FRISC-II, and FRAXIS) (24–29) have studied low-molecular-weight heparins in more than 15,000 patients with unstable angina and non-ST-elevation MI. The trials were heterogeneous: 3 different LMWH preparations (dalteparin, enoxaparin, nadroparin) were studied; therapy was administered for varying durations (2 days to 6 months); different primary endpoints were evaluated; highly variable study designs were utilized, including placebo control, active UFH control, or both, depending on the acute or chronic phase of a study. Thus, a brief review summarizing the key findings of each of these trials is in order.

1. FRIC

In the FRIC study (24), 1506 patients presenting with unstable angina received aspirin and were randomized in a double-blind fashion to either subcutaneous

Table 1 Comparison of LMWHs

Generic name (trade name or synonym)	Company	MW	Xa:lla	FDA approval
Enoxaparin (Lovenox, Clexane)	Aventis	4200	3.8	Yes
Nadroparin (Fraxiparine, Sleparina)	Sanofi	4500	3.6	No
Reviparin (Clivaparine)	Knoll	4000	3.5	No
Dalteparin (Fragmin)	Pharmacia & Upjohn	6000	2.7	Yes
Parnaparin (Fluxum, Minidalton)	Opocrin	4500–5000	2.4	No
Ardeparin (Normiflo)	Wyeth-Ayerst	6000	1.9	Yes (DVT prophylaxis)
Tinzaparin (Innohep, Logiparin)	Leo, Dupont	4500	1.9	Yes
Certoparin (Alphaparin)	Alpha Therapeutic	4200–6200	NA	No
Bioparin	Bioberica	NA	NA	No
Miniparin	Syntex	NA	NA	No
Sandoparin (Monoembolex)	Sandoz	NA	NA	No
Unfractionated heparin.	—	15,000	1.2	Yes

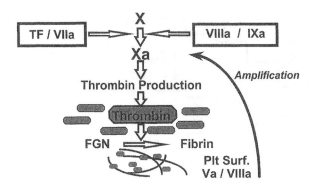

Figure 2 Amplification process of thrombin generation. Following rupture of a vulnerable plaque, tissue factor is exposed, and factor VIIa levels increase, ultimately leading to the conversion of factor X to factor Xa. This is an important step in stimulation of the coagulation cascade because of a multiplier effect such that a single molecule of factor Xa leads to the reduction of many molecules of thrombin. As compared with UFH, LMWH preparations are clinically attractive because of enriched anti-Xa activity, which interferes with the coagulation pathway further upstream, resulting in a marked reduction in thrombin production.

dalteparin (120 IU/kg body weight [maximum 10,000 IU] twice daily for 6 days then 7500 IU once daily for the next 35 to 45 days) or placebo injections. During the first 6 days, the rate of death and new myocardial infarction was lower in the dalteparin group than in the placebo group (13 [1.8%] vs.36 [4.8%]; risk ratio 0.37 [95% CI 0.20 to 0.68]) (Fig. 3). Among patients randomized to dalteparin, there was also less need for revascularization (3 [0.4%] vs. 9 [1.2%]; 0.33 [0.10 to 1.10]). The composite endpoint (death, myocardial infarction, revascularization)

Table 2 Potential Clinical Advantages of LMWH over UFH

	UFH	LMWH
1. Dosing	Continuous infusion	Twice daily
2. Route of administration	Intravenous	Subcutaneous
3. aPTT monitoring	Required	Unnecessary
4. Dose adjustment	Yes, frequently	No
5. Uninterrupted therapy	No	Yes
6. Antithrombotic effect	Lower	Higher
7. Ease of outpatient use	Complex	Easy
8. Overall cost to health-care system	Higher	Lower

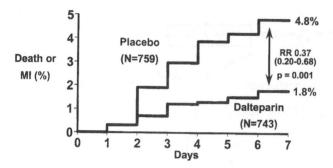

Figure 3 Primary results of the FRISC trial comparing dalteparin with placebo among patients with unstable angina or non-ST-elevation MI treated with aspirin.

favored dalteparin (40 [5.4%] vs.78 [10.3%]; 0.52 [0.37 to 0.75]). This trial demonstrated the benefit of adding a LMWH to aspirin monotherapy in patients presenting with unstable angina. Note, however, that half the patients with unstable angina received no heparin of any type.

2. FRISC-I

The FRISC-I trial (25) was the first large study to directly compare a LMWH with UFH. Included in the study were 1482 patients presenting with unstable angina. There were two phases: in an open, acute phase (days 1 to 6), patients were assigned either twice-daily weight-adjusted subcutaneous injections of dalteparin (120 IU/kg) or dose-adjusted intravenous infusion of UFH. In the double-blind, prolonged treatment phase (days 6 to 45), patients received either dalteparin (7500 IU once daily) or placebo administered as subcutaneous injections. During the first 6 days (open, acute phase), the rate of death, myocardial infarction, or recurrence of angina was 7.6% among the patients randomized to UFH and 9.3% in patients randomized to dalteparin (relative risk, 1.18 [0.84 to 1.66]). The corresponding rates in the two treatment groups for the composite endpoint of death or myocardial infarction were 3.6% and 3.9%, respectively (relative risk, 1.07 [0.63 to 1.80]). Between days 6 and 45, the rate of death, myocardial infarction, or recurrence of angina was 12.3% in both the placebo and dalteparin groups (relative risk, 1.01 [0.74 to 1.38]). The corresponding rates for death or myocardial infarction were 4.7% and 4.3% (relative risk, 0.92 [0.54 to 1.57]). Thus, there were no statistically significant differences in important clinical outcomes when dalteparin was substituted for UFH in the acute treatment phase, while prolonged therapy (days 6 to 45) with a fixed dose of dalteparin once daily did not appear to confer any benefit over placebo.

3. ESSENCE

The ESSENCE study (26) was a double-blind, placebo-controlled trial that randomly assigned 3171 patients with angina at rest or non-Q-wave myocardial infarction to receive 2 to 8 days therapy with either 1 mg/kg of enoxaparin subcutaneously twice daily or continuous intravenous UFH. At 14 days, the risk of death, myocardial infarction, or recurrent angina was significantly lower in the patients assigned to enoxaparin than in those assigned to UFH (16.6% vs. 19.8%; $p = 0.019$). At 30 days, the risk of this composite endpoint remained significantly lower in the enoxaparin group (19.8% vs. 23.3%; $p = 0.016$). The need for revascularization procedures at 30 days was also significantly less frequent in the patients assigned to enoxaparin (27.1% vs. 32.2%; $p = 0.001$). The 30-day incidence of major bleeding complications was 6.5% in the enoxaparin group and 7.0% in the unfractionated-heparin group, but the incidence of bleeding overall was significantly higher in the enoxaparin group (18.4% vs. 14.2%; $p = 0.001$), primarily because of ecchymoses at injection sites. Thus, the ESSENCE trial indicates that enoxaparin plus aspirin is more effective than UFH plus aspirin in reducing the incidence of ischemic events in patients with unstable angina or non-Q-wave myocardial infarction in the early phase. This benefit was associated with an increase in minor, but not major, bleeding.

4. TIMI-11B

In TIMI-11B (27), 3910 patients with unstable angina or non-Q-wave MI were randomized to either intravenous UFH for 3 to 8 days followed by subcutaneous placebo injections, or enoxaparin during both the acute phase (initial 30-mg IV bolus followed by injections of 1.0 mg/kg every 12 h for 3 to 8 days) and outpatient phase (injections every 12 h for up to 43 days of 40 mg for patients weighing $\geq$65 kg and 60 mg for those weighing $<$65 kg). The primary endpoint (death, myocardial infarction, or urgent revascularization) occurred by 8 days in 14.5% of patients in the UFH group and 12.4% of patients in the enoxaparin group (OR 0.83 [0.69 to 1.00]; $p = 0.048$) and by 43 days in 19.7% of the UFH group and 17.3% of the enoxaparin group (OR 0.85 [0.72 to 1.00]; $p = 0.048$). During the first 72 h and also throughout the entire initial hospitalization, there was no difference in the rate of major hemorrhage in the treatment groups. During the outpatient phase, major hemorrhage occurred in 1.5% of the group treated with placebo and 2.9% of the group treated with enoxaparin ($p = 0.021$). Consistent with the ESSENCE findings described above, the results of the TIMI-11B study demonstrate that enoxaparin is superior to UFH in reducing a composite of death and serious cardiac ischemic events during the acute management of patients presenting with unstable angina, but does not cause a significant increase in the rate of major hemorrhage. The outpatient phase of TIMI-11B suggests that continued therapy with enoxaparin does not further decrease the rate of cardiac events, but is associated with an increase in the rate of major hemorrhage.

5. FRISC-II

In FRISC-II (28), 2267 patients with unstable coronary artery disease were randomly assigned to continue double-blind subcutaneous dalteparin twice daily or placebo for 3 months, after at least 5 days of treatment with open-label dalteparin. During the 3 months of double-blind treatment, there was a nonsignificant decrease in the composite endpoint of death or myocardial infarction of 6.7% and 8.0% in the dalteparin and placebo groups, respectively (risk ratio 0.81 [0.60 to 1.10]; $p = 0.17$). At 30 days, this decrease was significant (3.1 vs. 5.9%, 0.53 [0.35 to 0.80]; $p = 0.002$). In the total cohort, at 3 months there was a decrease in death, myocardial infarction, or revascularization (29.1 vs. 33.4%, 0.87 [0.77 to 0.99]; $p = 0.031$). These initial benefits were not sustained at 6-month follow-up. Thus, continued therapy with dalteparin beyond the initial 5 days may be of benefit during the first month of therapy, particularly as a bridge in patients awaiting revascularization; however, the benefit attenuates with time despite continued treatment.

6. FRAXIS

Last, the FRAXIS trial (29) randomized 3468 patients in a double-blind fashion to one of three treatment regimens: UFH (5000 IU bolus, followed by an infusion for 6 ± 2 days); nadroparin for 6 days (nadroparin 86 anti-Xa IU/kg IV bolus, followed by twice-daily subcutaneous injections for 6 ± 2 days); or nadroparin for 14 days (same dose as the prior group for 14 days). No statistically significant differences were observed among the three treatment regimens with respect to the primary outcome (cardiac death, myocardial infarction, refractory angina, or recurrence of unstable angina at day 14). The absolute differences between the groups in the incidence of the primary outcome were: -0.3% ($p = 0.85$) for the nadroparin 6-day group vs. the UFH group, and $+1.9\%$ ($p = 0.24$) for the nadroparin 14-day group vs. the unfractionated heparin group. Furthermore, there were no significant intergroup differences regarding any of the secondary efficacy outcomes. However, there was an increased risk of major hemorrhage in the nadroparin 14-day group compared with UFH (3.5% vs. 1.6%; $p = 0.0035$). Thus, similar to the FRISC-I trial findings with dalteparin, treatment with nadroparin for 6 days provides similar efficacy and safety to treatment with UFH for the same period. A prolonged regimen of nadroparin (14 days) does not provide any additional clinical benefit and is associated with an increase risk of major hemorrhage.

7. Overview

Several important conclusions emerge from review of the data from the six unstable angina trials above. First, in the acute phase, when added to aspirin dalteparin further reduces the early risk of death or MI when compared to placebo plus aspirin (24). Second, in two studies (26,27) using active controls, enoxaparin was superior to UFH in reducing the combined triple endpoint of death, MI, or recurrent ischemia by 12 to 25% at various timepoints between 48 h and 43 days. However, two other similar trials, one with dalteparin (25) and one with nadroparin (29), demonstrated no benefit of LMWH over UFH. Despite the temptation to ascribe these different outcomes to the specific formulation of LMWH, the many heterogeneities between the trials need to be recognized as equally important potential explanations. Last, these trials were generally underpowered to evaluate "harder" clinical endpoints, such as death and MI; however, a metanalysis of the two phase-III enoxaparin studies did demonstrate an 18 to 23% reduction in the rate of death or MI at 8, 14, and 43 days (Fig. 4) (30).

Overviews of clinical trials of LMWH in acute coronary syndromes (with the caveats noted above regarding the heterogeneity of the studies) have also concluded that the LMWHs are at least as efficacious as UFH at reducing death or myocardial infarction and appear to have a similar safety profile (31,32). When

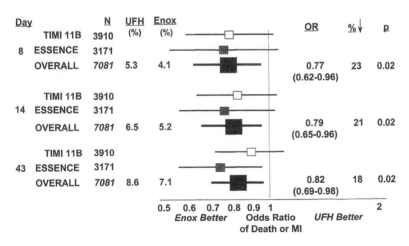

Figure 4 Metanalysis of two phase-III studies comparing enoxaparin with UFH. A consistent reduction of approximately 20% in the odds of death or myocardial infarction occurred in both trials at 8, 14, and 43 days.

"softer" clinical endpoints such as recurrent angina, rehospitalization, or need for revascularization are considered, the totality of the evidence supports a benefit for LMWHs over UFH.

Data supporting the use of LMWH after hospital discharge are less convincing. No additional benefit of continued therapy with dalteparin was noted in the FRISC (24), FRIC (25), and FRISC-II (28) trials when treatment was extended for 45 to 180 days, compared to placebo. Similarly, in the TIMI-11B chronic phase (27), the absolute event rates in the placebo and enoxaparin arms were nearly identical (5.2% vs. 4.9%; p = NS) between 8 and 43 days, while the rates of major hemorrhage were increased during this period (2.9% vs. 1.5%; p = 0.02). A metanalysis (32) of long-term LMWH use concluded that the likelihood of a major hemorrhage was more than doubled (OR 2.26 [1.63 to 3.14]; $p <$ 0.0001), translating into an excess of approximately 12 major bleeds per 1000 patients treated after the acute phase.

C. Adjunctive Therapy with Fibrinolysis for ST-Elevation MI

The use of LMWH as an adjunct to fibrinolytic therapy is actively under investigation (33–37). Preliminary results from the HART-II angiographic study (37) demonstrated slightly higher rates of infarct artery patency (80.1% vs. 75.1%; p = NS) and TIMI grade 3 flow rates (52.9% vs. 47.6%; p = NS) at 90 min among 200 patients receiving tPA and enoxaparin (30 mg IV bolus followed by 1 mg/ kg SQ twice daily for ≥72 h) compared to tPA and UFH. Clinical event rates were similar and reocclusion among patients with a patent artery at 90 min tended to be less frequent in those randomized to enoxaparin (5.9 vs. 9.8%; p = NS). In another angiographic study (36), dalteparin was compared with placebo in patients receiving streptokinase. TIMI grade 3 flow 20 to 28 h later tended to be higher in patients treated with dalteparin (68% vs. 51%; p = 0.10) and the number of ischemic episodes on continuous ECG monitoring was lower (16% vs. 38%; p = 0.04) (36).

One recent study (35) found a significant reduction in the rate of death, MI, or readmission for an acute coronary syndrome among 300 patients treated with fibrinolytic therapy (predominantly streptokinase) who were randomized to enoxaparin (40-mg IV bolus, followed by 40 mg SQ every 8 h) compared to UFH for 4 days. The rate of the composite endpoint at 3 months was 36.4% for heparin vs. 25.5% for enoxaparin (p = 0.04) (35). It appeared that "rebound" thrombosis was reduced by enoxaparin, as the rate of reinfarction from day 4 to 6 was only 2.2% for enoxaparin compared to 6.6% for heparin (p = 0.05) (35). Other studies of LMWH as adjunctive therapy for fibrinolysis, such as the ENTIRE-TIMI 23 trial studying TNK-tPA, abciximab, and enoxaparin vs. UFH, are ongoing.

D. Combination with Glycoprotein IIb/IIIa Inhibitors

Limited data are available on the combination of LMWH with glycoprotein IIb/ IIIa inhibitors (38,39). A small pilot trial (38) studied 54 patients with an acute coronary syndrome for 48 to 96 h prior to coronary angiography treated with standard-dose tirofiban and either enoxaparin 1 mg/kg SQ every 12 h or UFH. No major or minor hemorrhagic events (using the TIMI criteria) were noted. Mean levels of platelet inhibition were slightly higher in the tirofiban-enoxaparin group, and the range of platelet inhibition was less compared to tirofiban-UFH.

Preliminary results from the National Investigators Collaborating on Enoxaparin (NICE) 4 Registry (39) suggest that 75% of the usual enoxaparin dose (0.75 mg/kg) administered intravenously in combination with a standard dose of abciximab is efficacious and safe in patients undergoing percutaneous coronary intervention. Rates of major hemorrhage (0.6%), transfusion (1.8%), and thrombocytopenia (2.3%) among the 817 patients in NICE 4 were similar or lower than those reported in other contemporary interventional trials with abciximab and UFH (40,41). Similarly, rates of important clinical events (death 0.4%, MI 1.7%, urgent revascularization 0.6%) were quite low.

E. Future Considerations

Five issues regarding the use of LMWH in acute coronary syndromes include safety, preparation, interface with the catheterization laboratory, combination with glycoprotein IIb/IIIa inhibitors, and cost effectiveness. Hemorrhage and thrombocytopenia are the two major safety issues that arose during clinical testing. However, the totality of the evidence suggests that LMWH are as safe, if not safer, than UFH. There was no difference in the risk of major hemorrhage during treatment with unfractionated heparin compared to LMWH (OR 1.00, 95% CI 0.64 to 1.57; $p = 0.99$) in data from five trials comparing these agents head to head (32). Post-marketing surveillance suggests that the combination of LMWH and neuraxial anesthesia (e.g., epidural catheters) should be avoided whenever possible to minimize the risk of epidural hematoma (42) (a potential complication shared by all anticoagulants in this setting). Because LMWH bind less avidly to platelets (and hence do not activate platelets to the same degree as UFH), the risk of thrombocytopenia with LMWH is much less than that associated with UFH (43).

Little data exist comparing different LMWH preparations to one another Whether differences in mean molecular weight, anti-Xa:IIa activity, pharmacokinetics, and dosing administration of the various LMWHs translate into important clinical differences will have to await such head-to-head comparisons.

The interface of LMWHs with the catheterization laboratory is under investigation and use of LMWH during angiography and percutaneous coronary intervention appears promising (39,44,45). Likewise, use of LMWHs in combination with GP IIb/IIIa inhibitors is being tested, although considerably more study is required to investigate the various combinations of drugs from both classes. Last, formal economic analyses of the use of LMWHs are needed to help guide the use of this more expensive agent. One such analysis from the ESSENCE trial (23) suggests that despite a twofold increase in drug costs, use of enoxaparin resulted in a net savings per patient during hospitalization ($763) and through 30 days ($1172).

III. DIRECT THROMBIN INHIBITORS

A. Pharmacology

Direct thrombin inhibitors, as indicated by the class name, do not require anti-thrombin or another cofactor to inhibit the function of thrombin. Direct thrombin inhibitors inhibit all the major actions of thrombin, including thrombin-induced generation of fibrin, thrombin-induced platelet activation, as well as thrombin's autocatalytic reaction (46,47). Potential advantages of direct thrombin inhibitors over heparin include: (1) inhibition of clot-bound thrombin (48); (2) lack of inhibition by activated platelets (49); and (3) stable anticoagulant response since no cofactor is required (46).

The prototypic direct thrombin inhibitor is hirudin, a polypeptide consisting of 65 amino acids derived from the leech *Hirudo medicinalis* (47). Hirudin selectively binds thrombin in a 1:1 fashion at two locations: (1) the carboxy terminus of hirudin binds to the substrate recognition site, the domain of thrombin that recognizes fibrinogen (50) or the platelet (51) and (2) the amino terminus of hirudin binds to the catalytic site of thrombin (50). Hirudin does not inhibit factor Xa, IX, kallikrein, activated protein C, plasmin, tissue plasminogen activator, or other enzymes in the coagulation or fibrinolytic pathways (47). Although hirudin does not bind covalently to thrombin, the dissociation rate is extremely slow; thus, hirudin essentially irreversibly inhibits thrombin (47,52).

Hirudin is produced in yeast by recombinant DNA technology. Several different hirudin preparations are available, including desirudin (53–55) and lepirudin (56). Other available analogs include bivaluridin (Hirulog) (57,58), argatroban (59), efegatran (60), and inogatran (61).

B. Use in Unstable Angina and Non-ST-Elevation MI

Desirudin was studied in the GUSTO-IIb trial (55) involving 12,142 patients with unstable angina/non-ST-elevation MI as well as patients with ST-elevation MI (most of the latter group received fibrinolytic therapy). In the entire cohort, the 30-day rate of death or MI tended to be lower, 8.9% vs. 9.8% ($p = 0.06$), with no difference in mortality and a modest reduction in reinfarction (5.4% vs. 6.3%

for heparin; $p = 0.04$). Among the 8011 patients with unstable angina or non-ST-elevation MI, the rate of death or MI was not significantly reduced at 30 days (8.3% vs. 9.1%; $p = 0.22$) (55).

Lepirudin was compared to heparin in the OASIS-2 trial (56). While there were trends toward a reduction in cardiovascular death or MI at 72 h (2.0% vs. 2.6%; $p = 0.04$) and at 7 days (3.6% vs. 4.2%; $p = 0.08$), there was an attenuation of this benefit by day 35, in contrast to the sustained superiority of enoxaparin over UFH (30). Furthermore, major bleeding requiring transfusion was more frequent with lepirudin (1.2% vs. 0.7% for heparin; $p = 0.01$). The authors performed a metanalysis of all the hirudin trials and observed a modest 10% benefit favoring hirudin, although this was not statistically significant for patients with unstable angina/non-ST-elevation MI at 35 days (56). The Food and Drug Administration (FDA) recently reviewed the available clinical data and did not approve hirudin for use in unstable angina/non-ST-elevation MI, citing the lack of sustained benefit and increased risk of bleeding.

Other synthetic direct thrombin inhibitors have also been tested (e.g., argatroban, inogatran, and bivaluridin [Hirulog]) and, again, only modest or no improvements were observed compared with heparin (61–63), although lower rates of bleeding have been observed with bivalirudin (63). The direct thrombin inhibitors have been observed to provide a very stable level of anticoagulation, as measured by aPTT (55,64,65), and no episodes of thrombocytopenia were reported for the hirudin class. Of note, lepirudin is approved by the FDA for use as an anticoagulant in patients with heparin-induced thrombocytopenia, and has been demonstrated to prevent death, limb amputation, and new thromboembolic complications (66).

C. Adjunctive Therapy with Fibrinolysis for ST-Elevation MI

The effects of desirudin in the setting of fibrinolysis were tested in the TIMI-5, -6 and -9 and GUSTO-II trials (53–55,67). Hirudin provided a more stable aPTT, and was within the target range almost twice as frequently as UFH. No episodes of thrombocytopenia were reported for hirudin.

In TIMI-5, a lower rate of recurrent MI was observed (4.3% vs. 11.9%, for hirudin and UFH respectively; $p = 0.03$) as well as a trend toward lower reocclusion 1.6% vs. 6.7% ($p = 0.07$) when hirudin was administered as an adjunct to tPA in comparison to UFH (53). In the phase III TIMI-9B trial, a similar trend in lower reinfarction with hirudin was observed in-hospital (2.3% vs. 3.4%; $p = 0.07$), but no difference was observed in the primary endpoint, death, MI, or severe CHF/shock at 30 days (12.9% for hirudin vs. 11.9% for heparin; $p = $ NS) (54). Similarly, rates of death or MI did not differ between the two anticoagulants (9.7% vs. 9.5%; $p = $ NS) (54).

In the GUSTO-IIb trial (55), among 4131 patients with ST-elevation MI, hirudin was associated with a slightly lower rate of death or MI (9.9% vs. 11.3%; $p = 0.13$) compared to UFH. Benefit was observed in the subgroup of patients receiving streptokinase in GUSTO-II (68), but not in TIMI-9B (54), making this isolated subgroup finding questionable. In a prospectively planned metanalysis of the TIMI-9B and GUSTO-IIb data, mortality rates were similar at 30 days in both treatment groups (hirudin and UFH) (OR 1.00, 95% CI 0.87 to 1.17), while a generally consistent reduction in the rate of reinfarction of approximately 14% (OR 0.86, 95% CI 0.75 to 0.98) was observed with hirudin (69).

In the HIT-3 trial (70), excess intracranial hemorrhage was observed with lepirudin (0.4 mg/kg bolus, 0.15 mg/kg/h infusion) compared to UFH (3.4% vs. 0%) among 302 patients receiving tPA. In the subsequent HIT-4 trial (71), involving 1208 patients and using a lower dose of lepirudin (0.2 mg/kg bolus, 0.5 mg/kg subcutaneously b.i.d.) in combination with streptokinase, TIMI flow grade 3 was observed in 40.7% in the lepirudin and in 33.5% in the heparin group ($p = 0.16$). No difference were seen between lepirudin and heparin in the rate of hemorrhagic stroke (0.2% vs. 0.3%), reinfarction (4.6% vs. 5.1%), or mortality (6.8% vs. 6.4%) at 30 days. Thus, intravenous lepirudin (as administered in HIT-3) as an adjunct to tPA appears to be unsafe, and lower dose lepirudin in combination with streptokinase does not significantly improve reperfusion or clinical outcomes.

Angiographic trials with other direct thrombin inhibitors in conjunction with fibrinolytic therapy have also been conducted. In a pilot study and the HERO trial, a trend toward improved early (90 to 120 min) TIMI grade 3 flow was observed with the higher dose of Hirulog as compared with heparin in patients receiving streptokinase (57,58). Testing with other agents found modest or no improvements compared with heparin (59,60). HERO-II, an international phase III trial of approximately 17,000 patients with ST-elevation MI treated with streptokinase, is randomizing patients to either Hirulog or UFH and should complete enrollment in the latter half of 2000.

D. FDA Update

The Food and Drug Administration has approved the anticoagulant argatroban (Novastan, SmithKline Beecham) for the prevention or treatment of thrombosis associated with heparin-induced thrombocytopenia (HIT). Argatroban is the first synthetic direct thrombin inhibitor approved for the prevention and treatment of thrombosis in patients with HIT.

The FDA has sent an approvable letter to The Medicines Company for bivalirudin (Angiomax) for use as an anticoagulant in patients with unstable angina undergoing percutaneous transluminal coronary angioplasty (PTCA). Final approval is pending.

DuPont Pharmaceuticals' once-daily low-molecular-weight heparin (LMWH) tinzaparin sodium injection (Innohep) has been approved by the FDA for the treatment of acute symptomatic deep vein thrombosis with or without pulmonary embolism when administered with warfarin sodium.

E. Future of Direct Thrombin Inhibitors

Despite tremendous initial enthusiasm for the direct thrombin inhibitors, their current role in clinical practice is limited to use as an anticoagulant in patients with heparin allergy, or in the treatment of heparin-induced thrombocytopenia and thrombotic syndrome. Ongoing and future research, particularly as adjunctive therapy in patients receiving fibrinolysis or percutaneous coronary intervention, may identify other clinical situations in which these drugs could play a useful role. However, studies to date have identified a narrow therapeutic window, marginal evidence of incremental, sustained efficacy over UFH, and the possibility of a "rebound" effect. These problems represent challenges to this class of antithrombotic drugs.

IV. CONCLUSIONS

Standard management of acute coronary syndromes includes the combined use of antiplatelet and antithrombotic therapy. UFH has been the standard antithrombotic drug for decades. However, newer agents have been developed and widely tested. In patients with unstable angina and non-ST-elevation MI, the totality of the evidence suggests that LMWHs are at least as efficacious as UFH, equally safe, and much easier to administer. Further studies are needed to define the role of LWMH in patients receiving GP IIb/IIIa inhibitors, fibrinolytic therapy, angiography, and coronary intervention. Also, additional research comparing different LMWH preparations and examining the cost effectiveness of these drugs is required. The clinical role of direct thrombin inhibitors is currently limited to patients who have a heparin allergy or heparin-induced thrombocytopenia, although efforts to identify other groups of patients who might benefit from direct thrombin inhibition are ongoing.

REFERENCES

1. Fuster V, Badimon L, Badimon JJ, Chesebro JH. The pathogenesis of coronary artery disease and the acute coronary syndromes (1). N Engl J Med 1992; 326:242–250.
2. Theroux P, Fuster V. Acute coronary syndromes: unstable angina and non-Q-wave myocardial infarction. Circulation 1998; 97:1195–1206.

3.   Collaborative overview of randomised trials of antiplatelet therapy—I: Prevention of death, myocardial infarction, and stroke by prolonged antiplatelet therapy in various categories of patients. Antiplatelet Trialists' Collaboration [see comments] [published erratum appears in BMJ 1994 Jun 11; 308(6943):1540]. BMJ 1994; 308:81–106.

4.   Williams DO, Kirby MG, McPherson K, Phear DN. Anticoagulant treatment of unstable angina. Br J Clin Pract 1986; 40:114–116.

5.   Telford AM, Wilson C. Trial of heparin versus atenolol in prevention of myocardial infarction in intermediate coronary syndrome. Lancet 1981; 1:1225–1228.

6.   Lewis HD Jr., Davis JW, Archibald DG, et al. Protective effects of aspirin against acute myocardial infarction and death in men with unstable angina. Results of a Veterans Administration Cooperative Study. N Engl J Med 1983; 309:396–403.

7.   Theroux P, Ouimet H, McCans J, et al. Aspirin, heparin, or both to treat acute unstable angina [see comments]. N Engl J Med 1988; 319:1105–1111.

8.   Theroux P, Waters D, Qiu S, McCans J, de Guise P, Juneau M. Aspirin versus heparin to prevent myocardial infarction during the acute phase of unstable angina [see comments]. Circulation 1993; 88:2045–2048.

9.   Cohen M, Adams PC, Parry G, et al. Combination antithrombotic therapy in unstable rest angina and non-Q-wave infraction in nonprior aspirin users. Primary end points analysis from the ATACS trial. Antithrombotic Therapy in Acute Coronary Syndromes Research Group. Circulation 1994; 89:81–88.

10. Oler A, Whooley MA, Oler J, Grady D. Adding heparin to aspirin reduces the incidence of myocardial infarction and death in patients with unstable angina. A meta-analysis [see comments]. JAMA 1996; 276:811–815.

11. Hsia J, Hamilton WP, Kleiman N, Roberts R, Chaitman BR, Ross AM. A comparison between heparin and low-dose aspirin as adjunctive therapy with tissue plasminogen activator for acute myocardial infarction. Heparin-Aspirin Reperfusion Trial (HART) Investigators [see comments]. N Engl J Med 1990; 323:1433–1437.

12. de Bono DP, Simoons ML, Tijssen J, et al. Effect of early intravenous heparin on coronary patency, infarct size, and bleeding complications after alteplase thrombolysis: results of a randomised double blind European Cooperative Study Group trial [see comments]. Br Heart J 1992; 67:122–1228.

13. Bleich SD, Nichols TC, Schumacher RR, Cooke DH, Tate DA, Teichman SL. Effect of heparin on coronary arterial patency after thrombolysis with tissue plasminogen activator in acute myocardial infarction. Am J Cardiol 1990; 66:1412–1417.

14. O'Connor CM, Meese R, Carney R, et al. A randomized trial of intravenous heparin in conjunction with anistreplase (anisoylated plasminogen streptokinase activator complex) in acute myocardial infarction: the Duke University Clinical Cardiology Study (DUCCS) 1. J Am Coll Cardiol 1994; 23:11–18.

15. The effects of tissue plasminogen activator, streptokinase, or both on coronary-artery patency, ventricular function, and survival after acute myocardial infarction. The GUSTO Angiographic Investigators [see comments] [published erratum appears in N Engl J Med 1994 Feb 17;330(7):516]. N Engl J Med 1993; 329:1615–1622.

16. GISSI-2: a factorial randomised trial of alteplase versus streptokinase and heparin versus no heparin among 12,490 patients with acute myocardial infarction. Gruppo

Italiano per lo Studio della Sopravvivenza nell'Infarto Miocardico [see comments]. Lancet 1990; 336:65–71.

17. ISIS-3: a randomised comparison of streptokinase vs tissue plasminogen activator vs anistreplase and of aspirin plus heparin vs aspirin alone among 41,299 cases of suspected acute myocardial infarction. ISIS-3 (Third International Study of Infarct Survival) Collaborative Group [see comments]. Lancet 1992; 339:753–770.

18. An international randomized trial comparing four thrombolytic strategies for acute myocardial infarction. The GUSTO investigators [see comments]. N Engl J Med 1993; 329:673–682.

19. Weitz JI. Low-molecular-weight heparins [published erratum appears in N Engl J Med 1997 Nov 20;337(21):1567] [see comments]. N Engl J Med 1997; 337:688–698.

20. Rosenberg RD, Bauer KA. The heparin-antithrombin system: a natural anticoagulant mechanism. In: Colman RW, Hirsch J, Marder VJ, Salzman EW, eds. Hemostasis and Thrombosis: Basic Principles and Clinical Practice. Philadelphia: J.B. Lippincott, 1994:837–860.

21. Danielsson A, Raub E, Lindahl U, Bjork I. Role of ternary complexes, in which heparin binds both antithrombin and proteinase, in the acceleration of the reactions between antithrombin and thrombin or factor Xa. J Biol Chem 1986; 261:15467–15473.

22. Jordan RE, Oosta GM, Gardner WT, Rosenberg RD. The kinetics of hemostatic enzyme-antithrombin interactions in the presence of low molecular weight heparin. J Biol Chem 1980; 255:10081–10090.

23. Mark DB, Cowper PA, Berkowitz SD, et al. Economic assessment of low-molecular-weight heparin (enoxaparin) versus unfractionated heparin in acute coronary syndrome patients: results from the ESSENCE randomized trial. Efficacy and Safety of Subcutaneous Enoxaparin in Non-Q wave Coronary Events [unstable angina or non-Q-wave myocardial infarction]. Circulation 1998; 97:1702–1707.

24. Low-molecular-weight heparin during instability in coronary artery disease, Fragmin during Instability in Coronary Artery Disease (FRISC) study group [see comments]. Lancet 1996; 347:561–568.

25. Klein W, Buchwald A, Hillis SE, et al. Comparison of low-molecular-weight heparin with unfractionated heparin acutely and with placebo for 6 weeks in the management of unstable coronary artery disease. Fragmin in unstable coronary artery disease study (FRIC) [see comments] [published erratum appears in Circulation 1998 Feb 3;97(4):413]. Circulation 1997; 96:61–68.

26. Cohen M, Demers C, Gurfinkel EP, et al. A comparison of low-molecular-weight heparin with unfractionated heparin for unstable coronary artery disease. Efficacy and Safety of Subcutaneous Enoxaparin in Non-Q-Wave Coronary Events Study Group [see comments]. N Engl J Med 1997; 337:447–452.

27. Antman EM, McCabe CH, Gurfinkel EP, et al. Enoxaparin prevents death and cardiac ischemic events in unstable angina/non-Q-wave myocardial infarction. Results of the thrombolysis in myocardial infarction (TIMI) 11B trial [see comments]. Circulation 1999; 100:1593–1601.

28. Long-term low-molecular-mass heparin in unstable coronary-artery disease: FRISC II prospective randomised multicentre study. FRagmin and Fast Revascularisation

during InStability in Coronary artery disease. Investigators [see comments] [published erratum appears in Lancet 1999 Oct 23;354(9188):1478]. Lancet 1999; 354: 701–707.

29. Comparison of two treatment durations (6 days and 14 days) of a low molecular weight heparin with a 6-day treatment of unfractionated heparin in the initial management of unstable angina or non-Q wave myocardial infarction: FRAX.I.S. (FRAxiparine in Ischaemic Syndrome) [see comments]. Eur Heart J 1999; 20:1553–1562.

30. Antman EM, Cohen M, Radley D, et al. Assessment of the treatment effect of enoxaparin for unstable angina/non-Q-wave myocardial infarction. TIMI 11B-ESSENCE meta-analysis [see comments]. Circulation 1999; 100:1602–1608.

31. Kaul S, Shah PK. Low molecular weight heparin in acute coronary syndrome: evidence for superior or equivalent efficacy compared with unfractionated heparin? J Am Coll Cardiol 2000; 35:1699–1712.

32. Eikelboom JW, Anand SS, Malmberg K, Weitz JI, Ginsberg JS, Yusuf S. Unfractionated heparin and low-molecular-weight heparin in acute coronary syndrome without ST elevation: a meta-analysis [see comments]. Lancet 2000; 355:1936–1942.

33. Strandberg LE, Kahan T, Lundin P, Svensson J, Erhardt L. Anticoagulant effects of low-molecular-weight heparin following thrombolytic therapy in acute myocardial infarction: a dose-finding study. Haemostasis 1996; 26:247–257.

34. Nesvold A, Kontny F, Abildgaard U, Dale J. Safety of high doses of low molecular weight heparin (Fragmin) in acute myocardial infarction. A dose-finding study. Thromb Res 1991; 64:579–587.

35. Baird SH, McBride SJ, Trouton TG, Wilson C. Low Molecular Weight Heparin Versus Unfractionated Heparin Following Thrombolysis in Myocardial Infarction. J Am Coll Cardiol 1998; 31:1–191A (abstr).

36. Frostfeldt G, Ahlberg G, Gustafsson G, et al. Low molecular weight heparin (dalteparin) as adjuvant treatment of thrombolysis in acute myocardial infarction-a pilot study: biochemical markers in acute coronary syndromes (BIOMACS II). J Am Coll Cardiol 1999; 33:627–633.

37. Ross AM. A Randomized Comparison of Low-Molecular-Weight Heparin and Unfractionated Heparin Adjunctive to t-PA Thrombolysis and Aspirin (HART-II), American College of Cardiology 49th Annual Scientific Sessions, Anaheim, CA, March 12–15, 2000, 2000.

38. Cohen M, Theroux P, Weber S, et al. Combination therapy with tirofiban and enoxaparin in acute coronary syndromes. Int J Cardiol 1999; 71:273–81.

39. Kereiakes DJ, Grines C, Fry E, et al. Abciximab-Enoxaparin Interaction During Percutaneous Coronary Intervention: Results of the NICE 1 and 4 Trials. J Am Coll Cardiol 2000; 35:1–92A.

40. Platelet glycoprotein IIb/IIIa receptor blockade and low-dose heparin during percutaneous coronary revascularization. The EPILOG Investigators [see comments]. N Engl J Med 1997; 336:1689–1696.

41. Randomised placebo-controlled and balloon-angioplasty-controlled trial to assess safety of coronary stenting with use of platelet glycoprotein-IIb/IIIa blockade. The EPISTENT Investigators. Evaluation of Platelet IIb/IIIa Inhibitor for Stenting [see comments]. Lancet 1998; 352:87–92.

42. Horlocker TT, Heit JA. Low molecular weight heparin: biochemistry, pharmacology, perioperative prophylaxis regimens, and guidelines for regional anesthetic management. Anesth Analg 1997; 85:874–85.
43. Warkentin TE, Levine MN, Hirsh J, et al. Heparin-induced thrombocytopenia in patients treated with low-molecular-weight heparin or unfractionated heparin [see comments]. N Engl J Med 1995; 332:1330–1335.
44. Invasive compared with non-invasive treatment in unstable coronary-artery disease: FRISC II prospective randomised multicentre study. FRagmin and Fast Revascularisation during InStability in Coronary artery disease Investigators [see comments]. Lancet 1999; 354:708–715.
45. Cannon CP, Weintraub WS, Demopoulos LA, Robertson DH, Gormley GJ, Braunwald E. Invasive versus conservative strategies in unstable angina and non-Q-wave myocardial infarction following treatment with tirofiban: rationale and study design of the international TACTICS-TIMI 18 Trial. Treat Angina with Aggrastat and determine Cost of Therapy with an Invasive or Conservative Strategy. Thrombolysis In Myocardial Infarction. Am J Cardiol 1998; 82:731–736.
46. Talbot M. Biology of recombinant hirudin (CGP 39393): a new prospect in the treatment of thrombosis. Semin Thromb Hemost 1989; 15:293–301.
47. Markwardt F. Hirudin and derivatives as anticoagulant agents. Thromb Haemost 1991; 66:141–152.
48. Weitz JI, Hudoba M, Massel D, Maraganore J, Hirsh J. Clot-bound thrombin is protected from inhibition by heparin-antithrombin III but is susceptible to inactivation by antithrombin III-independent inhibitors. J Clin Invest 1990; 86:385–391.
49. Fareed J, Walenga JM, Pifarre R, Hoppensteadt D, Koza M. Some objective considerations for the neutralization of the anticoagulant actions of recombinant hirudin. Haemostasis 1991; 21:64–72.
50. Rydel TJ, Ravichandran KG, Tulinsky A, et al. The structure of a complex of recombinant hirudin and human alpha-thrombin. Science 1990; 249:277–280.
51. Vu TK, Wheaton VI, Hung DT, Charo I, Coughlin SR. Domains specifying thrombin-receptor interaction. Nature 1991; 353:674–677.
52. Stone SR, Hofsteenge J. Kinetics of the inhibition of thrombin by hirudin. Biochemistry 1986; 25:4622–4628.
53. Cannon CP, McCabe CH, Henry TD, et al. A pilot trial of recombinant desulfatohirudin compared with heparin in conjunction with tissue-type plasminogen activator and aspirin for acute myocardial infarction: results of the Thrombolysis in Myocardial Infarction (TIMI) 5 trial. J Am Coll Cardiol 1994; 23:993–1003.
54. Antman EM. Hirudin in acute myocardial infarction. Thrombolysis and Thrombin Inhibition in Myocardial Infarction (TIMI) 9B trial [see comments]. Circulation 1996; 94:911–921.
55. A comparison of recombinant hirudin with heparin for the treatment of acute coronary syndromes. The Global Use of Strategies to Open Occluded Coronary Arteries (GUSTO) IIb investigators [see comments]. N Engl J Med 1996; 335:775–782.
56. Effects of recombinant hirudin (lepirudin) compared with heparin on death, myocardial infarction, refractory angina, and revascularisation procedures in patients with acute myocardial ischaemia without ST elevation: a randomised trial. Organisation

to Assess Strategies for Ischemic Syndromes (OASIS-2) Investigators [see comments]. Lancet 1999; 353:429–438.

57. White HD, Aylward PE, Frey MJ, et al. Randomized, double-blind comparison of hirulog versus heparin in patients receiving streptokinase and aspirin for acute myocardial infarction (HERO). Hirulog Early Reperfusion/Occlusion (HERO) Trial Investigators [see comments]. Circulation 1997; 96:2155–2161.

58. Theroux P, Perez-Villa F, Waters D, Lesperance J, Shabani F, Bonan R. Randomized double-blind comparison of two doses of Hirulog with heparin as adjunctive therapy to streptokinase to promote early patency of the infarct-related artery in acute myocardial infarction. Circulation 1995; 91:2132–2139.

59. Jang IK, Brown DF, Giugliano RP, et al. A multicenter, randomized study of argatroban versus heparin as adjunct to tissue plasminogen activator (TPA) in acute myocardial infarction: myocardial infarction with novastan and TPA (MINT) study. J Am Coll Cardiol 1999; 33:1879–1885.

60. Fung AY, Lorch G, Cambier PA, et al. Efegatran sulfate as an adjunct to streptokinase versus heparin as an adjunct to tissue plasminogen activator in patients with acute myocardial infarction. ESCALAT Investigators. Am Heart J 1999; 138:696–704.

61. A low molecular weight, selective thrombin inhibitor, inogatran, vs heparin, in unstable coronary artery disease in 1209 patients. A double-blind, randomized, dose-finding study. Thrombin inhibition in Myocardial Ischaemia (TRIM) study group [see comments]. Eur Heart J 1997; 18:1416–1425.

62. Gold HK, Torres FW, Garabedian HD, et al. Evidence for a rebound coagulation phenomenon after cessation of a 4-hour infusion of a specific thrombin inhibitor in patients with unstable angina pectoris [see comments]. J Am Coll Cardiol 1993; 21:1039–1047.

63. Kong DF, Topol EJ, Bittl JA, et al. Clinical outcomes of bivalirudin for ischemic heart disease. Circulation 1999; 100:2049–2053.

64. Cannon CP. Thrombin inhibitors in acute myocardial infarction. Cardiol Clin 1995; 13:421–433.

65. Fuchs J, Cannon CP. Hirulog in the treatment of unstable angina. Results of the Thrombin Inhibition in Myocardial Ischemia (TIMI) 7 trial. Circulation 1995; 92:727–733.

66. Greinacher A, Janssens U, Berg G, et al. Lepirudin (recombinant hirudin) for parenteral anticoagulation in patients with heparin-induced thrombocytopenia. Heparin-Associated Thrombocytopenia Study (HAT) investigators. Circulation 1999; 100:587–593.

67. Lee LV. Initial experience with hirudin and streptokinase in acute myocardial infarction: results of the Thrombolysis in Myocardial Infarction (TIMI) 6 trial. Am J Cardiol 1995; 75:7–13.

68. Metz BK, White HD, Granger CB, et al. Randomized comparison of direct thrombin inhibition versus heparin in conjunction with fibrinolytic therapy for acute myocardial infarction: results from the GUSTO-IIb Trial. Global Use of Strategies to Open Occluded Coronary Arteries in Acute Coronary Syndromes (GUSTO-IIb) Investigators. J Am Coll Cardiol 1998; 31:1493–1498.

69. Antman EM, Bittl JA. Direct Thrombin Inhibitors. In: Hennekens CH, ed. Clinical

Trials in Cardiovascular Disease. Philadelphia: W.B. Saunders Company, 1999: 145–165.

70. Neuhaus KL, von Essen R, Tebbe U, et al. Safety observations from the pilot phase of the randomized r-Hirudin for Improvement of Thrombolysis (HIT-III) study. A study of the Arbeitsgemeinschaft Leitender Kardiologischer Krankenhausarzte (ALKK) [see comments]. Circulation 1994; 90:1638–1642.

71. Neuhaus KL, Molhoek GP, Zeymer U, et al. Recombinant hirudin (lepirudin) for the improvement of thrombolysis with streptokinase in patients with acute myocardial infarction: results of the HIT-4 trial. J Am Coll Cardiol 1999; 34:966–973.

6

Platelet Glycoprotein IIb/IIIa Inhibition in Acute Coronary Syndromes

Christopher P. Cannon
Brigham and Women's Hospital and Harvard Medical School, Boston, Massachusetts

Because approximately 4 million patients each year are admitted to hospitals worldwide with unstable angina or acute myocardial infarction (MI), and nearly 1 million patients annually worldwide undergo percutaneous coronary intervention (PCI), physicians have focused a great deal of attention on developing new treatments for these acute coronary syndromes (ACS). The initiating event of these acute coronary syndromes is rupture of an atherosclerotic plaque followed by local thrombosis. Similar pathophysiology is present during PCI, which is essentially a "planned" plaque disruption.

Antiplatelet therapy is the cornerstone of treatment in ACS. Aspirin has been shown to have dramatic effects in reducing both mortality and nonfatal events in patients across the spectrum of acute coronary syndromes (1–8). In addition, the newer agents clopidogrel and ticlopidine have been shown to be beneficial in reducing clinical events compared with aspirin alone in coronary stenting (9–13) and in symptomatic patients with atherosclerosis (1,14,15). The newest class of drugs is the platelet glycoprotein (GP) IIb/IIIa receptor inhibitor group of agents, which directly inhibit platelet aggregation.

I. MECHANISM OF ACTION

GP IIb/IIIa inhibitors bind directly to the IIb/IIIa receptor, thereby preventing the binding of fibrinogen to the platelet and preventing formation (or progression) of a platelet aggregate. Thus, regardless of which stimuli lead to platelet activation, the IIb/IIIa inhibitor inhibits platelet aggregation. The doses of the IIb/IIIa inhibitors being tested clinically inhibit 20-μM adenosine diphosphate (ADP)–induced platelet aggregation by approximately 80 to 90%.

II. TYPES OF GP IIb/IIIa INHIBITORS

There are three broad categories of IIb/IIIa inhibitors: (1) monoclonal antibody fragment to the IIb/IIIa receptor, abciximab (ReoPro); (2) intravenous peptide and nonpeptide small molecule inhibitors, such as eptifibatide (Integrilin) and tirofiban (Aggrastat); and (3) oral IIb/IIIa inhibitors, such as xemilofiban, orbofiban, and sibrafiban.

Abciximab is a monoclonal antibody fragment that binds very tightly to the IIb/IIIa receptor, with a long half-life of dissociation from the receptor (approximately 40 min) (16). Thus, the antiplatelet effect lasts much longer than the infusion period—a potential benefit on improving efficacy. Thus, most drug circulates bound to platelets. To reverse the effect, transfusion of platelets will allow the drug to redistribute among all the platelets, thereby reducing the level of platelet inhibition. Abciximab also binds to other integrins on the platelet receptor, such as the vitronectin ($\alpha_v\beta_3$) receptor (17).

The peptide and peptidomimetic inhibitors (e.g., tirofiban and eptifibatide) are competitive inhibitors of the IIb/IIIa receptor, with very rapid half-lives of dissociation from the IIb/IIIa receptor (10–20 s) (18,19). Thus, the level of platelet inhibition is directly related to the drug level in the blood. Since both inhibitors have short half-lives, when the drug infusion is stopped (18,19) the antiplatelet activity reverses after a few hours, which is a potential benefit for avoiding bleeding complications.

The third group of GP IIb/IIIa inhibitors are the oral agents. Within this group, there are also the two broad types of agents, those that are competitive inhibitors, and those that bind tightly to the receptor. The oral drugs are usually prodrugs, which are absorbed and then converted to active compounds in the blood (20–22). The oral agents all have longer half-lives, such that they can be given once, twice, or three times daily in order to achieve relatively steady levels of IIb/IIIa inhibition.

III. IIb/IIIa INHIBITION DURING PCI ANGIOPLASTY

A. Abciximab

In the Evaluation of c7E3 for the Prevention of Ischemic Complication (EPIC) trial of patients undergoing high-risk PCI, abciximab bolus and infusion had a 35% lower rate of death, MI, or urgent revascularization at 30 days compared to the placebo group, 8.3% vs. 12.8% ($p = 0.008$) (23). In long-term follow-up, significant reduction in death or MI has been observed at 6 months and 3 years (24,25). Similar reductions in major cardiac events were observed in elective PCI in the Evaluation in PTCA to Improve Long-term Outcome with Abciximab Glycoprotein IIb/IIIa Blockade (EPILOG) trial. Death, MI, or urgent revascularization at 30 days for the abciximab plus low-dose heparin group was 5.2% vs. 11.7% for heparin alone, a 58% risk reduction ($p < 0.001$) (26). Death or MI was similarly reduced by more than 50% when adding abciximab. When using a lower dose of heparin with abciximab, there was no difference in the incidence of major bleeding or the need for transfusion between abciximab-treated patients and placebo. Thus, the low-dose heparin regimen is the current recommendation with abciximab (and other agents): 70-U/kg initial bolus of heparin with additional 20-U/kg boluses if the activated clotting time is <200 s.

Abciximab was also found to be beneficial when started 24 h *prior* to a PCI in the c7E3 Fab Antiplatelet Therapy in Unstable Refractory Angina (CAPTURE) trial: death, MI, or urgent revascularization was reduced by abciximab from 15.9 to 11.3% ($p = 0.012$) (27). In the Evaluation of IIb/IIIa inhibitor for Stenting (EPISTENT) trial (28), compared with stenting with only aspirin and heparin, the rate of death, MI, or urgent revascularization at 30 days was significantly reduced in both abciximab groups—from 10.8 to 5.3% for stent plus abciximab ($p < 0.001$) and 6.9% for balloon angioplasty with abciximab ($p = 0.007$) (28). Benefits were maintained at 6 months (29) and 1 year, with a significant reduction in 1 year mortality in patients treated with stent plus abciximab compared with stent alone (30). In addition, a metanalysis of abciximab trials has shown that there is a significant reduction in *mortality* when GP IIb/IIIa inhibition is used (31,32) (Fig. 1).

B. Eptifibatide

Eptifibatide has been studied in three PCI trials and one large unstable angina trial. In the Integrilin to Minimise Platelet Aggregation and Coronary Thrombosis (IM-PACT) II trial, there was a trend toward a lower composite event rate in each of the doses of eptifibatide vs. placebo, 9.2% and 9.9% vs. 11.4%, respectively ($p = 0.063$) for low-dose eptifibatide. However, the eptifibatide infusion rates of 0.5 µg/kg/min and 0.75 µg/kg/h were later found to achieve only 50 to 60% platelet inhibition. In the subsequent Platelet Glycoprotein IIb/IIIa in Unstable Angina Receptor Suppression Using Integrilin therapy (PURSUIT) trial of eptifibatide in ACS, which used a higher dose (180 µg/kg bolus followed by a 2.0-mg/kg/h infusion) among patients undergoing early angioplasty or stenting while on study drug, benefits were more dramatic: 16.7% for placebo vs. 11.6% for eptifibatide ($p = 0.01$) (33,34).

More recently, the Enhanced Suppression of the Platelet Receptor IIb/IIIa with Eptifibatide Therapy (ESPRIT) trial tested a higher dose, 180-µg/kg bolus

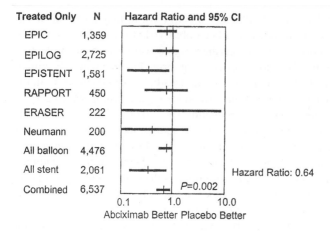

Figure 1 Metanalysis of mortality through follow-up in trials of percutaneous coronary intervention comparing abciximab and placebo. (Data from Ref. 31; reproduced from Ref. 32.)

followed by a 2.0-µg/kg/min infusion, with a second bolus of 180 µg/kg given 10 min after the first bolus. This dose was targeted to achieve 85 to 95% platelet inhibition, with the second bolus to ensure no fall in the level of inhibition of platelet aggregation at the early periprocedural time point. In this trial, patients enrolled had either stable angina or unstable angina or a recent, but not acute, MI. The primary endpoint—death, MI, urgent revascularization, or thrombotic bailout at 48 h—was reduced by 37% (10.5 vs. 6.6%; $p = 0.0017$) (35). Death or MI at 48 h was reduced from 9.2 to 5.5% ($p = 0.0013$), a relative 40% reduction. Death, MI, or target vessel revascularization was reduced from 9.3 to 6.0%; $p = 0.0045$) (35). Thus, eptifibatide in the new double bolus and infusion regimen led to a substantial reduction in early complications from PCI.

The 30-day data showed durability of the results (Fig. 2). The rate of death, MI, or urgent target vessel revascularization was reduced by 35% with eptifibatide ($p = 0.003$), and there was a 38% relative reduction in the rate of death or MI (6.3% with eptifibatide vs. 10.2% with placebo; $p = 0.002$, representing an absolute 3.9% reduction). Again, the individual endpoints each showed similar relative reductions, including a nonsignificant trend for reduced mortality, 0.4% eptifibatide vs. 0.6% for placebo.

Overall, the rates of bleeding were relatively low. Severe bleeding occurred in 0.7% of eptifibatide patients vs. 0.5% of placebo ($p = $ NS). Moderate bleeding, as coded by the investigator, occurred in 1.3 and 1.1%, respectively. Major bleeding using Thrombolysis in Myocardial Infarction (TIMI) criteria (greater than 15% absolute drop in hematocrit or 5 g/dL drop in hemoglobin) (36) did show a small increase in bleeding (1.4 vs. 0.4%, eptifibatide vs. placebo). Most of these events involved the vascular access site for the cardiac catheterization. These

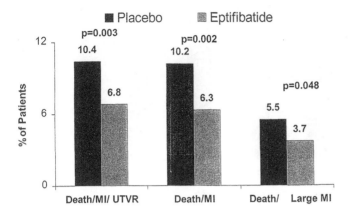

Figure 2   Thirty-day results from the ESPRIT trial. (Data from Ref. 35.)

rates compare favorably with prior IIb/IIIa inhibitor trials and may be due in part to the low-dose, weight-adjusted heparin that was used in both the placebo and eptifibatide groups.

C. Tirofiban

Tirofiban is a nonpeptide GPIIb/IIIa receptor antagonist with a short half-life (approximately 2 h). The RESTORE trial enrolled 2139 patients undergoing high-risk PCI, and randomized patients to tirofiban (10-mg/kg bolus followed by 0.15-mg/kg/h infusion for 36 h). Tirofiban led to a lower but not statistically significant reduction in the primary composite endpoint of death, MI, revascularization for target vessel ischemia, or stent placement for abrupt vessel closure at 30 days (10.3 vs. 12.2%, a 16% risk reduction; $p = 0.16$) (37). Death, MI, or urgent revascularization to 30 days was reduced by tirofiban by 24% (8.0 vs. 10.5%; $p = 0.052$). In this trial, however, systematic collection of cardiac enzymes peri-procedurally was not carried out, and thus uniform ascertainment of a major endpoint was not carried out as in the other trials. The TARGET trial directly compared abciximab and tirofiban in PCI and found a lower death rate, MI, or urgent revascularization at 30 days (6.0 vs. 7.5%) favoring abciximab (37a). However, at 6 months there was no significant difference in death, MI, or target vessel revascularization, or in mortality.

D. Primary PCI

In the setting of "primary" PCI for acute ST-elevation MI, favorable results were first observed in a subgroup of the EPIC trial, with more than 50% reductions in

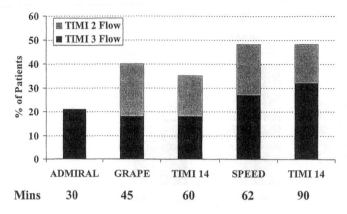

Figure 3   Facilitation of early reperfusion with IIb/IIIa inhibition prior to primary PCI. Mins = time in minutes from start of IIb/IIIa inhibitor to angiogram. (Data from Refs. 41–44.)

cardiac events (38). Subsequently, the ReoPro and Primary Angioplasty Organization and Randomized Trial (RAPPORT) trial found that abciximab reduced death, MI, or urgent revascularization at 30 days by 48%, from 11.2 to 5.8% ($p = 0.03$). This beneficial effect was sustained at 6 months (17.8% vs. 11.6%; $p = 0.05$) (39). Two other randomized trials have also shown benefit of abciximab in primary PCI, each with a similar 50% reduction in death, MI, or urgent revascularization at 30 days (40,41).

Another important finding has been observed from treatment of patients with ST-elevation MI with GP IIb/IIIa inhibitors in the Emergency Department 30 to 90 min *prior* to carrying out the PCI. Early TIMI grade 3 flow is achieved in 20 to 30% of patients, with TIMI grade 2 or 3 flow of approximately 50% (Fig. 3) (41–44). Thus, use of GP IIb/IIIa inhibitors can "facilitate" the PCI by providing better preprocedural flow and consequently better procedural outcomes. Thus, given this broad experience with GP IIb/IIIa inhibitors in PCI, and with reductions in death or MI of approximately 50%, their use has become a new therapeutic standard for "primary" PCI.

IV.   IIb/IIIa INHIBITION IN UNSTABLE ANGINA AND NON-ST-ELEVATION MI

The three IIb/IIIa inhibitors discussed above have also been shown to be beneficial in treating patients with unstable angina and non-ST-elevation MI.

A. Tirofiban

The PRISM-PLUS trial enrolled 1915 patients with unstable angina/non-ST-elevation MI with either electrocardiographic changes or positive enzymes. The combination of tirofiban, heparin, and aspirin led to a 32% reduction in the rate of death, MI, or recurrent refractory ischemia at 7 days (the primary endpoint) compared with aspirin plus heparin, 12.9 vs. 17.9%, respectively ($p = 0.004$) (45). This benefit was due to a 47% reduction in MI ($p = 0.006$) and a 30% reduction in refractory ischemia ($p = 0.02$). Early benefits were observed: there was a significant 66% reduction in death or MI by 48 h (0.9% vs. 2.6%; $p = 0.01$). These benefits were preserved during follow-up, with a 30% reduction in the rate of death or MI (11.9 to 8.7%; $p = 0.03$) and a significant reduction in the composite event rate at 6 months (45).

All subgroups had similar relative benefits of the combination therapy, but the *absolute* benefit, in terms of the number of events prevented, was greater in higher risk patient subgroups, such as the elderly, diabetics, those who were already taking aspirin, and with ST segment changes or positive cardiac markers (Fig. 4). The benefit of the combination of tirofiban plus heparin and aspirin was observed across all management strategies: death or MI at 30 days was reduced by 25% in patients managed medically, by 34% in those who had angioplasty, and by 30% in those who subsequently went on to bypass surgery.

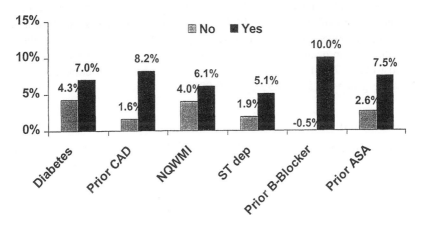

Figure 4 Absolute reduction in the primary endpoint (death, MI, or refractory angina at 7 days) in various subgroups in the PRISM-PLUS trial when treated with tirofiban, aspirin, and heparin as compared with aspirin and heparin alone. As shown, there is, with the addition of tirofiban, an absolute benefit of 6 to 8 fewer patients per 100 treated who suffer a primary event in the various high-risk subgroups. (Data from Ref. 45.)

The PRISM trial, involving 3232 patients with unstable angina/non-ST-elevation MI, randomized patients to receive either heparin or tirofiban (not the combination of both as in PRISM PLUS), with all patients receiving aspirin (46). The goal of the trial was to determine whether the IIb/IIIa inhibitor could reduce events during medical therapy only. Accordingly, the primary endpoint was a composite of death, MI, and refractory ischemic conditions at 48 h, and coronary procedures were not permitted during the first 48 h unless required by refractory ischemia. Tirofiban-treated patients had a significant 32% lower composite event rate than the placebo group, 3.8 vs. 5.6% ($p = 0.01$) (46). At 30 days, the improvement on the composite endpoint or death or MI was a trend toward reduction only (death or MI, risk ratio 0.80; $p = 0.11$). Thus, the effects of GP IIb/IIIa inhibition appeared to have greater long-term effects when used in conjunction with heparin (as was the case in PRISM-PLUS).

B. Eptifibatide

Eptifibatide was studied in the PURSUIT trial, which involved 10,948 patients with unstable angina and non-ST-elevation MI. Patients received aspirin and were recommended to receive heparin, and were randomized to receive eptifibatide or placebo. Of two initial doses, eptifibatide 180-μg/kg bolus and 2.0-μg/kg/h infusion significantly reduced the rate of death or MI at 30 days from 15.7 to 14.2% ($p = 0.042$) (33). This reduction of 15 events per 1000 patients treated was achieved after only 72 h (i.e., while the patients were receiving study drug), 7.6% for placebo vs. 5.9% for eptifibatide ($p = 0.001$). The benefits were more dramatic among patients undergoing PCI within 72 h (i.e., while on study drug), 16.7% for placebo vs. 11.6% for eptifibatide ($p = 0.01$) (33). In this group, there were reductions in death or MI observed prior to PCI and during the first 24 to 48 h post-PCI (47). Moderate or severe hemorrhage was more common in the eptifibatide group (12.8 vs. 9.9%; $p < 0.001$).

C. Abciximab

Abciximab was tested in the Global Use of Strategies to Open Occluded Coronary Arteries (GUSTO) IV–ACS trial for the medical management of patients with unstable angina and non-ST-elevation MI. The results were surprisingly negative.

A total of 7800 patients were enrolled at 458 hospitals in 24 countries around the world, with 48% coming from western Europe, 31% from eastern Europe, and only 14% from North America. Patients received aspirin and heparin, and were randomized to receive in a double-blind fashion, a 24-h infusion of abciximab, a 48-h infusion of abciximab, or placebo. The dose was similar to the dose used in the more recent PCI trials, with a 0.25-mg/kg bolus and a 0.125-μg/kg/min (weight-adjusted) infusion for 24 or 48 h.

The primary endpoint was death or MI, defined as either new Q-waves or positive creatine kinase (CK)–MB, with a peak CK-MB $\geq$ 3 times the upper limit of normal (ULN), with at least two measurements showing a CK-MB $>$ ULN, which was a higher threshold from prior ACS trials. The primary endpoint, death or MI at 30 days, occurred in 8.0% of the placebo group vs. 8.2% in the 24-h abciximab group, 9.1% in the 48-h group (p = NS). Events to 48 h (at the end of the study drug infusion) were also not different: 1.5%, 1.9%, and 2.2%, respectively (p = NS). Morality at 48 h was 0.3 vs. 0.7 vs. 0.9% in the three groups, respectively. Similarly, the results at 7 days were not different: death or MI occurred in 4.5, 4.0, and 4.1%, respectively. The percentage of patients who underwent revascularization by 30 days was approximately 35% in each group, with the percentage who underwent PCI approximately 20%, without differences between the groups.

The rate of intracranial hemorrhage was low in all groups: 0.08% in the placebo group, 0.19% for the 24-h abciximab group, and 0.15% for the 48-h abciximab group. Major bleeding was also low but more common in abciximab-treated patients, occurring in 0.3, 0.6 (p = NS), and 1.0% ($p < 0.001$), respectively. Low rates of blood transfusion were also seen: 0.7, 0.8 (p = NS), and 1.3% ($p < 0.05$) in the three groups. Minor bleeding was also rare, occurring in 1.5, 2.5 ($p < 0.05$), and 3.6% ($p < 0.001$), respectively. Thrombocytopenia with platelet count falling below 50,000 cells/dL occurred in 0.04, 1.6, and 1.4% in the three groups, respectively.

In contrast to Gusto IV–ACS abciximab has been shown to improve outcomes dramatically among patients with unstable angina/non-ST-elevation MI who undergo PCI (i.e., those managed with an early invasive strategy). In CAPTURE, involving 1265 patients, death, MI or urgent revascularization was reduced by abciximab from 15.9 to 11.3% (p = 0.012) (27). Similar reductions have been seen in unstable angina patients in the EPIC trial (48).

D. Lamifiban

Lamifiban is another IIb/IIIa inhibitor not approved by the Food and Drug Administration for use. Following encouraging results from the Platelet IIb/IIIa Antagonism for the Reduction of Acute Coronary Syndromes in a Global Organization Network (PARAGON) A study, the PARAGON B trial evaluated lamifiban in 5225 patients. Overall, death, MI, or severe recurrent ischemia was not significantly reduced: 12.8% for placebo vs. 11.8% for lamifiban; p = 0.33 (49). However, among those with positive troponin T at baseline, there was a significant reduction in events, from 19 to 11% (p = 0.018), which is consistent with the benefit seen in PRISM and CAPTURE based on troponin levels (Fig. 5) (50,51). Thus, this study emphasized the importance of risk stratification in identifying the appropriate patients to treat with these agents.

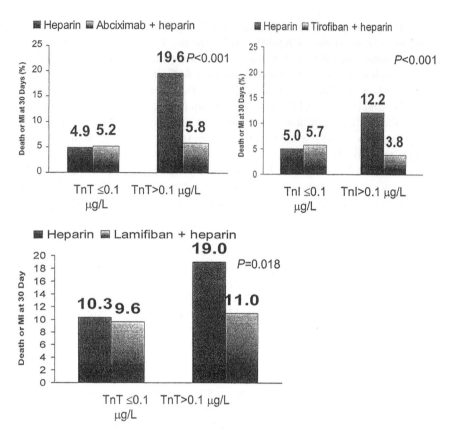

Figure 5 Benefit of IIb/IIIa inhibitors vs. placebo is accentuated in patients with positive vs. negative troponin T at study entry in the CAPTURE, PRISM (top panel), and PARAGON B (bottom panel) trials. (Data from Refs. 49–51.)

V. ANGIOGRAPHIC OBSERVATIONS: ESTABLISHING THE PARADIGM OF BENEFIT

The benefit of IIb/IIIa inhibitors on resolution of coronary thrombus has been observed in two trials, PRISM-PLUS and CAPTURE. The angiographic substudy of the PRISM-PLUS trial found that the coronary thrombus was significantly smaller in patients treated with tirofiban plus heparin and aspirin compared with heparin and aspirin alone. There was a 23% improvement in overall thrombus grade ($p = 0.02$) and the percentage of patients who had definite thrombus was reduced from 24 to 17% (52). Similar observations were made in the CAP-

TURE trial (53). Most dramatically, and for the first time in an unstable angina trial, the rate of TIMI grade 3 flow was significantly improved, from 74.5 to 81.9%, which represented a 35% overall improvement in TIMI flow grade ($p = 0.002$) (52). Together these data establish the pathophysiological link between the potent platelet inhibition, a reduction in coronary thrombus, improvement in coronary blood flow, and consequent improvement in clinical outcomes for patients (54).

VI. REDUCING INFARCT SIZE WITH IIb/IIIa INHIBITION

An emerging concept of GP IIb/IIIa inhibition, based on evidence from two trials (55,58), is that these agents appear to be able to reduce the size of an evolving non-ST-elevation MI, and potentially prevent the development of myocardial necrosis. In the troponin substudy of PRISM-PLUS, patients randomized to tirofiban plus heparin and aspirin had a significantly lower peak troponin level as compared with patients who received heparin and aspirin alone (Fig. 6) (56). This observation was made among patients who had a negative CK-MB on admission (Fig. 6). In PURSUIT, using peak CK-MB as a measure of infarct size, it was observed that infarct size, either the index MI or a recurrent MI, was significantly smaller in patients treated with eptifibatide (55). Thus, when using these potent antiplatelet therapies early in the course of treatment, there appears to be an immediate reduction of the severity of the presenting illness, which is similar to the beneficial effect of chronic aspirin use in reducing the severity of the presenting acute coronary syndrome (57–59).

Another new concept in GP IIb/IIIa inhibition is that there appears to be a greater benefit with more rapid time to treatment. In a preliminary analysis from PURSUIT, the absolute reduction in death or MI with eptifibatide was 2.8% for patients treated within 6 h from the onset of pain, 2.3% for those treated between 6 to 12 h, 1.7% for those treated between 12 to 24 h and no benefit in patients treated more than 24 h after the onset of pain (60). Similar unpublished data have been observed in PRISM-PLUS.

A. Potential Risks

The two major side effects of this class of agents, which fortunately are rare, are bleeding and thrombocytopenia. Although the initial EPIC trial found increased bleeding using abciximab plus heparin compared with heparin alone (23), a strong interaction with the dose of heparin was observed. In the EPILOG trial, which tested low-dose heparin, the rate of major bleeding was identical between heparin control patients and those receiving abciximab and low-dose heparin (28). Similarly, the rate of major bleeding has generally not been significantly increased

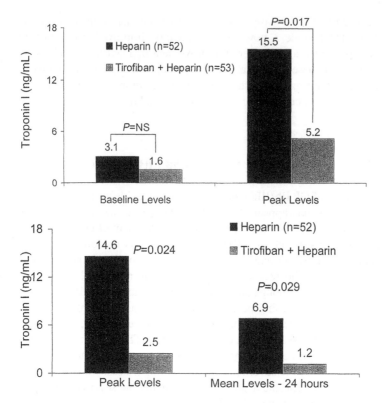

Figure 6 PRISM PLUS troponin substudy: Peak levels of troponin I (TnI) were reduced in patients treated with the GP IIb/IIIa inhibitor tirofiban compared with aspirin and heparin in the trial. (Data from all patients in the substudy on top panel, and among patients with a negative baseline troponin in bottom panel.) These data demonstrate that early treatment (within 12 h from the onset of chest pain in this study) led to a reduced infarct size among patients with unstable angina/non-ST-elevation MI (top) and also *prevented* myocardial necrosis in some patients (bottom). (Data from Ref. 56.)

in other trials (37,61). Thus, use of lower doses of heparin and careful monitoring of the level of anticoagulation will avoid bleeding complications in patients receiving IIb/IIIa inhibitors.

Thrombocytopenia, with platelet counts falling below 100,000 cells/mL occurs in approximately 1 to 2% of patients treated with IIb/IIIa inhibitors, and platelet counts falling to <50,000 occurs in <0.5% of patients (26,45,61). Thrombocytopenia is associated with increased bleeding and, in some patients, thrombotic events (62,62a,63). This syndrome bears some resemblance to heparin-induced thrombocytopenia, and indicates a need to monitor platelet counts carefully during the GP IIb/IIIa infusion.

B. Potential Role for IIb/IIIa Inhibition with Thrombolysis in Acute MI

Thrombolytic therapy has dramatically reduced mortality following acute myocardial infarction. Its benefit is due to *early* achievement of infarct-related artery patency, which limits myocardial infarct size, decreases left ventricular dysfunction, and improves survival (64,65). While thrombolytic therapy has proved to be a major advance in the treatment of patients with acute myocardial infarction, current regimens are limited by failure of initial reperfusion, inadequate perfusion with delayed flow (TIMI grade 2 flow) (66), reocclusion, and reinfarction in significant percentages of patients (66,67). Because these problems are associated with increased subsequent mortality (68–70), and because platelets play a central role in failed reperfusion, reocclusion, and reinfarction, attention has turned to the promising glycoprotein IIb/IIIa inhibitors.

C. Clinical Trials of IIb/IIIa Inhibition with Thrombolysis

In the setting of ST-elevation MI, IIb/IIIa inhibition was first used following thrombolysis in the Thrombolysis and Angioplasty in Myocardial Infarction (TAMI)-8 trial using abciximab following tissue plasminogen activator (tPA) (71). A consistent dose-dependent inhibition of platelet aggregation was observed and major bleeding was not increased.

Eptifibatide was tested in the Integrilin to Manage Platelet Aggregation and Combat Acute Myocardial Infarction (IMPACT-AMI) trial (72). In addition to accelerated, full-dose tPA, aspirin, and heparin, patients were randomized to eptifibatide, at one of six doses, or placebo. The highest dose of eptifibatide appeared to improve the 90-min rate of TIMI grade 3 flow (66 vs. 39% for placebo; $p = 0.006$) (72). More recently, a pilot study combined full-dose streptokinase (1.5 million U/h) and three doses of eptifibatide (180-μg/kg bolus and either 0.75-, 1.33-, or 2.0-μg/kg/min infusion for 24 h) or placebo (73). Adding the IIb/IIIa inhibitor led to a modest improvement in early complete reperfusion (TIMI grade flow 3 at 90 min) from 38% with placebo to approximately 50% with eptifibatide (73). The highest dose of eptifibatide was associated with increased bleeding and was discontinued. Further testing of eptifibatide is planned with reduced-dose thrombolytic agents.

D. Reduced-Dose Fibrinolysis Plus GP IIb/IIIa Inhibition

The combination of a *reduced*-dose fibrinolytic agent and a GP IIb/IIIa inhibitor was tested in the TIMI-14 trial, using tPA, streptokinase, and reteplase; in SPEED (Strategies for Patency Enhancement in the Emergency Department) using reteplase; and in INTRO-AMI and several ongoing trials.

In the TIMI-14 trial dose-ranging phase, 681 patients with ST-segment-elevation MI meeting with standard eligibility criteria were randomized within 12 h of onset of chest pain to receive one of four reperfusion regimens (each with several dose levels): accelerated (full-dose) tPA alone (the control arm); reduced-dose tPA plus abciximab; reduced-dose streptokinase plus abciximab; or abciximab alone. All patients received aspirin and heparin, with the initial heparin dosage being 70-U/kg bolus and a 15-U/kg/h infusion in the tPA control arm, and 60-U/kg bolus and a 7-U/kg/h infusion in the abciximab groups.

Abciximab alone was associated with a rate of TIMI grade 3 flow at 90 min of 32% and patency rate of 48% (43). The combination of streptokinase and abciximab produced only slight improvement in 90-min TIMI grade 3 flow: 42% in the 0.5-MU group; 39% in the 0.75-MU group; and 47% in the 1.25-MU group. The 1.5-MU regimen plus abciximab was discontinued after four of six patients developed a major hemorrhage, one of whom had an ICH.

Of the various dosing regimens of tPA tested, the best angiographic results were obtained using a 50-mg dose given as a 15-mg bolus and a 35-mg infusion over 60 min. The rate of TIMI grade 3 flow at 90 min was 77% compared with 62% for tPA alone ($p = 0.02$) (Fig. 7). Overall patency was achieved in 93% of patients with the combination of abciximab and half-dose tPA compared with 78% for full-dose tPA alone ($p = 0.09$). An even greater difference was observed at 60 min: accelerated tPA achieved only 43% TIMI grade 3 flow at 60 min compared with 72% for 50-mg tPA plus abciximab ($p = 0.0009$) (Fig. 7). Major hemorrhage was similar (approximately 6%) among the tPA plus abciximab and control groups. In-hospital mortality was low in all groups, ranging from 3 to 5%.

Thus, the addition of the GP IIb/IIIa receptor inhibitor abciximab to half-dose tPA was able to increase the rate of TIMI grade 3 flow at 60 min by an absolute 29%, which represents a relative 67% improvement over standard tPA. At 90 min, the combination regimen improved TIMI grade 3 flow by an absolute 15% (a relative 25% improvement). These results indicate that the combination of GP IIb/IIIa receptor inhibition with reduced-dose fibrinolytic therapy is a promising new regimen for enhancing the speed and extent of reperfusion in acute ST-elevation MI.

Results from the SPEED trial similarly demonstrated improvements in early TIMI grade 3 flow with reteplase (rPA). The combination of half-dose rPA (5U + 5U) and abciximab achieved 60-min TIMI grade 3 flow in 62% of patients (44). The GUSTO V and ASSENT III trials each found that the combination

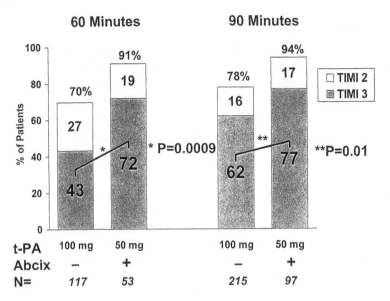

Figure 7   Results from the Thrombolysis in Myocardial Infarction (TIMI)-14 Trial. Comparison of 90-min accelerated tissue plasminogen activator (tPA) with combination therapy using abciximab (abcix) and reduced-dose tPA (15-mg bolus and 35-mg infusion over 60 min) (tPA = flow grade). (Data from Ref. 43; reproduced from Ref. 54.)

regimen did not reduce mortality, but appeared to reduce infarction, at the cost of increased major bleeding (44a,b). Thus these regimens are a modest improvement over current thrombolytic regimens.

VII.   ORAL IIb/IIIa INHIBITORS

Given the dramatic benefits observed with the intravenous IIb/IIIa inhibitors observed to date, great optimism has existed for the potential to extend the window of benefit using long-term oral IIb/IIIa inhibitors. The oral agents all have longer half-lives, such that they can be given once, twice, or three times daily in order to achieve relatively steady levels of IIb/IIIa inhibition. As with the intravenous compounds, two major groups of drugs exist in the oral class: those with competitive inhibition and short "off time" from the receptor, where a high drug level is critical to achieving high levels of platelet inhibition, and those with "tight" binding (i.e., high affinity) to the platelet (similar to abciximab) with the majority of the drug circulating in the bound state.

A. OPUS–TIMI-16 Trial

The Orbofiban in Patients with Unstable Coronary Syndromes (OPUS-TIMI)-16 trial tested the oral II/IIIa inhibitor, orbofiban, in patients with acute coronary syndromes. This trial enrolled 10,288 patients at 888 hospitals in 28 countries. The inclusion criteria were onset of an acute coronary syndromes within 72 h, defined as an episode of rest ischemic pain lasting at least 5 min associated with either positive cardiac enzymes (i.e., an acute MI), ECG changes, or a prior history of coronary or vascular disease. Exclusion criteria included renal insufficiency (creatinine >1.6 mg/dL, increased high bleeding risk, or need for oral anticoagulation.

All patients received 150 to 162 mg of ASA daily and were randomized, in double-blind fashion, to one of two doses of orbofiban or placebo. In one group, orbofiban was administered as 50 mg twice daily throughout the trial (50/50 group); in the other group, 50 mg was given twice daily for the first 30 days (the highest risk period), and was reduced to 30 mg twice daily for the remainder of the trial (50/30 group). Other treatments were at the discretion of the patient's physician. The primary endpoint was a composite of death, MI, recurrent ischemia leading to rehospitalization or urgent revascularization, or stroke. The planned sample size was 12,000 patients, but the trial was terminated early after an unexpected finding of increased mortality at 30 days in one of the orbofiban groups (22).

Mortality through 10 months was 3.7% for the placebo group versus 5.1% in the 50/30 group ($p = 0.008$) and 4.5% in the 50/50 group ($p = 0.11$). There were no differences in the primary composite endpoint at 10 months (22.9, 23.1, and 22.8%, for the placebo, 50/30, and 50/50 groups, respectively). Major or severe bleeding (but not intracranial hemorrhage) was higher with orbofiban; it occurred in 2.0, 3.7 ($p = 0.0004$), and 4.5% ($p < 0.0001$) of patients, respectively. Exploratory subgroup analyses did identify that patients who underwent percutaneous coronary intervention had a lower mortality and a significant reduction in the composite endpoint ($p = 0.001$) with orbofiban.

Two substudies from OPUS–TIMI-16 found that orbofiban led to increases in measures of platelet activation, notably P-selectin (74,75). These data are consistent with observations of other agents, which induced an apparent prothrombotic effect, with increases in measures of platelet activation and increases in platelet aggregation when drug levels were low (76). Interestingly, in the TIMI-12 trial, no increase in P-selectin was observed with sibrafiban therapy (77). Active research is ongoing, but these initial studies suggest that there may be differences among the various oral IIb/IIIa inhibitors with regard to potential prothrombotic effects.

Many lessons were learned from the OPUS–TIMI-16 trial that will be useful in planning future trials with other agents. First, optimization of the dosing strategy used with the oral agents is important, potentially to mimic the stable antiplatelet effect achieved by the intravenous drugs. Thus, the goal would be to reduce the inter- and intrapatient variability by using a dose adjusted to the patient's weight and/or renal function. Use of plasma drug level and/or bedside platelet function tests would be an even more accurate way to adjust the dose. Second, one could target stabilized patients rather than more unstable patients.

B. EXCITE Trial

The Evaluation of oral Xemilofiban in Controlling Thrombotic Events (EXCITE) trial studied xemilofiban in 7232 patients undergoing PCI with either stenting or balloon angioplasty without adjunctive intravenous IIb/IIIa inhibition. Patients were randomized in a double-blind fashion to receive one of two doses of xemilofiban or placebo: All the xemilofiban patients received a first 20-mg dose 30 to 90 min prior to PCI, followed by either 10 or 20 mg three times daily for 6 months (78).

The primary endpoint—death, MI, or urgent revascularization at 6 months—occurred in 13.6% of patients in the placebo group, 14.1% of patients in the xemilofiban 10-mg group, and 12.6% of patients in the xemilofiban 20-mg group (p = NS) (78). There was a trend toward fewer periprocedural MIs over the first 48 h following PCI, but this benefit was not sustained at 30 days or 6 months (78). Mortality at 6 months was 1.0% for placebo, 1.6% for the 10-mg xemilofiban dose group, and 1.1% in the 20-mg dose group (78). Major bleeding was significantly more common in the xemilofiban-treated patients (78). Thus, xemilofiban did not significantly reduce cardiac events in this patient population.

C. Symphony I

Following the Phase II trial of sibrafiban (TIMI-12) (21), the first SYMPHONY (Sibrafiban versus aspirin to Yield Maximum Protection from ischemic Heart events post-acute cOroNary syndromes) trial was a large double-blind, aspirin-controlled trial of two regimens of sibrafiban for the treatment of patients stabilized following an acute coronary syndrome (79). A total of 9233 patients with either acute myocardial infarction or high-risk unstable angina (with ST deviation of $\geq$ 0.5 mm) who were clinically stable for at least 12 h were randomized to receive either aspirin (80 mg twice daily) or one of two doses of sibrafiban (without aspirin) every 12 h for a total of 3 months. The dose of sibrafiban was either 3, 4.5, or 6 mg based on body weight and renal function. The primary endpoint was a composite of death, MI, and severe recurrent ischemia.

There was no difference in the primary endpoint between aspirin (9.8%), low-dose sibrafiban (10.1%), and high-dose sibrafiban (10.1%) (79). The individual components of the endpoint were also not different between the groups. There was a higher rate of major bleeding in the two sibrafiban groups, high-dose (5.7%), low-dose (5.2%) vs. aspirin (3.9%) (79). In conclusion, sibrafiban without aspirin was not superior to aspirin for prevention of cardiac events following acute coronary syndromes.

D. Symphony II

The second Symphony trial was terminated prematurely at the time the results from the first Symphony trial were available (and not due to safety issues). It compared the combination of low-dose sibrafiban *plus* aspirin vs. high-dose sibrafiban (without aspirin) vs. aspirin alone in 6671 patients with stabilized acute coronary syndromes. With an average follow-up of 90 days, the primary endpoint, death, MI, or severe recurrent ischemia, was not different among the three groups: 10.5% in the high-dose sibrafiban group; 9.2% for low-dose sibrafiban plus aspirin vs. 9.3% for aspirin alone. In this trial (but not in the larger first Symphony trial), mortality was significantly higher with the high-dose sibrafiban group: 2.4 vs. 1.7% for the low-dose sibrafiban plus aspirin group vs. 1.3% for placebo. Recurrent MI followed a similar pattern: 6.9% for high-dose sibrafiban, 5.3% for the low-dose plus aspirin group, and 5.3% for aspirin. Major bleeding was more common with high-dose sibrafiban (4.6%), and higher still for the combination of low-dose sibrafiban plus aspirin (5.7%) vs. 4.0% for aspirin alone.

Some potential reasons for these failures of the first-generation oral IIb/IIIa inhibitors include a higher amount of variability in the drug level and a lower degree of platelet inhibition achieved with oral as compared with intravenous drugs (21). It also appears that some of the agents may have intrinsic proaggregatory effects (74). Trials are continuing to evaluate "second-generation" oral IIb/IIIa inhibitors, which have longer half-lives and tighter binding to the IIb/IIIa receptor similar to that of abciximab (81, 82). Thus, for the oral IIb/IIIa inhibitors, we need to "stay tuned."

VIII. CURRENT STATUS

It is an exciting time for the practicing physician given the availability of this important new therapy that can significantly reduce death, MI, or refractory ischemia/urgent revascularization. The benefits apply to essentially all patients undergoing PCI, thereby becoming a new standard of care in this setting. For the huge number of patients with unstable angina and non-ST-elevation MI, IIb/IIIa inhibition will significantly reduce recurrent ischemic events. The trials to date have targeted the higher risk unstable angina patients—those with ECG changes or positive cardiac enzymes, and thus these are the patients in clinical practice who should be targeted for early use of IIb/IIIa inhibitors. Research is continuing to define the appropriate dosing strategy for the oral agents. In acute MI, the combination of IIb/IIIa inhibition and reduced-dose fibrinolytic therapy is very promising. It is a rapidly evolving field, with many significant advances that should translate into improved clinical outcomes for our patients with acute coronary syndromes.

REFERENCES

1. Antiplatelet Trialist' Collaboration. Collaborative overview of randomised trials of antiplatelet therapy—I: prevention of death myocardial infarction and stroke by prolongued antiplatelet therapy in various categories of patients. BMJ 1994; 308:81–106.

2. Steering Committee of the Physicians' Health Study Research Group. Final report on the aspirin component of the ongoing Physicians' Health Study. N Engl J Med 1989; 321:129–35.

3. Ridker PM, Manson JE, Gaziano JM, Buring JE, Hennekens CH. Low-dose aspirin therapy for chronic stable angina. A randomized, placebo-controlled clinical trial. Ann Intern Med 1991; 114:835–839.

4. Lewis HD, Davis JW, Archibald DG, et al. Protective effects of aspirin against acute myocardial infarction and death in men with unstable angina. N Engl J Med 1983; 309:396–403.

5. Cairns JA, Gent M, Singer J, et al. Aspirin, sulfinpyrazone, or both in unstable angina. N Engl J Med 1985; 313:1369–1375.

6. Theroux P, Ouimet H, McCans J, et al. Aspirin, heparin or both to treat unstable angina. N Engl J Med 1988; 319:1105–1111.

7. The RISC Group. Risk of myocardial infarction and death during treatment with low dose aspirin and intravenous heparin in men with unstable coronary artery disease. Lancet 1990; 336:827–830.

8. ISIS-2 (Second International Study of Infarct Survival) Collaborative Group. Randomised trial of intravenous streptokinase, oral aspirin, both, or neither among 17,187 cases of suspected acute myocardial infarction: ISIS-2. Lancet 1988; 2:349–360.

9. Schömig A, Neumann F-J, Kastrati A, et al. A randomized comparison of antiplatelet and anticoagulant therapy after the placement of coronary-artery stents. N Engl J Med 1996; 334:1084–1089.

10. Bertrand ME, Legrand V, Boland J, et al. Randomized multicenter comparison of conventional anticoagulation versus antiplatelet therapy in unplanned and elective coronary stenting. The full anticoagulation versus aspirin and ticlopidine (FANTASTIC) study. Circulation 1998; 98:1597–1603.

11. Leon MB, Baim DS, Popma JJ, et al. A clinical trial comparing three antithrombotic drug regimens after coronary-artery stenting. Stent Anticoagulation Restenosis Study Investigators. N Engl J Med 1998; 339:1665–1671.

12. Berger PB, Bell MR, Rihal CS, et al. Clopidogrel versus ticlopidine after intracoronary stent placement. J Am Coll Cardiol 1999; 34:1891–1894.

13. Muller C, Buttner HJ, Petersen J, Roskamm H. A randomized comparison of clopidogrel and aspirin versus ticlopidine and aspirin after the placement of coronary-artery stents. Circulation 2000; 101:590–593.

14. Clopidogrel in Unstable Angina to Prevent Recurrent Events Trial Investigators. Effects of clopidogrel in addition to aspirin in patients with acute coronary syndromes without ST-segment elevation. N Engl J Med 2001; 345:494–502.

15. CAPRIE Steering Committee. A randomised, blinded, trial of clopidogrel versus aspirin in patients at risk of ischaemic events (CAPRIE). Lancet 1996; 348:1329–1339.

16. Coller BS, Folts JD, Scutter LE, Smith SR. Antithrombotic effect of a monoclonal antibody to the platelet glycoprotein IIb/IIIa receptor in an experimental model. Blood 1986; 68:783–786.

17. Lefkovits J, Plow EF, Topol EJ. Platelet glycoprotein IIb/IIIa receptors in cardiovascular medicine. N Engl J Med 1995; 332:1553–1559.

18. Kereiakes DJ, Kleiman NS, Ambrose J, et al. Randomized, double-blind, placebo-controlled dose-ranging study of tirofiban (MK-383) platelet IIb/IIIa blockade in high risk patients undergoing coronary angioplasty. J Am Coll Cardiol 1996; 27:536–642.

19. Tcheng JE, Harrington RA, Kottke-Marchant K, et al. Multicenter, randomized, double-blind, placebo-controlled trial of the platelet integrin glycoprotein IIb/IIIa blocker integrelin in elective coronary intervention. Circulation 1995; 91:2151–2157.

20. Kereiakes DJ, Runyon JP, Kleiman NS, et al. Differential dose-response to oral xemilofiban after antecedant intravenous abciximab. Administration for complex coronary intervention. Circulation 1996; 94:906–910.

21. Cannon CP, McCabe CH, Borzak S, et al. A randomized trial of an oral platelet glycoprotein IIb/IIIa antagonist, sibrafiban, in patients after an acute coronary syndrome: Results of the TIMI 12 trial. Circulation 1998; 97:340–349.

22. Cannon CP, McCabe CH, Wilcox RG, et al. Oral glycoprotein IIb/IIIa inhibition with orbofiban in patients with unstable coronary syndromes (OPUS-TIMI 16) trial. Circulation 2000; 102:149–156.

23. The EPIC Investigators. Use of a monoclonal antibody directed against the platelet glycoprotein IIb/IIIa receptor in high risk angioplasty. N Engl J Med 1994; 330:956–61.

24. Topol EJ, Califf RM, Weisman HF, et al. Randomised trial of coronary intervention with antibody against platelet IIb/IIIa integrin for reduction of clinical restenosis: results at six months. Lancet 1994; 343:881–886.

25. Topol EJ, Ferguson JJ, Weisman HF, et al. Long term protection from myocardial ischemic events after brief integrin B_3 blockade with percutaneous coronary intervention. JAMA 1997; 278:479–484.

26. The EPILOG Investigators. Platelet glycoprotein IIb/IIIa receptor blockade and low-dose heparin during percutaneous coronary revascularization. N Engl J Med 1997; 336:1689–1696.

27. The CAPTURE Investigators. Randomised placebo-controlled trial of abciximab before and during coronary intervention in refractory unstable angina: the CAPTURE study. Lancet 1997; 349:1429–1435 [published erratum appears in Lancet 1997; 350:744].

28. The EPISTENT Investigators. Randomised placebo-controlled and balloon-angioplasty-controlled trail to assess the safety of coronary stenting with use of platelet glycoprotein-IIb/IIIa blockade. Lancet 1998; 352:87–92.
29. Lincoff AM, Califf RM, Moliterno DJ, et al. Complementary clinical benefits of coronary-artery stenting and blockade of platelet glycoprotein IIb/IIIa receptors. Evaluation of Platelet IIb/IIIa Inhibition in Stenting Investigators. N Engl J Med 1999; 341:319–327.
30. Topol EJ, Mark DB, Lincoff AM, et al. Outcomes at 1 year and economic implications of platelet glycoprotein IIb/IIIa blockade in patients undergoing coronary stenting: results from a multicentre randomised trial. Lancet 1999; 354:2019–2024.
31. Anderson KM, Califf RM, Stone GW, et al. Long-term mortality benefit with abciximab in patients undergoing percutaneous coronary intervention. J Am Coll Cardiol 2001; 37:2059–2065.
32. Cannon CP. Incorporating platelet glycoprotein IIb/IIIa inhibition in critical pathways: unstable angina/non-ST-segment elevation myocardial infarction. Clin Cardiol 1999; 22(suppl IV):30–36.
33. The PURSUIT Trial Investigators. Inhibition of Platelet Glycoprotein IIb/IIIa with eptifibatide in patients with acute coronary syndromes. N Engl J Med 1998; 339: 436–443.
34. Kleiman NS, Lincoff AM, Flaker GC, et al. Early percutaneous coronary intervention, platelet inhibition with eptifibatide, and clinical outcomes in patients with acute coronary syndromes. Circulation 2000; 101:751–757.
35. Tcheng JE. ESPRIT, American College of Cardiology Scientific Sessions, Anaheim, CA, 2000.
36. Bovill EG, Terrin ML, Stump DC, et al. Hemorrhagic events during therapy with recombinant tissue-type plasminogen activator, heparin, and aspirin for acute myocardial infarction. Results of the Thrombolysis in Myocardial Infarction (TIMI), Phase II trial. Ann Intern Med 1991; 115:256–265.
37. The RESTORE Investigators. The effects of platelet glycoprotein IIb/IIIa blockade with tirofiban on adverse cardiac events in patients with unstable angina or acute myocardial infarction undergoing coronary angioplasty. Circulation 1997; 96:1445–1453.
37a. Topol EJ, Moliterno DJ, Herrmann HC, et al. Comparison of two platelet glycoprotein IIb/IIIa inhibitors, tirofiban and abciximab, for the prevention of ischemic events with percutaneous coronary revascularization. N Engl J Med 2001; 344:1888–1894.
38. Lefkovits J, Ivanhoe RJ, Califf RM, et al. Effects of platelet glycoprotein IIb/IIIa receptor blockade by a chimeric monoclonal antibody (abciximab) on acute and six-month outcomes after percutaneous transluminal coronary agioplasty for acute myocardial infarction. Am J Cardiol 1996; 77:1045–1051.
39. Brenner SJ, Barr LA, Burchenal JEB, et al. Randomized, placebo-controlled trial of platelet IIb/IIIa blockade with primary angioplasty for acute myocardial infarction. Circulation 1998; 98:734–741.
40. Neumann F-J, Blasini R, Schmitt C, et al. Effect of glycoprotein IIb/IIIa receptor blockade on recovery of coronary flow and left ventricular function after placement of coronary-artery stents in acute myocardial infarction. Circulation 1998; 98:2695–2701.

41. Montalescot G, Barragan P, Wittenberg O, et al. Platelet glycoprotein IIb/IIIa inhibition with coronary stenting for acute myocardial infarction. N Engl J Med 2001; 344:1895–1903.

42. van den Merkhof LF, Zijlstra F, Olsson H, et al. Abciximab in the treatment of acute myocardial infarction eligible for primary percutaneous transluminal coronary angioplasty. Results of the Glycoprotein Receptor Antagonist Patency Evaluation (GRAPE) pilot study. J Am Coll Cardiol 1999; 33:1528–1532.

43. Antman EM, Giugliano RP, Gibson CM, et al. Abciximab facilitates the rate and extent of thrombolysis: Results of TIMI 14 trial. Circulation 1999; 99:2720–2732.

44. Strategies for Patency Enhancement in the Emergency Department (SPEED) Group. Trial of abciximab with and without low-dose reteplase for acute myocardial infarction. Circulation 2000; 101:2788–2794.

45. The Platelet Receptor Inhibition for Ischemic Syndrome Management in Patients Limited by Unstable Signs and Symptoms (PRISM-PLUS) Trial Investigators. Inhibition of the platelet glycoprotein IIb/IIIa receptor with tirofiban in unstable angina and non-Q-wave myocardial infarction. N Engl J Med 1998; 338:1488–1497.

46. The Platelet Receptor Inhibition For Ischemic Syndrome Management (PRISM) Study Investigators. A comparison of aspirin plus tirofiban with aspirin plus heparin for unstable angina. N Engl J Med 1998; 338:1498–1505.

47. Kleiman NS, Tracy RP, Talley JD, et al. Inhibition of platelet aggregation with a glycoprotein IIb-IIIa antagonist does not prevent thrombin generation in patients undergoing thrombolysis for acute myocardial infarction. J Thromb Thrombolysis 2000; 9:5–12.

48. Lincoff AM, Califf RM, Anderson KM, et al. Evidence for prevention of death and myocardial infarction with platelet membrane glycoprotein IIb/IIIa receptor blockade by abciximab (c7E3 Fab) among patients with unstable angina undergoing percutaneous coronary revascularization. J Am Coll Cardiol 1997; 30:149–156.

49. Newby LK, Ohman EM, Christenson RH, et al. Benefit of glycoprotein IIb/IIIa inhibition in patients with acute coronary syndromes and troponin t-positive status: the paragon-B troponin T substudy. Circulation 2001; 103:2891–2896.

50. Hamm CW, Heeschen C, Goldmann B, et al. Benefit of abciximab in patients with refractory unstable angina in relation to serum troponin T levels. c7E3 Fab Antiplatelet Therapy in Unstable Refractory Angina (CAPTURE) Study Investigators. N Engl J Med 1999; 340:1623–9.

51. Heeschen C, Hamm CW, Goldmann B, et al. Troponin concentrations for stratification of patients with acute coronary syndromes in relation to therapeutic efficacy of tirofiban. Lancet 1999; 354:1757–1762.

52. Zhao X-Q, Theroux P, Snapinn SM, Sax FL, for the PRISM-PLUS Investigators. Intracoronary thrombus and platelet glycoprotein IIb/IIIa receptor blockade with tirofiban in unstable angina or non-Q-wave myocardial infarction. Angiographic results from the PRISM-PLUS trial (Platelet Receptor Inhibition for Ischemic Syndrome Management in Patients Limited by Unstable Signs and Symptoms). Circulation 1999; 100:1609–1615.

53. van den Brand M, Laarman GJ, Steg PG, et al. Assessment of coronary angiograms prior to and after treatment with abciximab, and the outcome of angioplasty in refractory unstable angina patients. Angiographic results from the CAPTURE trial. Eur Heart J 1999; 20:1572–1578.

54. Cannon CP. Overcoming thrombolytic resistance: Rationale and initial clinical experience combining thrombolytic therapy and glycoprotein IIb/IIIa receptor inhibition for acute myocardial infarction. J Am Coll Cardiol 1999; 34:1395–1402.

55. Alexander JH, Sparapani RA, Mahaffey KW, et al. Eptifibatide reduces the size and incidence of myocardial infarction in patients with non-ST-elevation acute coronary syndromes. J Am Coll Cardiol 1999; 33(suppl A):331A.

56. Januzzi JL, Hahn SS, Chae CU, et al. Effects of tirofiban plus heparin versus heparin alone on Troponin I levels in patients with acute coronary syndromes. Am J Cardiol 2000; 86:713–717.

57. Cannon CP, Thompson B, McCabe CH, et al. Predictors of non-Q-wave acute myocardial infarction in patients with acute ischemic syndromes: An analysis from the Thrombolysis in Myocardial Ischemia (TIMI) III Trials. Am J Cardiol 1995; 75: 977–981.

58. Borzak S, Cannon CP, Kraft PL, et al. Effects of prior aspirin and anti-ischemic therapy on outcome of patients with unstable angina. Am J Cardiol 1998; 81:678–681.

59. Garcia-Dorado D, Theroux P, Tomos P, et al. Previous aspirin use may attenuate the severity of the manifestation of acute ischemic syndromes. Circulation 1995; 92:1743–1748.

60. Bhatt DL, Marso SP, Houghtaling P, Labinaz M, Lauer MA. Does earlier administration of eptifibatide reduce death and MI in patients with acute coronary syndromes? Circulation 1998; 98(suppl I):I-561.

61. The IMPACT-II investigators. Randomised placebo-controlled trial of effect of eptifibatide on complications of percutaneous coronary intervention: IMPACT-II. Lancet 1997; 349:1422–1428.

62. Berkowitz SD, Sane DC, Sigmon KN, et al. Occurrence and clinical significance of thrombocytopenia in a population undergoing high-risk percutaneous coronary revascularization. Evaluation of c7E3 for the Prevention of Ischemic Complications (EPIC) Study Group. J Am Coll Cardiol 1998; 32:311–319.

62a. Dasgupta H, Blankenship JC, Wood GC, Frey CM, Demko SL, Menapace FJ. Thrombocytopenia complicating treatment with intravenous glycoprotein IIb/IIIa receptor inhibitors: A pooled analysis. Am Heart J 2000; 140:206–211.

63. Mahaffey KW, Harrington RA, Simoons ML, et al. Stroke in patients with acute coronary syndromes: incidence and outcomes in the Platelet glycoprotein IIb/IIIa in Unstable angina Receptor suppression using integrilin therapy (PURSUIT) trial. Circulation 1999; 99:2371–2377.

64. Braunwald E. Myocardial reperfusion, limitation of infarct size, reduction of left ventricular dysfunction, and improved survival: Should the paradigm be expanded? Circulation 1989; 79:441–444.

65. Braunwald E. The open-artery theory is alive and well—again. N Engl J Med 1993; 329:1650–1652.

66. TIMI Study Group. The Thrombolysis in Myocardial Infarction (TIMI) Trial; Phase I findings. N Engl J Med 1985; 312:932–936.

67. Braunwald E. Enhancing thrombolytic efficacy by means of "front-loaded" administration of tissue plasminogen activator. J Am Coll Cardiol 1989; 14:1570–1571.

68. The GUSTO Angiographic Investigators. The comparative effects of tissue plasminogen activator, streptokinase, or both on coronary artery patency, ventricular func-

tion and survival after acute myocardial infarction. N Engl J Med 1993; 329:1615–1622.

69. Ohman EM, Califf RM, Topol EJ, et al. Consequences of reocclusion after successful reperfusion therapy in acute myocardial infarction. Circulation 1990; 82:781–791.

70. Cannon CP, Sharis PJ, Schweiger MJ, et al. Prospective validation of a composite end point in thrombolytic trial of acute myocardial infarction (TIMI 4 and 5). Am J Cardiol 1997; 80:696–699.

71. Kleiman N, Ohman EM, Califf RM, et al. Profound inhibition of platelet aggregation with monoclonal antibody 7E3 Fab after thrombolytic therapy. Results of the Thrombolysis and Angioplasty in Myocardial Infarction (TAMI) 8 pilot study. J Am Coll Cardiol 1993; 22:381–389.

72. Ohman EM, Kleiman NS, Gacioch G, et al. Combined accelerated tissue-plasminogen activator and platelet glycoprotein IIb/IIIa integrin receptor blockade with integrilin in acute myocardial infarction. Circulation 1997; 95:846–854.

73. Ronner E, van Kesteren HA, Zijnen P, et al. Safety and efficacy of eptifibatide vs. placebo in patients receiving thrombolytic therapy with streptokinase for acute myocardial infarction; a phase II dose escalation, randomized, double-blind study. Eur Heart J 2000; 21:1530–1536.

74. Holmes MB, Sobel BE, Cannon CP, Schneider DJ. Increased platelet reactivity in patients given orbofiban after an acute coronary syndrome. An OPUS-TIMI 16 substudy. Am J Cardiol 2000; 85:491–493.

75. Casey M, Fornari C, Bozovich G, Iglesias Varela ML, Mautner B, Cannon CP. Increased expression of platelet P-selectin in patients treated with oral orbofiban in the OPUS TIMI 16 study. Circulation 1999; 100(suppl I):I-681.

76. Peter K, Schwarz M, Ylanne J, et al. Induction of fibrinogen binding and platelet aggregation as a potential intrinsic property of various glycoprotein IIb/IIIa ($a_{IIb}B_3$) inhibitors. Blood 1998; 92:3240–3249.

77. Ault K, Cannon CP, Mitchell J, et al. Platelet activation in patients after an acute coronary: Results from the TIMI 12 trial. J Am Coll Cardiol 1999; 33:634–639.

78. O'Neill WW, Serruys P, Knudtson M, et al. Long-term treatment with a platelet glycoprotein-receptor antagonist after percutaneous coronary revascularization. N Engl J Med 2000; 342:1316–1324.

79. The SYMPHONY Investigators. Comparison of sibrafiban with aspirin for prevention of cardiovascular events after acute coronary syndromes: a randomised trial. Lancet 2000; 355:337–345.

80. Second Symphony Investigators. Randomized trial of aspirin, sibrafiban, or both for secondary prevention after acute coronary syndromes. Circulation 2001; 103:1727–1733.

81. Mousa SA, Bozarth JM, Lorelli W, et al. Antiplatelet efficacy of XV459, a novel nonpeptide platelet GPIIb/IIIa antagonist: comparative platelet binding profiles with c7E3. J Pharmacol Exp Ther 1998; 286:1277–1284.

82. Mousa SA, Khurana S, Forsythe MS. Comparative in vitro efficacy of different platelet glycoprotein IIb/IIIa antagonists on platelet-mediated clot strength induced by tissue factor with use of thromboelastography: differentiation among glycoprotein IIb/IIIa antagonists. Arterioscler Thromb Vasc Biol 2000; 20:1162–1167.

7

Aspirin, Ticlopidine, and Clopidogrel

Mark A. Creager
Brigham and Women's Hospital and Harvard Medical School,
Boston, Massachusetts

Platelets are integrally involved in the thrombotic complications of atherosclerosis. Their contribution to thrombosis complicating a ruptured atherosclerotic plaque is well established. Interference with platelet function, therefore, should help to prevent thrombotic occlusion of arteries affected by atherosclerosis. Indeed, numerous studies have demonstrated that antiplatelet agents decrease adverse cardiovascular events in patients with atherosclerosis. This chapter will focus on three such antiplatelet agents: aspirin, ticlopidine, and clopidogrel. It will include a brief review of platelet function followed by a discussion of the mechanisms of action of these antiplatelet drugs. Thereafter, clinical evidence supporting the notion that antiplatelet agents reduce adverse cardiovascular events in patients with atherosclerosis will be presented.

I. PLATELET FUNCTION

The three principal events in the formation of a platelet plug include platelet adhesion, activation, and aggregation. Platelets normally circulate in an inactivated state. Vascular injury and disruption of the endothelial lining initiates the process of platelet adhesion, in which platelets are deposited on the intimal surface of blood vessels. Among the most important substances to mediate platelet adhesion to the vascular surface is von Willebrand factor. It binds subendothelial collagen to the platelet glycoprotein Ib-IX-V receptor. Binding of platelets to the vascular surface prompts an intracellular signaling mechanism, including the metabolism of arachidonic acid to thromboxane A_2. In addition, the platelets release constituents of their alpha and dense granules such as p-selectin, platelet factor IV, fibronectin, von Willebrand factor, adenosine diphosphate (ADP), and serotonin, among others (1). ADP activates platelet surface receptors to induce conformational changes in the glycoprotein IIb/IIIa complex. The glycoprotein IIb/IIIa complex, in turn, binds fibrinogen, which acts to bridge one platelet with another, thus causing platelet aggregation and formation of a platelet plug.

II. MECHANISMS OF ACTION OF ANTIPLATELET AGENTS

Aspirin inhibits arachidonic acid metabolism and prevents the formation of thromboxane A_2 by irreversibly inhibiting cyclooxygenase via acetylation of a serine moiety. Platelet inhibition occurs approximately 60 min following the oral ingestion of aspirin. The inhibitory effects of platelets last the life of a platelet, which is approximately 10 days. Hemostatic recovery following a single dose of aspirin occurs as new platelets are formed and enter the circulation.

Both ticlopidine and clopidogrel are thienopyridines. These inhibit the function of platelet ADP receptors and thereby limit conformational changes in the glycoprotein IIb/IIIa receptor. Inhibition of platelet aggregation occurs approximately 1 to 2 days following administration of these drugs, and 40 to 60% inhibition of ADP-induced aggregation is observed 3 to 5 days following ingestion (2). Platelet function is restored approximately 3 to 4 days after discontinuation of ticlopidine or clopidogrel.

III. ASPIRIN

The beneficial effects of aspirin on cardiovascular outcome in patients with atherosclerosis is well established (3). The Antiplatelet Trialists' Collaboration performed a metanalysis of over 73,000 patients with clinical manifestations of atherosclerosis such as acute myocardial infarction, prior myocardial infarction, or prior stroke or transient ischemic attack, in which patients were treated with either antiplatelet therapy or a control (4). The most widely studied antiplatelet drug was aspirin. Overall, antiplatelet therapy was associated with a 25% odds reduction for the aggregate endpoint of stroke, myocardial infarction, or vascular death (Fig. 1). The studies included in this metanalysis, as well as some more recent studies, highlight the efficacy of aspirin in reducing cardiovascular morbidity and mortality in patients with atherosclerosis. Some of the larger studies involving patients with coronary artery disease, cerebrovascular disease, or peripheral arterial disease are described below.

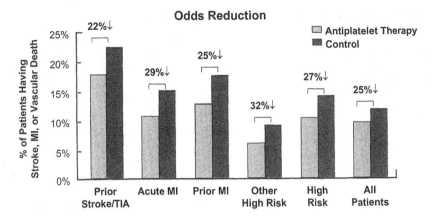

Figure 1 Antiplatelet Trialists' Collaboration: Prevention of ischemic events in patients with prior stroke/TIA, acute myocardial infarction, prior myocardial infarction, and other high-risk patients. Antiplatelet therapy, compared to control treatment, was consistently associated with a significant odds reduction in the percent of patients having stroke, myocardial infarction, or vascular death. (Reproduced from Ref. 4.)

A. Coronary Artery Disease

In the Antiplatelet Trialists' Collaboration, antiplatelet therapy, primarily aspirin, was associated with a 29% odds reduction for stroke, myocardial, or vascular death among approximately 20,000 patients with acute myocardial infarction and a 25% odds reduction for these adverse events among approximately 20,000 patients with prior myocardial infarction (4). The largest trial for acute myocardial infarction included in the Antiplatelet Trialists' Collaboration was the Second International Study of Infarct Survival (ISIS-2), which randomized over 17,000 patients with acute myocardial infarction to aspirin, streptokinase, both, or neither (5). Compared to placebo, aspirin was associated with a 23% risk reduction for vascular death, a 50% reduction for nonfatal reinfarction, and a 46% reduction for nonfatal stroke 5 weeks after randomization (Table 1). The combination of streptokinase and aspirin was more effective than either agent alone in reducing vascular death. The efficacy of aspirin in preventing coronary reocclusion following thrombolysis for acute myocardial infarction is supported by a metanalysis of 32 studies (6). Reocclusion occurred in 11% of 419 patients treated with aspirin versus 25% of 513 patients not treated with aspirin, and recurrent ischemic events occurred in 25% of 2977 patients treated with aspirin compared to 41% of 721 patients who were not treated with aspirin.

Table 1   Second International Study of Infarct Survival (ISIS-2)

Endpoint (5 weeks)	Aspirin ($n = 8{,}587$)	Placebo ($n = 8{,}600$)	Risk reduction (%)
Nonfatal reinfarction	83	170	50
Nonfatal stroke	27	51	46
Vascular death	804	1016	23
Any vascular event	914	1237	23

Source: Ref. 5.

Several large trials have demonstrated the efficacy of aspirin in preventing myocardial infarction and death in patients with unstable angina. A Veterans Administration Cooperative study randomized 1256 men with unstable angina to aspirin or placebo for 12 weeks (7). The incidence of fatal or nonfatal myocardial infarction was reduced by 51% in the group treated with aspirin compared to the group treated with placebo. A Canadian multicenter trial randomized 555 patients with unstable angina to aspirin, sulfinpyrizone, both, or neither to 24 months of treatment. The incidence of fatal or nonfatal myocardial infarction was 8.6% in the groups receiving aspirin compared to 17% in the groups not receiving aspirin, resulting in a 51% risk reduction with aspirin (8). Theroux et al. compared the efficacy of aspirin, intravenous heparin, both, or neither in 479 patients with unstable angina. Approximately 6 days following randomization, myocardial infarction had occurred in 11.9% of patients who received neither aspirin nor heparin, in 3.3% who received any aspirin, in 0.8% of those who received only heparin, and in 1.6% of patients who received both aspirin and heparin (8a). The Research Group on Instability in Coronary Artery Disease in Southeast Sweden (R.I.S.C.) randomized 796 men with unstable angina or non-Q-wave myocardial infarction to aspirin or placebo. After 1 year, myocardial infarction occurred in 21.4% of patients treated with placebo and in 11% of patients treated with aspirin. Thus, aspirin treatment reduced the risk of nonfatal or fatal myocardial infarction by 48% (9).

B. Cerebrovascular Disease

The Antiplatelet Trialists' Collaboration evaluated the efficacy of antiplatelet therapy, primarily with aspirin in 12 randomized trials, consisting of over 10,000 patients with previous stroke or transient ischemic attack (4). Antiplatelet therapy was associated with a 22% odds reduction for the risk of stroke, myocardial infarction, or vascular death. A more recent metanalysis evaluated the effect of low (50 to 100 mg), medium (250 to 500 mg), and high (1000 to 1500 mg) doses of aspirin based on 10 randomized trials consisting of over 9000 patients (10). Compared to placebo, aspirin was associated with a 13% relative risk reduction for stroke, myocardial infarction, and vascular death, and no difference in efficacy was found among the three dose ranges.

Two recent large trials have studied the efficacy and safety of aspirin in patients with acute ischemic strokes (Fig. 2). The International Stroke Trial randomized 19,435 patients with acute ischemic stroke to unfractionated heparin, either 5,000 or 12,500 units twice daily, aspirin 300 mg daily, or both heparin and aspirin (11). Among the patients treated with aspirin, there were 2.8% recurrent ischemic strokes within 14 days, compared to 3.9% in the groups not receiving aspirin, and no excess of hemorrhagic strokes. There was a nonsignificant trend for decreased mortality in patients treated with aspirin compared to those not treated with aspirin at 14 days (9% vs. 9.4%). At 14 days, therefore, there was a significant reduction in death or any nonfatal recurrent stroke in the aspirin-treated group (11.3% vs. 12.4%). In patients treated with heparin, there were 2.9% recurrent ischemic strokes within 14 days compared to 3.8% in the groups not receiving heparin, but an increase in hemorrhagic strokes (1.2% vs. 0.4%). As a consequence, there was no significant difference in the incidence of nonfatal recurrent stroke or death between the heparin and nonheparin groups (11.7% vs. 12%, respectively). The Chinese Acute Stroke Trial studied the effect of 160 mg

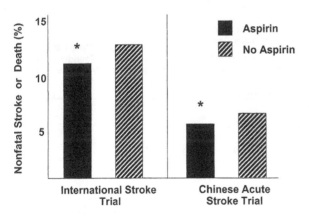

Figure 2   The effect of aspirin treatment versus no aspirin treatment on recurrent nonfatal stroke or death. The left panel demonstrates the findings from the International Stroke Trial where the risk of nonfatal recurrent stroke or death at 14 days was 11.3% in the aspirin-treated group and 12.4% in the group not treated with aspirin ($p = 0.02$). The right panel demonstrates the findings in the Chinese Acute Stroke Trial. At 4 weeks, the risk of recurrent nonfatal stroke or death was 5.3% in the aspirin-treated group and in 5.9% in the placebo-treated group ($p = 0.03$). (Adapted from Refs. 11 and 12.)

aspirin per day versus placebo in 21,106 patients with acute ischemic stroke (12). At 4 weeks, there were significantly fewer recurrent ischemic strokes in the aspirin-treated group compared to the placebo-treated group (1.6% vs. 2.1%), but slightly, though not significantly, more hemorrhagic strokes (1.1% vs. 0.9%). Overall, there was a 12% reduction (5.3% vs. 5.9%) in the risk of death or nonfatal stroke at 4 weeks.

C. Peripheral Arterial Disease

The Antiplatelet Trialists' Collaboration included a set of patients with peripheral arterial disease comprising 22 trials of patients with intermittent claudication, nine trials of patients with peripheral grafts, and two trials of patients with peripheral angioplasty (Fig. 3) (4). The subset of 3295 patients with claudication were treated with antiplatelet therapy, primarily aspirin, versus control. There was a nonsignificant, 16% odds reduction in the risk for myocardial infarction, stroke, or vascular death in claudicants receiving antiplatelet therapy compared to a control group. Moreover, antiplatelet therapy did not significantly reduce these adverse cardiovascular events in patients who received peripheral grafts or peripheral angioplasty. However, these trials consisted of relatively few patients. The Antiplatelet Trialists' Collaboration also evaluated 14 trials of patients with pe-

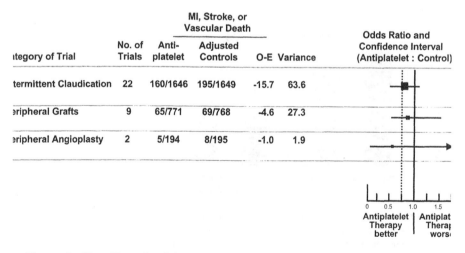

Figure 3 The effect of antiplatelet therapy versus control treatment in patients with peripheral arterial disease based on analysis from the Antiplatelet Trialists' Collaboration involving trials of patients with intermittent claudication, peripheral grafts, or peripheral angioplasty. (Reproduced from Ref. 4.)

ripheral arterial disease, including 11 involving peripheral grafts and two involving peripheral angioplasty and found that antiplatelet therapy was associated with a 43% reduction in vascular occlusion (13).

D. Primary Prevention

Several trials have studied the efficacy of aspirin as primary prevention for myocardial infarction, stroke, and death, but the results have not been consistent. The Physicians' Health Study compared aspirin to placebo in 22,071 male physicians over the age of 40 and followed them for 5 years (14). Myocardial infarction occurred in 139 persons assigned to aspirin and 239 assigned to placebo. Thus, aspirin was associated with a 44% reduction in the risk of myocardial infarction. Cardiovascular death occurred in 81 persons assigned to aspirin and 83 assigned to placebo. Thus, there was no significant reduction in total cardiovascular mortality. The reduction in the risk of myocardial infarction occurred only among men 50 years of age and older. There was a nonsignificant, slightly increased risk of stroke among those taking aspirin compared to those taking placebo. A separate study of 5139 healthy British male physicians compared aspirin to placebo (15). Total mortality was slightly, but not significantly, less in the control group compared to the aspirin-treated group. There was no significant difference in the incidence of nonfatal myocardial infarction or stroke.

Another British trial, the Thrombosis Prevention Trial, evaluated the effect of low-dose aspirin (75 mg/day) as well as oral anticoagulation with warfarin (average INR = 1.47) in 5499 healthy men aged 45 to 69 years who were randomized to warfarin, aspirin, both, or neither (16). The average International Normalized Ratio (INR) for those receiving warfarin was 1.47. Warfarin was associated with a 21% reduction in coronary death, fatal, and nonfatal myocardial infarction, and aspirin was associated with a 20% reduction in coronary death and myocardial infarction. The risk of hemorrhagic and fatal strokes was increased in the warfarin-treated patients. The principal effect of aspirin was primarily a 32% reduction in nonfatal myocardial infarction; aspirin did not reduce total cardiovascular mortality. The effect of aspirin as primary prevention was also evaluated in 87,678 U.S. registered nurses who had been participating in a prospective cohort study (17). Among women taking one to six aspirin per week, there was a significant, 32% relative risk reduction for myocardial infarction, a nonsignificant, 11% relative risk reduction for cardiovascular death, and no decrease in the risk of stroke.

E. Adverse Effects of Aspirin

Gastrointestinal symptoms and hemorrhage are the most frequent adverse effects encountered with aspirin. Indigestion, nausea, vomiting, peptic ulcer, and major gastrointestinal bleeding occur more commonly among persons using aspirin. An analysis of 21 trials included in the Antiplatelet Trialists' Collaboration found that the odds ratio among persons using aspirin for upper gastrointestinal bleeding was 1.7; for peptic ulcer, 1.3; and for all gastrointestinal bleeding, 1.5 to 2.0 (18).

The risk of cerebral hemorrhage is increased by aspirin. A recent metanalysis of 16 trials constituting 55,462 persons found that the absolute risk of hemorrhagic stroke in groups treated with aspirin was 1.2 per thousand individuals accounting for a relative risk of 1.84 (19). Hypersensitivity reactions to aspirin, including nasal congestion, urticaria, and bronchospasm may occur (20). The frequency of these adverse effects in patients with chronic urticaria is 23%, in patients with asthma is 4 to 19%, and in patients with nasal polyps is approximately 23% (21).

IV. TICLOPIDINE

The efficacy of ticlopidine has been evaluated in patients with coronary artery disease, cerebrovascular disease, and peripheral vascular disease (2). Data derived from the Antiplatelet Trialists' Collaboration suggests that there is a relative odds reduction of 10% for an adverse cardiovascular event such as myocardial infarction, stroke, or vascular death in patients treated with ticlopidine compared to those treated with aspirin (4).

A. Coronary Artery Disease

The Studio della Ticlopidinia nell'Angina Instabile Groupe evaluated the efficacy of ticlopidine in 652 patients with unstable angina (Fig. 4) (22). Following treatment for 6 months, 7.3% of the patients receiving ticlopidine had a nonfatal myocardial infarction or vascular death compared to 13.6% of patients who did not receive ticlopidine, accounting for a 46.3% relative risk reduction.

Several trials have evaluated the efficacy of ticlopidine in preventing thrombosis or ischemic events subsequent to placement of an intracoronary stent. The Full Anticoagulation versus Aspirin and Ticlopidine (FANTASTIC) study randomized patients to aspirin and ticlopidine or to aspirin and conventional anticoagulation with heparin or oral anticoagulants (23). The primary endpoint of bleeding or peripheral vascular complications occurred in 13.5% of patients treated with aspirin and ticlopidine and 21% of patients treated with aspirin and anticoagulants. The overall incidence of stent occlusion was similar in each group; yet, acute stent occlusion occurred more frequently in the antiplatelet group (2.4 vs. 0.4%), whereas subacute stent occlusion within 1 week occurred more frequently in the anticoagulant group (3.5 vs. 0.4%). Among electively stented patients, major cardiac events, including death, myocardial infarction, or stent occlusion

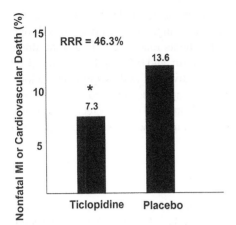

Figure 4 The effect of ticlopidine compared to placebo on nonfatal myocardial infarction or cardiovascular death at 6 months in patients presenting with unstable angina based on findings in 652 patients studied by the Studio della Ticlopdinia nell'Angina Instabile Groupe. (Adapted from Ref. 22.)

occurred in 2.4% of the aspirin and ticlopidine group compared to 9.9% of the aspirin and anticoagulant group.

The Multicenter Aspirin and Ticlopidine Trial after Intracoronary Stenting (MATTIS) study randomized 350 high-risk patients following stent implantation to aspirin and ticlopidine or to aspirin and oral anticoagulation (24). After 30 days, the primary cardiac endpoint of cardiovascular death, myocardial infarction, or repeated revascularization occurred in 5.6% of the aspirin and ticlopidine group compared to 11% of the aspirin and anticoagulant group, accounting for approximately 50% reduction in the risk of an adverse event with the former compared to the latter group.

Schomig et al. randomized 257 patients undergoing placement of coronary artery stents to aspirin and ticlopidine, or to aspirin plus anticoagulation with heparin or phenprocoumon (25). The primary cardiac endpoint of cardiac death, nonfatal myocardial infarction, coronary artery bypass surgery, or repeat angioplasty occurred in 1.6% of patients randomized to aspirin plus ticlopidine as compared to 6.2% of those randomized to aspirin plus anticoagulation, accounting for a relative risk of 0.25 in those randomized to antiplatelet therapy alone. Moreover, hemorrhagic complications occurred in 6.5% of the anticoagulant therapy group, but in none of the antiplatelet therapy group.

Leon et al. reported the results of a multicenter trial of 1965 patients who underwent coronary artery stenting and who were randomized to one of three antithrombotic drug regimens, including aspirin alone, aspirin plus warfarin, or aspirin plus ticlopidine (26). The primary endpoint of death, myocardial infarction, revascularization of the target lesion, or angiographically evident thrombosis within 30 days occurred in 3.6% of patients randomized to aspirin alone, 2.7% of those randomized to aspirin plus warfarin, and 0.5% of those randomized to aspirin and ticlopidine, accounting for a relative risk in the aspirin and ticlopidine group of 0.15 compared to aspirin alone and 0.20 compared to aspirin plus warfarin. Hemorrhagic complications occurred in 1.8% of those receiving aspirin alone, 6.2% of those receiving aspirin and warfarin, and 5.5% of those receiving aspirin and ticlopidine.

B. Cerebrovascular Disease

Two large clinical trials evaluated the efficacy of ticlopidine in patients with symptomatic cerebrovascular disease. The Canadian American Ticlopidine Studies (CATS) randomized 1072 with recent thromboembolic stroke to ticlopidine or placebo and followed them for an average of 24 months (27). The primary endpoint of stroke, myocardial infarction, or vascular death occurred in 15.3% per year of those treated with placebo and 10.8% per year of those treated with ticlopidine, accounting for a relative risk reduction with ticlopidine of 30.2%. There was no significant difference in the total mortality rate, which was 4.5% per year in those receiving placebo and 4.1% per year in those receiving ticlopidine.

The Ticlopidine Aspirin Stroke Study (TASS) randomized 3069 patients with recent transient ischemic attack, amaurosis fugax, or minor stroke to aspirin or ticlopidine (Fig. 5) (28). The primary endpoint of nonfatal stroke or death by 3 years occurred in 17% of patients randomized to ticlopidine and 19% of those randomized to aspirin, accounting for a significant 12% risk reduction in favor

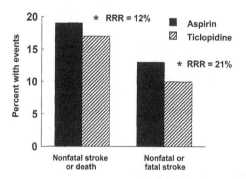

Figure 5 The effect of ticlopidine compared to aspirin in the 3069 patients with recent transient ischemic attack, amaurosis fugax, or minor stroke, who participated in the Ticlopidine, Aspirin, Stroke Study (TASS). (Adapted from Ref. 28.)

of ticlopidine. Fatal and nonfatal stroke at 3 years occurred in 10% of patients randomized to ticlopidine and 13% of those randomized to aspirin, accounting for a 21% risk reduction.

C. Peripheral Arterial Disease

Several studies have examined the efficacy of ticlopidine in patients with peripheral arterial disease. Balsano et al. studied 151 patients with intermittent claudication who were randomized to treatment with ticlopidine or placebo (29). Improvement in pain-free and maximal walking distance was greater in the ticlopidine than in the placebo group. The Swedish Ticlopidine Multicenter Study (STIMS) assessed the effect of ticlopidine on cardiovascular events in 687 patients with intermittent claudication followed for a median duration of 5.6 years (Fig. 6) (30,31). The incidence of myocardial infarction, stroke, and transient ischemic attack was 29% in patients treated with placebo compared to 25% among those treated with ticlopidine, accounting for a risk reduction of 11.4% in favor of ticlopidine. Mortality was 26.1% in the placebo group and 18.5% in the ticlopidine group, accounting for a relative risk reduction of 29%. A recent metanalysis involving studies of patients with intermittent claudication found that mortality was significantly decreased by ticlopidine compared to placebo, with an odds ratio of 0.68 (32). The efficacy of ticlopidine compared to placebo for maintaining

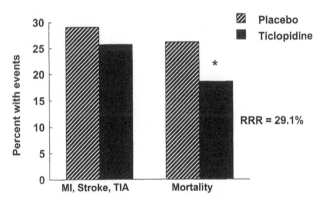

Figure 6 The effect of ticlopidine compared to placebo on adverse cardiovascular events in patients with intermittent claudication participating in the Swedish Ticlopidine Multicenter Study. There was a nonsignificant trend for reduction in myocardial infarction, stroke, and transient ischemic attack in favor of ticlopidine and a significant 29.1% risk reduction for mortality in the group treated with ticlopidine compared to placebo. (Adapted from Ref. 30.)

graft patency was studied in 243 patients with infrainguinal bypass grafts (33). Two years after randomization, 66% of patients randomized to ticlopidine were alive with a patent graft compared to 51% of those randomized to placebo; the 2-year cumulative patency rate was 82% in the ticlopidine group compared to 63% in the placebo group.

D. Adverse Effects of Ticlopidine

The most important adverse effect related to ticlopidine is neutropenia. Ticlopidine also is associated with an increased incidence of skin rash. In one study, 12% of the patients developed dermatological reactions, the most common of which were urticaria, pruritus, and maculopapular eruption (34). In CATS and TASS, neutropenia occurred in 2.1% of the patients receiving ticlopidine and was severe, defined as less than 450 neutrophils/μL in approximately 1% of patients (27,28). In patients treated with ticlopidine, diarrhea occurs in approximately 20%, and skin rash in approximately 12% (35). Severe diarrhea or severe skin rash each occur in approximately 2% of patients.

Severe thrombocytopenia has been related to several fatalities (36). An unusual, but life-threatening side effect of ticlopidine is thrombotic thrombocytopenic purpura. A recent review identified 60 cases (37). Ticlopidine had been administered for less than 1 month in 80% of these patients. The mortality rate among those not treated with plasmapheresis was 50% compared to 24% in those who were treated with plasmapheresis. Gastrointestinal side effects such as nausea, vomiting, and diarrhea occur in 30 to 50% of patients (2).

V. CLOPIDOGREL

The efficacy of clopidogrel compared to aspirin in preventing adverse cardiovascular events was evaluated in a clinical trial comprising 19,185 patients (38). Patients enrolled in this trial had evidence of vascular disease based on one of three clinical criteria: ischemic stroke occurring between 1 week and 6 months before randomization, myocardial infarction occurring within 35 days of randomization, and peripheral arterial disease manifested as claudication with an ankle/brachial index <0.85 or a history of claudication with previous revascularization procedure or leg amputation. Patients were randomized to clopidogrel 75 mg/day or to aspirin 325 mg/day. The average duration of follow-up was 1.9 years. The primary outcome measure in this study was a cluster of cardiovascular events defined as ischemic stroke, myocardial infarction, or vascular death.

The average rate of these adverse events in patients randomized to aspirin was 5.32% per year and in those randomized to clopidogrel 5.83% per year. This

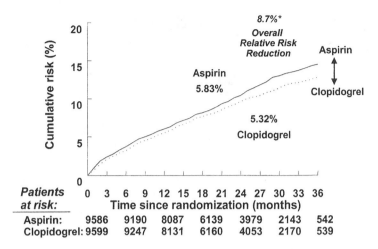

Figure 7   The effect of clopidogrel compared to aspirin in preventing adverse cardiovascular events was evaluated in the CAPRIE trial. The cumulative risk of ischemic stroke, myocardial infarction, or vascular death, was 5.83% in the patients randomized to aspirin and 5.32% in the patients randomized to clopidogrel, with a relative risk reduction of 8.7% in favor of clopidogrel. (Reproduced from Ref. 38.)

accounted for a relative risk reduction of 8.7% in favor of clopidogrel (Fig. 7). Subgroup analysis for the primary endpoint was determined. Of the patients enrolled with a recent ischemic stroke, the relative risk reduction was 7.3% (95% CI, -5.7 to 18.7; $p = 0.26$). Of the patients enrolled because of acute myocardial infarction, the event rate in those randomized to aspirin was 4.84% per year and those to clopidogrel 5.03% per year, accounting for a relative risk reduction of -3.7% (95% CI, -22.1 to 12.0; $p = 0.66$). Of the patients with peripheral arterial disease, those randomized to aspirin had an event rate of 4.86% per year and those randomized to clopidogrel 3.71% per year, accounting for a relative risk reduction of 23.8% (95% CI, 8.9 to 36.2; $p = 0.0028$) (Fig. 8). Much of the beneficial effect of clopidogrel compared to aspirin could be attributed to a reduction in fatal and nonfatal myocardial infarction. Myocardial infarction occurred in 3.6% of those randomized to aspirin and 2.9% of those randomized to clopidogrel, accounting for 19.2% relative risk reduction in favor of clopidogrel (39).

A recent trial examined the efficacy of clopidogrel plus aspirin compared to ticlopidine plus aspirin for 28 days in patients undergoing coronary stenting (40). Patients were randomized to clopidogrel as a 300-mg loading dose followed by 75 mg/day plus aspirin 325 mg/day, clopidogrel as 75 mg/day without a loading dose plus aspirin 325 mg/day, or ticlopidine 250 mg twice daily plus aspirin 325 mg/day. The primary endpoint of this safety trial was major periph-

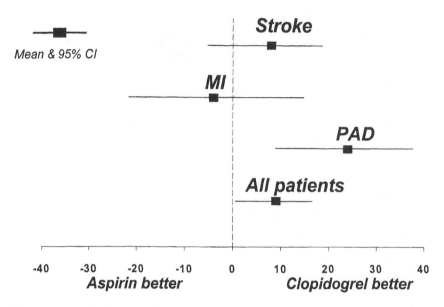

Figure 8 Subgroup analysis for the primary endpoint of ischemic stroke, myocardial infarction, or vascular death in the CAPRIE trial. Of the patients with peripheral arterial disease, those randomized to aspirin had an event rate of 4.86% per year and those randomized to clopidogrel had an event rate of 3.71% per year, accounting for relative risk reduction of 23.8%. (Reproduced from Ref. 38.)

eral arterial complications, bleeding, neutropenia, thrombocytopenia, or early drug discontinuation because of a noncardiac adverse event. This endpoint occurred in 4.6% of patients in the clopidogrel group compared to 9.1% of those assigned to ticlopidine. The incidence of major adverse cardiac events, defined as cardiac death, myocardial infarction, or target lesion revascularization occurred with a low, but similar, frequency in each treatment group, approximating 1.2% in those who received a clopidogrel loading dose plus maintenance therapy, 1.5% of those receiving maintenance clopidogrel without a load, and 0.9% of those receiving ticlopidine (Fig. 9). Thus, the efficacy of clopidogrel in preventing complications following coronary stenting was comparable to that of ticlopidine, yet there were fewer peripheral or bleeding complications with clopidogrel.

Given evidence that aspirin or clopidogrel given alone reduces vascular event rates, it became critical to evaluate whether the combination of these two agents might provide further benefit for high-risk patients. This issue was addressed in the recently completed Clopidogrel in Unstable angina to prevent Recurrent Events (CURE) trial, which included 12,562 patients with acute coronary

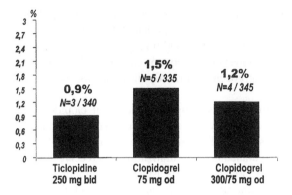

Figure 9   The CLASSICS trial. The effect of clopidogrel plus aspirin to ticlopidine plus aspirin in patients undergoing coronary stenting. The incidence of major adverse cardiovascular events, including cardiac death, myocardial infarction, or target lesion revascularization was comparable across treatment groups. (Adapted from Ref. 40.)

syndromes without ST segment elevation (i.e., unstable angina or non-Q-wave myocardial infarction) who presented within 24 h of chest pain onset (39a). Patients were required to have either ECG changes compatible with new ischemia (without ST segment elevation) or elevated cardiac enzymes or troponin I or T at least twice the upper limit of normal.

Patients were randomly allocated to clopidogrel (300 mg loading dose followed by 75 mg daily) or placebo, both given in combination with aspirin (75 to 325 mg daily) and other standard therapies. Patients were treated and followed for 1 year.

Overall, the combination of clopidogrel and aspirin resulted in a lower incidence of the primary trial outcome of cardiovascular death, MI, or stroke compared with the aspirin only group (9.3 vs. 11.4%; relative risk reduction 20%; 95% CI 10 to 28%; $p < 0.001$). When refractory ischemia was also included in this combined endpoint, there were 1040 events in the clopidogrel plus aspirin group as compared to 1196 events in the aspirin alone group, a relative risk reduction of 14 percent (95% CI 6 to 21%; $p < 0.001$). These benefits were seen in all major subgroups evaluated and were in addition to other standard treatments including heparin, glycoprotein IIb/IIIa inhibitors, beta-blockers, ACE inhibitors, and lipid-lowering agents. There was also a 25% reduction in severe ischemia during initial hospitalization and an 18% lower incidence of developing heart failure, although no difference was observed between treatment groups for refractory ischemia after hospital discharge.

The CURE trial data are likely to impact broadly on both the initial and long-term care of patients with acute coronary ischemia. Given the failure of oral glycoprotein IIb/IIIa inhibitors and the previously proven benefits of clopidogrel for initial management of in-stent thrombosis, it is probable that combined clopidogrel plus aspirin therapy will become a key addition to the care of high-risk patients. Compared with aspirin, however, the cost of clopidogrel is significant so the cost-effectiveness of this approach is currently uncertain for use beyond the first year.

Several additional trials that are assessing the efficacy of clopidogrel in preventing cardiovascular events are currently taking place. These include: the Clopidogrel Reduction of Events During Extending Observation (CREDO) trial in which patients undergoing percutaneous revascularization will receive clopidogrel with aspirin for 1 year versus clopidogrel plus aspirin for 1 month followed by aspirin for another 11 months and the Warfarin and Antiplatelet Therapy in Chronic Heart Failure (WATCH) trial in which patients with congestive heart failure will be randomized to warfarin (titrated to an INR of 2.5–3.0), clopidogrel 75 mg/day, or aspirin 160 mg/day, and followed for up to 5 years.

A. Adverse Effects of Clopidogrel

In the CAPRIE trial, bleeding occurred with comparable frequency in the patients receiving clopidogrel compared to aspirin (9.27% vs. 9.28%, respectively) (38). In patients receiving clopidogrel, intracranial hemorrhage occurred in 0.35% and gastrointestinal hemorrhage in 1.99%, the latter being less frequent than in patients receiving aspirin (38). In patients receiving clopidogrel, diarrhea occurred in 4.46% and rash occurred in 6.02%. Of patients receiving clopidogrel, neutropenia ($<1200/\mu L$) was present in 0.1%, severe neutropenia ($<450/\mu L$) in 0.05%, thrombocytopenia ($<100 \times 10^3/\mu L$) in 0.26%, and severe thrombocytopenia ($<80 \times 10^3/\mu L$) in 0.19% of patients receiving clopidogrel. A recent report highlighted the potential association of thrombotic thrombocytopenic purpura with clopidogrel (41). Eleven patients who had been treated with clopidogrel, 10 of whom had been treated for 14 days or less, were identified over a 2-year period by active surveillance of medical directors of blood banks, hematologists, and a surveillance overseen by pharmaceutical manufacturers. At the time of this report, the authors estimated that more than 3 million people had received clopidogrel. Idiopathic thrombotic thrombocytopenic purpura has been estimated to occur in approximately 3.7 per million persons per year (42).

The CURE trial provides important information on expected side effects that are associated with clopidogrel 75 mg daily given in addition to aspirin. During 1 year of therapy, there was a statistically significant increase in major bleeding between the clopidgrel plus aspirin–treated group compared to the aspirin-alone group (3.7 vs. 2.7%; $p = 0.003$). However, there was no statistically significant difference in the CURE trial for life-threatening bleeds between the two treatment groups.

Bleeding in the CURE trial was managed with either therapy interruption or transfusion; the principal sites for major bleeds were gastrointestinal and puncture sites.

VI. CONCLUSION

Platelets contribute to the thrombotic complications of atherosclerosis, and antiplatelet therapy reduces adverse cardiovascular events in patients with atherosclerosis. Both aspirin and clopidogrel are effective and relatively safe antiplatelet agents. Antiplatelet therapy should be incorporated into the treatment regimen of patients with atherosclerosis unless its use is contraindicated because of propensity to bleeding or adverse side effects. Recent trial evidence demonstrates efficacy of short-term therapy with clopidogrel to reduce in-stent thrombosis, as well as long-term use of this agent in combination with aspirin for patients with acute coronary syndromes.

REFERENCES

1. Hartwig JH. Platelet morphology. In Loscalzo J, Schafer AI, eds. Thrombosis and Hemorrhage, 2nd ed. Baltimore: Williams & Wilkins, 1998:207–228.
2. Quinn MJ, Fitzgerald DJ. Ticlopidine and clopidogrel. Circulation 1999; 100:1667–1672.
3. Awtry EH, Loscalzo J. Aspirin. Circulation 2000; 101:1206–1218.
4. Collaborative overview of randomised trials of antiplatelet therapy—I: Prevention of death, myocardial infarction, and stroke by prolonged antiplatelet therapy in various categories of patients. Antiplatelet Trialists' Collaboration [published erratum appears in BMJ 1994; 308(6943):1540]. BMJ 1994; 308:81–106.
5. Randomised trial of intravenous streptokinase, oral aspirin, both, or neither among 17,187 cases of suspected acute myocardial infarction: ISIS-2. ISIS-2 (Second International Study of Infarct Survival) Collaborative Group. Lancet 1988; 2:349–360.
6. Roux S, Christeller S, Ludin E. Effects of aspirin on coronary reocclusion and recurrent ischemia after thrombolysis: a meta-analysis. J Am Coll Cardiol 1992; 19:671–677.
7. Lewis HD, Jr, Davis JW, Archibald DG, Steinke WE, Smitherman TC, Doherty JEd, Schnaper HW, LeWinter MM, Linares E, Pouget JM, Sabharwal SC, Chesler E, DeMots H. Protective effects of aspirin against acute myocardial infarction and death in men with unstable angina. Results of a Veterans Administration Cooperative Study. N Engl J Med 1983; 309:396–403.
8. Cairns JA, Gent M, Singer J, Finnie KJ, Froggatt GM, Holder DA, Jablonsky G, Kostuk WJ, Melendez LJ, Myers MG, et al. Aspirin, sulfinpyrazone, or both in unstable angina. Results of a Canadian multicenter trial. N Engl J Med 1985; 313:1369–1375.

8a. Théroux P, Ouimet H, McCans J, et al. Aspirin, heparin, or both to treat acute unstable angina. N Engl J Med 1988; 319:1105–1111.

9. Wallentin LC. Aspirin (75 mg/day) after an episode of unstable coronary artery disease: long-term effects on the risk for myocardial infarction, occurrence of severe angina and the need for revascularization. Research Group on Instability in Coronary Artery Disease in Southeast Sweden. J Am Coll Cardiol 1991; 18:1587–1593.

10. Tijssen JG. Low-dose and high-dose acetylsalicylic acid, with and without dipyridamole: a review of clinical trial results. Neurology 1998; 51:S15–16.

11. The International Stroke Trial (IST): a randomised trial of aspirin, subcutaneous heparin, both, or neither among 19435 patients with acute ischaemic stroke. International Stroke Trial Collaborative Group. Lancet 1997; 349:1569–1581.

12. CAST: randomised placebo-controlled trial of early aspirin use in 20,000 patients with acute ischaemic stroke. CAST (Chinese Acute Stroke Trial) Collaborative Group. Lancet 1997; 349:1641–1649.

13. Collaborative overview of randomised trials of antiplatelet therapy—II: Maintenance of vascular graft or arterial patency by antiplatelet therapy. Antiplatelet Trialists' Collaboration. BMJ 1994; 308:159–168.

14. Final report on the aspirin component of the ongoing Physicians' Health Study. Steering Committee of the Physicians' Health Study Research Group. N Engl J Med 1989; 321:129–135.

15. Peto R, Gray R, Collins R, Wheatley K, Hennekens C, Jamrozik K, Warlow C, Hafner B, Thompson E, Norton S, et al. Randomised trial of prophylactic daily aspirin in British male doctors. Br Med J (Clin Res Ed) 1988; 296:313–316.

16. Thrombosis prevention trial: randomised trial of low-intensity oral anticoagulation with warfarin and low-dose aspirin in the primary prevention of ischaemic heart disease in men at increased risk. The Medical Research Council's General Practice Research Framework. Lancet 1998; 351:233–241.

17. Manson JE, Stampfer MJ, Colditz GA, Willett WC, Rosner B, Speizer FE, Hennekens CH. A prospective study of aspirin use and primary prevention of cardiovascular disease in women. JAMA 1991; 266:521–527.

18. Roderick PJ, Wilkes HC, Meade TW. The gastrointestinal toxicity of aspirin: an overview of randomised controlled trials. Br J Clin Pharmacol 1993; 35:219–226.

19. He J, Whelton PK, Vu B, Klag MJ. Aspirin and risk of hemorrhagic stroke: a meta-analysis of randomized controlled trials. JAMA 1998; 280:1930–1935.

20. Lee TH. Mechanism of aspirin sensitivity. Am Rev Respir Dis 1992; 145:S34–36.

21. Settipane GA. Aspirin and allergic diseases: a review. Am J Med 1983; 74:102–109.

22. Balsano F, Rizzon P, Violi F, Scrutinio D, Cimminiello C, Aguglia F, Pasotti C, Rudelli G. Antiplatelet treatment with ticlopidine in unstable angina. A controlled multicenter clinical trial. The Studio della Ticlopidina nell'Angina Instabile Group. Circulation 1990; 82:17–26.

23. Bertrand ME, Legrand V, Boland J, Fleck E, Bonnier J, Emmanuelson H, Vrolix M, Missault L, Chierchia S, Casaccia M, Niccoli L, Oto A, White C, Webb-Peploe M, Van Belle E, McFadden EP. Randomized multicenter comparison of conventional anticoagulation versus antiplatelet therapy in unplanned and elective coronary stenting. The full anticoagulation versus aspirin and ticlopidine (FANTASTIC) study. Circulation 1998; 98:1597–1603.

24. Urban P, Macaya C, Rupprecht HJ, Kiemeneij F, Emanuelsson H, Fontanelli A, Pieper M, Wesseling T, Sagnard L. Randomized evaluation of anticoagulation versus antiplatelet therapy after coronary stent implantation in high-risk patients: the multicenter aspirin and ticlopidine trial after intracoronary stenting (MATTIS). Circulation 1998; 98:2126–2132.

25. Schomig A, Neumann FJ, Kastrati A, Schuhlen H, Blasini R, Hadamitzky M, Walter H, Zitzmann-Roth EM, Richardt G, Alt E, Schmitt C, Ulm K. A randomized comparison of antiplatelet and anticoagulant therapy after the placement of coronary-artery stents. N Engl J Med 1996; 334:1084–1089.

26. Leon MB, Baim DS, Popma JJ, Gordon PC, Cutlip DE, Ho KK, Giambartolomei A, Diver DJ, Lasorda DM, Williams DO, Pocock SJ, Kuntz RE. A clinical trial comparing three antithrombotic-drug regimens after coronary-artery stenting. Stent Anticoagulation Restenosis Study Investigators. N Engl J Med 1998; 339:1665–1671.

27. Gent M, Blakely JA, Easton JD, Ellis DJ, Hachinski VC, Harbison JW, Panak E, Roberts RS, Sicurella J, Turpie AG. The Canadian American Ticlopidine Study (CATS) in thromboembolic stroke. Lancet 1989; 1:1215–1220.

28. Hass WK, Easton JD, Adams HP Jr., Pryse-Phillips W, Molony BA, Anderson S, Kamm B. A randomized trial comparing ticlopidine hydrochloride with aspirin for the prevention of stroke in high-risk patients. Ticlopidine Aspirin Stroke Study Group. N Engl J Med 1989; 321:501–507.

29. Balsano F, Coccheri S, Libretti A, Nenci GG, Catalano M, Fortunato G, Grasselli S, Violi F, Hellemans H, Vanhove P. Ticlopidine in the treatment of intermittent claudication: a 21-month double-blind trial. J Lab Clin Med 1989; 114:84–91.

30. Janzon L, Bergqvist D, Boberg J, Boberg M, Eriksson I, Lindgarde F, Persson G, Almgren B, Fagher B, Kjellstrom T, et al. Prevention of myocardial infarction and stroke in patients with intermittent claudication; effects of ticlopidine. Results from STIMS, the Swedish Ticlopidine Multicentre Study [published erratum appears in J Intern Med 1990 Dec; 228(6):659]. J Intern Med 1990; 227:301–308.

31. Janzon L. The STIMS trial: the ticlopidine experience and its clinical applications. Swedish Ticlopidine Multicenter Study. Vasc Med 1996; 1:141–143.

32. Girolami B, Bernardi E, Prins MH, ten Cate JW, Prandoni P, Hettiarachchi R, Marras E, Stefani PM, Girolami A, Buller HR. Antithrombotic drugs in the primary medical management of intermittent claudication: a meta-analysis. Thromb Haemost 1999; 81:715–722.

33. Becquemin JP. Effect of ticlopidine on the long-term patency of saphenous-vein bypass grafts in the legs. Etude de la Ticlopidine apres Pontage Femoro-Poplite and the Association Universitaire de Recherche en Chirurgie. N Engl J Med 1997; 337:1726–1731.

34. Yosipovitch G, Rechavia E, Feinmesser M, David M. Adverse cutaneous reactions to ticlopidine in patients with coronary stents. J Am Acad Dermatol 1999; 41:473–476.

35. Hankey GJ, Sudlow CL, Dunbabin DW. Thienopyridine derivatives (ticlopidine, clopidogrel) versus aspirin for preventing stroke and other serious vascular events in high-vascular risk patients. Cochrane Database Syst Rev 2; 2000.

36. Gill S, Majumdar S, Brown NE, Armstrong PW. Ticlopidine-associated pancytope-

nia: implications of an acetylsalicylic acid alternative. Can J Cardiol 1997; 13:909–913.

37. Bennett CL, Weinberg PD, Rozenberg-Ben-Dror K, Yarnold PR, Kwaan HC, Green D. Thrombotic thrombocytopenic purpura associated with ticlopidine. A review of 60 cases. Ann Intern Med 1998; 128:541–544.

38. A randomised, blinded, trial of clopidogrel versus aspirin in patients at risk of ischaemic events (CAPRIE). CAPRIE Steering Committee. Lancet 1996; 348:1329–1339.

39. Creager MA. Results of the CAPRIE trial: efficacy and safety of clopidogrel. Clopidogrel versus aspirin in patients at risk of ischaemic events. Vasc Med 1998; 3:257–260.

39a. Yusuf S et al., for the Clopidogrel in Unstable Angina to Prevent Recurrent Events (CURE) Investigators. Effects of clopidogrel in addition to aspirin in patients with acute coronary syndromes without ST elevation. N Engl J Med 2001; 365:494–502.

40. Bertrand ME, Rupprecht HJ, Urban P, Gershlick AH, Investigators. Double-blind study of the safety of clopidogrel with and without a loading dose in combination with aspirin compared with ticlopidine in combination with aspirin after coronary stenting: the clopidogrel aspirin stent international cooperative study (CLASSICS). Circulation 2000; 102:624–629.

41. Bennett CL, Connors JM, Carwile JM, Moake JL, Bell WR, Tarantolo SR, McCarthy LJ, Sarode R, Hatfield AJ, Feldman MD, Davidson CJ, Tsai HM. Thrombotic thrombocytopenic purpura associated with clopidogrel. N Engl J Med 2000; 342:1773–1777.

42. Torok TJ, Holman RC, Chorba TL. Increasing mortality from thrombotic thrombocytopenic purpura in the United States—analysis of national mortality data, 1968–1991. Am J Hematol 1995; 50:84–90.

8

Clinical Accomplishments of ACE Inhibition Therapy: With and Without Aspirin

Marc A. Pfeffer
Brigham and Women's Hospital and Harvard Medical School, Boston, Massachusetts

I. INTRODUCTION

Inhibitors of converting enzyme, or kininase II, commonly called angiotensin-converting enzyme (ACE) inhibitors, were first developed in the late 1970s as a specific pharmacological treatment to lower blood pressure in a subset of hypertensive patients with elevated renin (1). Over the past two decades, as a consequence of intense basic and clinical investigations, it has now become clear that these agents have a much greater therapeutic effect than originally conceived. Indeed, ACE inhibitors are currently considered as life-saving and morbidity-reducing therapies for patients with heart failure, asymptomatic left ventricular dysfunction, acute and chronic myocardial infarction, diabetes, and other forms of nephropathy. Most recently, this list of beneficiaries has been expanded to the broad population of patients with vascular disease or diabetes and a concomitant risk factor. These impressive accomplishments stem from a series of international multicenter trials generating consistent information regarding survival and other important clinical outcome benefits with the use of these compounds. This chapter will provide an overview of these accomplishments and then focus on one of the current issues that is particularly relevant to these proceedings on thrombosis and thromboembolism—the question of a potential aspirin–ACE-inhibitor negative interaction.

II. ACCOMPLISHMENTS OF ACE INHIBITORS

A. Heart Failure

Heart failure was the first major area in which ACE inhibitors have proven their undisputed role in improving clinical outcomes, indeed, survival. In the early 1980s, the "vasodilator era," then pioneering acute studies revealed that favorable hemodynamic improvements could be obtained by ACE inhibitors in patients with severe heart failure (2,3). The first demonstration of a survival benefit with the use of an ACE inhibitor in any cohort of patients can be attributed to the Cooperative North Scandinavian ENalapril SUrvival Study (CONSENSUS), which randomized patients with severe heart failure (4). In this trial, despite the use of digitalis, diuretics, and other vasodilators, the placebo mortality rate was exceedingly high, approaching 50% at 6 months. Those randomized to the active therapy (enalapril) had a pronounced reduction in the risk of death. Indeed, the combination of the high placebo event rate and the relative effectiveness of therapy led to conclusive results in a population of approximately 500 patients.

The Studies of Left Ventricular Dysfunction (SOLVD) greatly expanded the indications for ACE inhibitors as a consequence of their results in two parallel randomized trials collectively involving over 6000 patients (5,6). In the treatment arm, symptomatic heart failure patients with left ventricular dysfunction (ejection fraction <35%) of all etiologies were randomized to placebo or enalapril. Despite background therapy with digitalis or diuretics or both, the enalapril group experienced a 16% reduction in the risk of death and clear reductions in the need for rehospitalization for heart failure. The same screening procedures identified and randomized over 4000 patients who also had left ventricular dysfunction. However, the study investigators did not feel that these patients had sufficient symptoms to warrant therapy—the Prevention Arm. In this unique group, the randomization to enalapril showed a favorable trend for a reduction in fatal events with a clear reduction in the development of heart failure during the approximately 4 years of follow-up. As a consequence of these and other smaller studies, ACE inhibitors had proven themselves as an essential, indeed, "cornerstone" therapy for the management of patients with heart failure (7). In some respects, the V-HeFT-II study put the icing on the cake for the use of ACE inhibitors in heart failure. It showed that, in a group of symptomatic heart failure patients randomized to either the combination of hydralazine and nitrates (the first life-sustaining therapy for heart failure) versus enalapril, the ACE inhibitor resulted in superior survival even compared to a previously proven therapy for heart failure (8). Taken together, we now had clear evidence that the morbidity and mortality of heart failure could be effectively reduced by the use of an ACE inhibitor (9).

B. Myocardial Infarction

The rationale for the treatment of patients with myocardial infarction with an ACE inhibitor stems from the pioneering work of the late Dr. Janice Pfeffer, beginning when she was a fellow in the Braunwald laboratory. Experimental models of infarctions were readily utilized to determine whether infarct size could be favorably modified by pharmacological therapy. Pfeffer explored the relationship between infarct size and ventricular function and incorporated important lessons from her doctoral training in hypertension at Edward Frohlich's laboratory to determine the long-term consequences of abrupt loss of myocardium from coronary ligation. Indeed, she demonstrated in the animal model that the loss of myocytes should be viewed as the beginning of an insidious phase of progressive ventricular enlargement (remodeling), which is related both to the extent of the histological damage as well as to the duration of time from the infarct (10). Indeed, the enlargement itself is a central component in the progressive worsening of dysfunction. Ventricular remodeling could also involve the normal remaining myocardium, which, as a consequence of unfavorable geometry and wall stress, could suffer an abnormal hemodynamic burden (11).

These observations of ventricular remodeling provided a new therapeutic target for a novel use of ACE inhibition—to attenuate time-dependent ventricular enlargement following infarction. The use of ACE inhibitors was a natural extension of her work in hypertension, where these agents were particularly effective in preventing hypertrophy and left ventricular chamber enlargement (12). In the myocardial infarction model, long-term administration of an ACE inhibitor did indeed attenuate ventricular enlargement as treated animals had smaller left ventricular cavities and more preserved ventricular pump function (13). In a subsequent study, a prolongation of survival was demonstrated with ACE inhibitor treatment (14).

These animal studies provided the rationale for initially small mechanistic studies, which confirmed both the process of progressive enlargement post–myocardial infarction and the attenuation of enlargement with the use of an ACE inhibitor (15,16). These mechanistic studies were soon followed by an extensive series of international multicenter randomized trials testing the hypothesis that administration of an ACE inhibitor to patients in the acute and chronic phases of myocardial infarction would lead to improved survival. The Survival and Ventricular Enlargement (SAVE) study, as suggested by the trial's acronym, tested the hypothesis that attenuation of ventricular enlargement in high-risk patients post–myocardial infarction would lead to improved survival (17). The SAVE study demonstrated that the addition of captopril to a conventionally treated patient who survived a myocardial infarction with an ejection fraction less than 40% without overt heart failure would lead not only to a reduction in the risk of death, but also to a reduced risk of developing heart failure and experiencing a recurrent myocardial infarction. A detailed quantitative echocardiographic study did confirm an attenuation in remodeling in the ACE inhibitor group and, moreover, these investigators were able to demonstrate linkage between progressive enlargement, risk of an adverse cardiovascular event, and the favorable benefit of the ACE inhibitor therapy (18).

The Acute Infarction Ramipril Efficacy (AIRE) study administered the ACE inhibitor ramipril to patients starting in the acute phase of the infarct and continuing long term. The AIRE investigators identified high-risk patients based on clinical signs or symptoms of pulmonary congestion or transient heart failure. The long-term administration of the ACE inhibitor resulted in a 26% reduction in the risk of death and comparable reductions in other nonfatal cardiovascular endpoints (19).

The TRandolapril Cardiac Evaluation (TRACE) investigators employed echocardiographic assessment of wall motion to identify higher risk acute infarct patients. Here, again, the randomization to the ACE inhibitor resulted in an important reduction in the risk of death (20). In the Survival of Myocardial Infarction Long-term Evaluation (SMILE), the ACE inhibitor zofenopril was administered to patients with anterior myocardial infarction who had not received thrombolytic therapy (21). This randomized trial demonstrated a reduction in risk of death or development of heart failure during only 6 weeks of therapy. The TRACE and AIRE investigators have extended their observations beyond the formal trial period and demonstrated that the survival benefits persisted (22,23).

An overview of this selective approach to the use of ACE inhibitors for higher risk myocardial infarction patients indicates that approximately 20 to 30 lives are saved in the first month of treatment and that, with continued therapy, approximately 60 to 80 lives are saved per 1000 patients treated (24). It is important to underscore that the benefits of the use of an ACE inhibitor in myocardial infarct patients could be considered as additive to conventional therapy with thrombolytics, beta-blockade, and even aspirin. Therefore, it is fair to conclude that use of an ACE inhibitor in these patient populations results in a new and complementary modality to reduce risk of death and other major cardiovascular events (25).

Another approach for the use of ACE inhibitors in acute myocardial infarction that has been well studied utilized broad inclusion criteria and shorter duration of therapy. The International Studies of Infarct Survival (ISIS)-IV (26), Gruppo Italiano per lo Studio della Sopravvivenza nell'Infarto Miocardico (GISSI)-3 (27), and Chinese Captopril (28) studies all started an ACE inhibitor within the first 36 h of an infarct without selecting for either quantitative signs of left ventricular dysfunction or clinical symptoms of failure. In this broad use, it was possible to show collectively that the use of an oral ACE inhibitor led to statistical improvements in survival with approximately five lives saved per 1000 patients treated during the first 4 to 6 weeks (29).

The only "fly in the ointment" in the field of ACE inhibitors and acute myocardial infarction was from the CONSENSUS II study, which showed a negative trend when ACE inhibitor therapy was started intravenously in the first day of the infarct and then continued orally for the projected study duration of 6 months (30). With over 100,000 patients in randomized, placebo-controlled trials of different designs, agents and durations, the consensus of international experts strongly recommends the use of an ACE inhibitor starting early and continued long term for patients at higher risk (31). These authoritative guidelines do indicate that there are sufficient rationale and data for clinicians to adopt a more global approach for the use of ACE inhibitors in an even broader population.

C. Coronary Artery Disease

The independent and almost simultaneous reporting from the SAVE and SOLVD studies that the long-term use of two different ACE inhibitors (captopril and enalapril, respectively) resulted in a reduction in the incidence of myocardial infarction in their respective populations opened an entirely new area of research involving ACE inhibitors (5,6,17,32,33). Indeed, this reduction in atherosclerotic complications could not be solely attributed to the 3 mmHg blood pressure reduction observed in these two normotensive populations. Nor could the favorable mechanisms on left ventricular remodeling be readily used to evoke an explanation for the reduction in coronary atherosclerotic events.

Additional mechanisms to explain the ACE inhibitor influence on coronary events soon came from novel experimental studies that revealed an important interface between the renin-angiotensin system and the balance between thrombolysis and thrombosis. An infusion of angiotensin-II raised plasminogen activator inhibitor-1 (PAI-1), which would alter the fibrinolytic balance toward thrombosis (34). The randomized use of ACE inhibitors in patients with acute myocardial infarction did indeed lower PAI-1 levels and, particularly, the balance of PAI-1 to intrinsic tPA (35). Augmented PAI-1 levels had been associated with greater risk of infarct and others had speculated that reduced PAI-1 may be an indication of restoration of endothelial function (36). In the TREND study, the long-term treatment with the ACE inhibitor quinipril led to a better restoration of coronary endothelial function (37). Along these lines, it has been postulated that lowering angiotensin-II with an ACE inhibitor would reduce superoxide anions, promote nitric oxide, and limit further vascular damage (38). Despite all of these newly proposed mechanisms, an important limitation in the initial observation from both SAVE and SOLVD was that the finding of reduced coronary events was a secondary endpoint in populations selected for left ventricular dysfunction. It remained to be determined whether these observations would apply in a broader population, which would not be anticipated to have marked activation of the renin-angiotensin system.

In the mid-to-late 1990s, three major trials were initiated to determine whether an ACE inhibitor would reduce atherosclerotic events. The Heart Outcomes Prevention Evaluation (HOPE) study selected patients for clinical evidence of vascular disease with prior myocardial infarction, stroke, peripheral vascular disease, or diabetes plus another risk factor and randomized to conventional therapy plus placebo or ramipril. Patients with heart failure or known depressed ejection fraction were excluded (39). The Prevention of Events with Angiotensin Converting Enzyme Inhibition (PEACE) study, specifically designed as a follow-up of SAVE, included patients with documented coronary disease and an ejection fraction over 40% randomized to conventional therapy plus either trandolapril or placebo (40). The EUropean trial on Reduction Of cardiac events with Perindopril in stable coronary Artery disease (EUROPA) randomized patients with coronary disease regardless of their ejection fraction to either perindopril or placebo (41). Three large studies with about 9000, 8000, and 10,000 patients, respectively, and long-term follow-up will provide a definitive test of the ability of ACE inhibitors to favorably influence the atherosclerotic process.

HOPE was the first of these major studies to be completed. Randomization to ramipril resulted in a convincingly consistent 20% and greater reduction in atherosclerotic events, such as cardiovascular death, myocardial infarction, and stroke (42). The HOPE study results are based on a substantial number of clinical events and consistent findings were present in all predefined subgroups. Again, the small reduction in blood pressure with the ACE inhibitor in and of itself could not explain the magnitude of the clinical benefits in this patient population. Within the HOPE study, a mechanistic trial evaluating carotid arterial thickness as a surrogate marker of the atherosclerotic process did demonstrate a dose-dependent reduction in carotid thickness with the use of an ACE inhibitor (43). Other important mechanistic observations such as the reduction in the development of diabetes and diabetic complications may provide additional key insights. Indeed, the hemoglobin A1C levels in the subpopulation evaluated was reduced by chronic therapy with the ACE inhibitor. The HOPE study expands both the patient population who will receive benefits from ACE inhibitor therapy as well as the potential mechanisms that can be evoked to explain these impressive beneficial actions.

III. POTENTIAL ACE INHIBITOR ASPIRIN INTERACTION

The beneficial effect of ACE inhibitors in the wide range of patients is now indisputable and, as such, ACE inhibitors have become an important treatment for patients with cardiovascular disease. Similarly, in another impressive series of clinical trials, aspirin has proven to be an effective agent in lowering morbidity and mortality in patients with a wide range of coronary artery disease presentations from primary prevention through secondary prevention, including unstable angina and acute myocardial infarction (44,45). With the obvious broad overlap in patients who would benefit from both of these agents, a negative interaction with the concomitant use of these two agents would have major public health implications. At the outset, it must be acknowledged that there is yet to be a two-by-two trial of aspirin and ACE inhibitors as there was of thrombolytics and aspirin in ISIS-2 (46). Indeed, with the now established benefits of both of these agents, such a trial in which patients would have either of these life-saving therapies withheld would be deemed unethical. Decisions will have to be based on the experience of prior trials. Since most of the major aspirin trials were conducted prior to the knowledge of the survival benefit of ACE inhibitors, there are few data on concomitant use. On the other hand, there is extensive experience in the ACE inhibitor trials with patients on aspirin.

The initial hypothetical question of a possible interaction, whereby the concomitant use of both drugs offsets the potential benefits of an ACE inhibitor, was proposed by Donald Hall and his colleagues (47). A mechanistic study of patients with severe heart failure and marked neurohormone activation observed that the vasodilating effect of enalapril was offset by the concomitant use of aspirin (47). Since one of the important actions of an ACE inhibitor, aside from reducing the production of angiotensin-II, is to impede the breakdown of bradykinin, which also enhances the production of prostaglandins, it was reasoned that an aspirin effect on inhibiting prostaglandin synthesis could offset some of the hemodynamic benefits of administering an ACE inhibitor. Indeed, their work on the hemodynamics of severe heart failure was confirmed by others (48). This is similar to the use of nonsteroidal anti-inflammatory agents that had long been known to exacerbate signs and symptoms of heart failure, impairing renal function, and even offsetting antihypertensive effects of a variety of therapeutic compounds (49). Hall provided mechanistic underpinning and focus for important questions regarding a potential for aspirin to offset some of the clinical benefits of ACE inhibitor use in patients with severe heart failure (50).

Subsequently, a subgroup analysis from the SOLVD studies did indicate that there was a trend for less of a survival benefit in patients randomized to the ACE inhibitor who were reported to be on aspirin at baseline. Proponents of an important negative interaction whereby aspirin offsets some of the benefits of an ACE inhibitor could also turn to the CONSENSUS-II acute myocardial infarction study to bolster these positions (51). Conversely, subgroup analyses from other large studies appear to refute these observations (52). With the proven benefits of both of these agents independently and the overlapping clinical profile of patients that should be receiving these therapies simultaneously, this becomes a critical question to resolve.

Since we have not had (and are unlikely to have) a direct two-by-two test of these two proven agents, interpretation of the information from the existing studies must suffice to generate our clinical conclusions. Along these lines, it is fortunate that use of ACE inhibitors for reduction of cardiovascular events is an extremely well-studied area. Particularly so in patients with myocardial infarction, with over 100,000 patients in randomized trials and the majority on aspirin, providing a good data set from which to draw these conclusions. Just as the antiplatelet trialists have formed a collaboration to collectively extract more data from their individual studies (53), so have the ACE inhibitor myocardial infarction investigators. Representatives from eight major trials have pooled their individual data to provide more precise point estimates and to particularly probe prospective subgroup analyses for both efficacy and safety. The ACE Inhibitor Myocardial Infarction Collaborative group prospectively determined that the broad-inclusion, short-term studies should be analyzed separately from the elective-inclusion, long-term studies. Both of these systematic overviews (metanalysis) have been completed and recently published (54,24). In the short term, broad-inclusion analysis of 96,712 patients, aspirin was used at baseline in 86,884 (89.4%) and not in 10,228 patients (10.6%) (29). Aspirin use was not randomized and, as it turns out, there was a marked disparity in risk profile with respect to use of aspirin. Patients who did not receive aspirin were less likely to receive thrombolytics or beta-blockers, were older, and were more likely to have had pulmonary congestion as is manifested by Killip Class 2 and 3. Not surprisingly, regardless of ACE inhibitor status, the non-aspirin-treated patients had more than twice the mortality rate (14.4 vs. 6.5%, no aspirin vs. aspirin) in these short-term studies (29) (Fig. 1). The test for heterogeneity between the reductions in risk of death produced by randomization to the ACE inhibitor in the presence or absence of aspirin use at baseline was not significantly different. This analysis is inclusive of CONSENSUS-II, which is frequently cited as an example of an aspirin–ACE interaction where no benefit of the ACE inhibitor was observed in the presence of aspirin (51).

This overview provided additional information regarding safety and tolerability aspects of an ACE inhibitor in the presence or absence of aspirin (29). From the hemodynamic considerations, it could be speculated that there would be less hypotension in those on aspirin due to the inhibition of the vasodilator prostaglandins. In fact, this was not observed, nor was there any augmentation in reports of renal dysfunction.

The ACE Inhibitor Myocardial Infarction Collaborative Group also prospectively evaluated the cumulative experience of the long-term ACE inhibitor trials by pooling the individual data from the SAVE, AIRE, and TRACE trial experiences (24). To this experience, the two SOLVD studies were added where an aspirin and ACE inhibitor interaction was first observed. Once again, the clear 24% benefit in mortality reduction in those randomized to an ACE inhibitor were

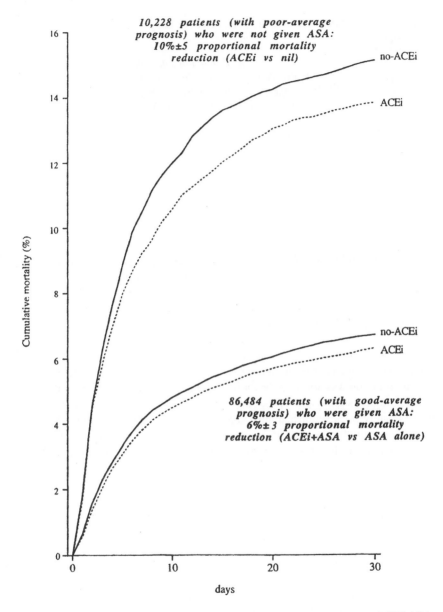

Figure 1 Metanalysis of aspirin use and mortality in the early broad use ACE inhibitor trials. (From Ref. 29.)

Table 1 SAVE, AIRE, TRACE, SOLVD (Selective Long-Term Trials)

Death		ACE inhibitor odds ratio
ASA: yes	1699/7597 (22.3%)	0.85 (0.76 − 0.95)
no	1457/5158 (28.6%)	0.75 (0.67 − 0.85)
	test for heterogeneity NS; $p = 0.23$	
Death, HF, MI		
ASA: yes	2571/7597 (33.8%)	0.76 (0.69 − 0.84)
no	2195/5158 (42.6%)	0.68 (0.60 − 0.76)
	test for heterogeneity NS; $p = 0.20$	

ASA use at baseline; ACE inhibitor odds ratio.
Source: From Ref. 29.

not statistically influenced by the use of aspirin. The appropriate test for a differential effect of an ACE inhibitor in the presence or absence of aspirin is the test for heterogeneity, which was not significant. When using the expanded endpoint of death, development of heart failure, or myocardial infarction that would favor a potential aspirin interaction by including development of heart failure and be a more statistically reliable evaluation of the concept since there were many more events, once again, there was no significant ACE inhibitor–aspirin interaction (Table 1). Indeed, the cumulative event rate of death, heart failure, or myocardial infarction was almost 34% for those on aspirin with a 24% risk reduction, which is highly significant. Those not on aspirin had a heightened event rate of approximately 43%, with a highly significant 32% reduction. Again, the test for heterogeneity for the specific question of whether the benefit of ACE inhibitor was influenced in the presence or absence of aspirin was not significant (Table 1).

IV. CONCLUSION

Like so many aspects of life, interpretation of subgroups is in the eyes of the beholder. The less definitive the data, the more likely we are to have reasonable differences of opinions. Subgroups by their very nature, and this aspirin–ACE-inhibitor potential interaction by the lack of randomization to aspirin, cannot give definitive data. Although investigators can clearly differ in providing rationale for new trials, the clinician has to make firm therapeutic decisions. In my view, the addition of an ACE inhibitor on top of aspirin therapy augments clinical benefits. Indeed, a fair and fitting conclusion to an impressive 20 years of research with ACE inhibitors is that their use in the appropriate patients produces important clinical benefits such as reduction in death, development of heart failure, myocardial infarction, and other coronary-related events, all of which should be viewed as additive to optimal conventional therapy (reperfusion strategies, beta-blockers, and, indeed, aspirin). If I were asked about an aspirin–ACE-inhibitor interaction, my response to the clinician would be: ''I do not believe that it is important enough for you to have to question which of these life-prolonging therapies you would *not* give your patient—use both.''

REFERENCES

1. Ondetti MA, Rubin B, Cushman DW. Design of specific inhibitors of angiotensin-converting enzyme: new class of orally active antihypertensive agents. Science 1975; 196:441–444.
2. Gavras H, Faxon DP, Berkoben J, Brunner HR, Ryan TJ. Angiotensin converting enzyme inhibition in patients with congestive heart failure. Circulation 1978; 58: 770–776.
3. Dzau VJ, Colucci WAS, Hollenberg NK, Williams GH. Relation of the renin-angio-tensin-aldosterone system to clinical state in congestive heart failure. Circulation 1981; 63:645–651.
4. CONSENSUS Trial Study Group. Effects of enalapril on mortality in severe conges-tive heart failure. Results of the Cooperative North Scandinavian Enalapril Survival Study (CONSENSUS). N Engl J Med 1987; 316:1429–1435.
5. The SOLVD Investigators Effect of enalapril on survival in patients with reduced left ventricular ejection fractions and congestive heart failure. N Engl J Med 1991; 325:293–302.
6. The SOLVD Investigators. Effect of enalapril on mortality and the development of heart failure in asymptomatic patients with reduced left ventricular ejection fractions. N Engl J Med 1992; 327:685–691.
7. Braunwald E. ACE inhibitors—a cornerstone of the treatment of heart failure. N Engl J Med 1991; 325:351–353.
8. Cohn JN, Johnson G, Ziesche S, Cobb F, Francis F, Tristani F, Smith R, Dunkman WB, Loeb H, Wong M, Bhat G, Goldman S, Fletcher RD, Doherty J, Hughes CV, Carson P, Cintron G, Shabetai R, Haakenson C. A comparison of enalapril with hydralazine—isosorbide dinitrate in the treatment of chronic congestive heart fail-ure. N Engl J Med 1991; 325:303–310.
9. Garg R, Yusuf S, for the Collaborative Group on ACE Inhibitor Trials. Overview of randomized trials of angiotensin-converting enzyme inhibitors on mortality and morbidity in patients with heart failure. JAMA 1995; 273:1450–1456.
10. Pfeffer JM, Pfeffer MA, Fletcher PJ, Braunwald E. Progressive ventricular remodel-ing in the rat with myocardial infarction. Am J Physiol 1991; 260 (Heart Circ. Phys-iol 29):H1406– H1414.
11. Pfeffer MA, Braunwald E. Ventricular remodeling after myocardial infarction: Experimental observations and clinical implications. Circulation 1990; 81:1161–1172.

12. Pfeffer JM, Pfeffer MA, Fletcher PJ, Fishbein MC, Braunwald E. Favorable effects of therapy on cardiac performance in spontaneously hypertensive rats. Am J Physiol 1982; 242:H766–H784.

13. Pfeffer JM, Pfeffer MA, Braunwald E. Influence of chronic captopril therapy on the infarcted left ventricle of the rat. Circ Res 1985; 57:84–95.

14. Pfeffer MA, Pfeffer JM, Steinberg C, Finn P. Survival after an experimental myocardial infarction: beneficial effects of long-term therapy with captopril. Circulation 1985; 72:406–412.

15. Pfeffer MA, Lamas GA, Vaughan DE, Parisi AF, Braunwald E. Effect of captopril on progressive ventricular dilatation after anterior myocardial infarction. N Engl J Med 1988; 319:80–86.

16. Sharpe N, Smith H, Murphy J, Hannan S. Treatment of patients with symptomless left ventricular dysfunction after myocardial infarction. Lancet 1988; 1:255–259.

17. Pfeffer MA, Braunwald E, Moyé LA, Basta L, Brown Jr EJ, Cuddy TE, Davis BR, Geltman EM, Goldman S, Flaker GC, Klein M, Lamas GA, Packer M, Rouleau J, Rouleau JL, Rutherford J, Wertheimer JH, Hawkins CM, on Behalf of the SAVE Investigators. Effect of captopril on mortality and morbidity in patients with left ventricular dysfunction after myocardial infarction. Results of the Survival and Ventricular Enlargement Trial. N Engl J Med 1992; 327:669–677.

18. St. John Sutton M, Pfeffer MA, Plappert T, Rouleau JL, Moyé LA, Dagenais GR, Lamas GA, Klein M, Sussex B, Goldman S, Menapace FJ, Parker JO, Lewis S, Sestier F, Gordon DF, McEwan P, Bernstein V, Braunwald E, for the SAVE investigators. Quantitative two dimensional echocardiographic measurements are major predictors of adverse cardiovascular events following acute myocardial infarction: The protective effects of captopril. Circulation 1984; 89:68–75.

19. Acute Infarction Ramipril Efficacy (AIRE) Study Investigators. Effect of ramipril on mortality and morbidity of survivors of acute myocardial infarction with clinical evidence of heart failure. Lancet 1993; 342:821–828.

20. Kober L, Torp-Pederson C, Carlsen JE, Bagger H, Eliasen P, Lyngborg K, Videbaek J, Cole DS, Auclert L, Pauly NC, Aliot E, Persson S, Camm AJA. A clinical trial of the angiotensin-converting-enzyme inhibitor trandolapril in patients with left ventricular dysfunction after myocardial infarction. N Engl J Med 1995; 333:1670–1676.

21. Ambrosioni E, Borghi C, Magnani B, for the Survival of Myocardial Infarction Long Term Evaluation (SMILE) Study Investigators. The effect of the angiotensin-converting-enzyme inhibitor zofenopril on mortality and morbidity after anterior myocardial infarction. N Engl J Med 1995; 332:80–85.

22. Torp-Pedersen C, Kober L. Effect of ACE inhibitor trandolapril on life expectancy of patients with reduced left-ventricular function after myocardial infarction. TRACE Study Group. Lancet 1999; 354:9–12.

23. Hall AS, Murray GD, Ball SG. Follow-up study of patients randomly allocated ramipril or placebo for heart failure after acute myocardial infarction: AIRE Extension (AIREX) Study. Lancet 1997; 349:1493–1497.

24. Flather MD, Yusuf S, Kober L, Pfeffer M, Hall A, Murray G, Torp-Pedersen C, Ball S, Pogue J, Moyé L, Braunwald E, for the ACE-inhibitor Myocardial Infarction Collaborative Group. Long-term ACE-inhibitor therapy in patients with heart failure

or left-ventricular dysfunction: a systematic overview of data from individual patients Lancet 2000; 355:1575–1581.

25. Pfeffer MA. ACE inhibitors in acute myocardial infarction: patient selection and timing [editorial]. Circulation 1998; 97:2192–2194.

26. ISIS-4 Collaborative Group ISIS-4. A randomised factorial trial assessing early oral captopril, oral mononitrate, and intravenous magnesium sulphate in 58,050 patients with suspected acute myocardial infarction. Lancet 1995; 345:669–685.

27. Gruppo Italiano per lo Studio della Sopravvivenza nell'Infarto Miocardico GISSI-3. Effects of lisinopril and transdermal glyceryl trinitrate singly and together on 6-week mortality and ventricular function after acute myocardial infarction. Lancet 1994; 343:1115–1122.

28. Chinese Cardiac Study Collaborative Group. Oral captopril versus placebo among 13,634 patients with suspected acute myocardial infarction: interim report from the Chinese Cardiac Study (CCS-1). Lancet 1995; 345:686–687.

29. Latini R, Tognoni G, Maggioni AP, Baigent C, Braunwald E, Chen ZM, Collins R, Flather M, Franzosi MG, Kjekshus J, Kober L, Liu LS, Peto R, Pfeffer M, Pizzetti F, Santoro E, Sleight P, Swedberg K, Tavazzi L, Wang W, Yusuf S, on behalf of the ACE Inhibitor Myocardial Infarction Collaborative Group. Clinical effects of early ACE inhibitor treatment for acute myocardial infarction are similar in the presence and absence of aspirin: systematic overview of individual data from 96,712 randomized patients. J Am Coll Cardiol 2000; 35:1801–1807.

30. Swedberg K, Held P, Kjekshus J, Rasmussen K, Rydén L, Wedel H, on Behalf of the CONSENSUS II Study Group. Effects of the early administration of enalapril on mortality in patients with acute myocardial infarction. Results of the Cooperative New Scandinavian Enalapril Survival Study II (CONSENSUS II). N Engl J Med 1992; 327:678–684.

31. Ryan TJ, Anderson JL, Antman EA, Braniff BA, Brooks NH, Califf RM, Hillis LD, Hiratzka LF, Rapaport E, Riegel BJ, Russell RO, Smith EE, III, Weaver WD. ACC/AHA Guidelines for the Management of Patients with Acute Myocardial Infarction: Executive Summary. A Report of the American College of Cardiology/American Heart Association Task Force on Practical Guidelines (Committee on Management of Acute Myocardial Infarction). J Am Coll Cardiol 1996; 28:1328–1428.

32. Yusuf S, Pepine CJ, Garces C, Pouleur H, Salem D, Kostis J, Benedict C, Rousseau M, Bourassa M, Pitt B. Effect of enalapril on myocardial infarction and unstable angina in patients with low ejection fractions. Lancet 1992; 340:1173–1178.

33. Rutherford JD, Pfeffer MA, Moyé LA, Davis BR, Flaker GC, Kowey PR, Lamas GA, Miller HS, Packer M, Rouleau JL, Braunwald E, on behalf of the SAVE investigators. Effects of captopril on ischemic events after myocardial infarction. Results of the Survival and Ventricular Enlargement Trial. Circulation 1994; 90:1731–1738.

34. Ridker PM, Gaboury CL, Conlin PR, Seely EW, Williams GH, Vaughan DE. Stimulation of plasminogen activator inhibitor in vivo by infusion of angiotensin II. Evidence of a potential interaction between the renin-angiotensin system and fibrinolytic function. Circulation 1993; 87:1969–1973.

35. Vaughan DE, Rouleau JL, Ridker PM, Arnold JMO, Menapace Jr FJ, Pfeffer MA, on behalf of the HEART Study Investigators. Effects of ramipril on plasma fibrinolytic

balance in patients with acute anterior myocardial infarction. Circulation 1997; 96: 442–447.

36. Brown NJ, Agirbasli MA, Williams GH, Litchfield WR, Vaughan DE. Effect of activation and inhibition of the renin-angiotensin system on plasma PAI-1. Hypertension 1998; 32:965–971.

37. Mancini GB, Henry GC, Macaya C, O'Neill BJ, Pucillo AL, Carere RG, Wargovich TJ, Mudra H, Luscher TF, Klibaner MI, Haber HE, Uprichard AC, Pepine CJ, Pitt B. Angiotensin-converting enzyme inhibition with quinapril improves endothelial vasomotor dysfunction in patients with coronary artery disease. The TREND (Trial on Reversing Endothelial Dysfunction) Study. Circulation 1996; 94:258–265.

38. Warnholtz A, Nickenig G, Schulz E, Macharzina R, Brasen JH, Skatchkov M, Heitzer T, Stasch JP, Griendling KK, Harrison DG, Bohm M, Meinertz T, Munzel T. Increased NADH-Oxidase-Mediated superoxide production in the early stages of atherosclerosis: evidence for involvement of the renin-angiotensin-system. Circulation 1999; 99:2027–2033.

39. The HOPE Study Investigators. The HOPE (Heart Outcomes Prevention Evaluation) Study: The design of a large, simple randomized trial of an angiotensin-converting enzyme inhibitor (ramipril) and vitamin E in patients at high risk of cardiovascular events. Can J Cardiol 1996; 12:27–136.

40. Pfeffer MA, Domanski M, Rosenberg Y, Verter J, Geller N, Albert P, Hsia J, Braunwald E. Prevention of Events with Angiotensin Converting Enzyme Inhibition (The PEACE Study Design). Am J Cardiol 1998; 82:25H–30H.

41. Fox KM, Henderson JR, Bertrand ME, Ferrari R, Remme WJ, Simoons ML. The European trial on reduction of cardiac events with perindopril in stable coronary artery disease (EUROPA). Eur Heart J 1998; 19:J52–J55.

42. Yusuf S, Sleight P, Pogue J, Bosch J, Davies R, Dagenais G. Effects of an angiotensin-converting-enzyme inhibitor, ramipril, on cardiovascular events in high-risk patients. The Heart Outcomes Prevention Evaluation Study Investigators. N Engl J Med 2000; 342:145–153.

43. Lonn E, Yusuf S, Dzavik V, Doris C, Yi Q, Smith S, Moore-Cox A, Bosch J, Riley W, Teo K. Effects of ramipril and Vitamin E on atherosclerosis: Results of the study to evaluate carotid ultrasound changes in patients treated with ramipril and vitamin E (SECURE). Circulation 2001; 103:919–925.

44. Hennekens CH, Buring JE, Sandercock P, Collins R, Peto R. Aspirin and other antiplatelet agents in the secondary and primary prevention of cardiovascular disease. Circulation 1989; 80:749–756.

45. Hennekens CH, Dyken ML, Fuster V. Aspirin as a therapeutic agent in cardiovascular disease. Circulation 1997; 96:2751–2753.

46. ISIS-2 (Second International Study of Infarct Survival) Collaborative Group. Randomised trial of intravenous streptokinase, oral aspirin, both, or neither among 17 187 cases of suspected acute myocardial infarction: ISIS-2. Lancet 1988; 2:349–360.

47. Hall D, Zeitler H, Rudolph W. Counteraction of the vasodilator effects of enalapril by aspirin in severe heart failure. J Am Coll Cardiol 1992; 20:1549–1555.

48. Spaulding C, Charbonnier B, Cohen-Solal A, Juilliere Y, Kromer EP, Benhamda K, Cador R, Weber S. Acute hemodynamic interaction of aspirin and ticlopidine

with enalapril. Results of a double-blind, randomized comparative trial. Circulation 1998; 98:757–765.

49. Brown J, Dollery C, Valdes G. Interaction of nonsteroidal anti-inflammatory drugs with antihypertensive and diuretic agents. Control of vascular reactivity by endogenous prostanoids. Am J Med 1986; 25:43–57.

50. Hall D. The aspirin-angiotensin-converting enzyme inhibitor tradeoff: to halve and halve not [editorial]. J Am Coll Cardiol 2000; 35:1808–1812.

51. Nguyen KN, Aursnes I, Kjekshus J. Interaction between enalapril and aspirin on mortality after acute myocardial infarction: subgroup analysis of the Cooperative New Scandinavian Enalapril Survival Study II (CONSENSUS II). Am J Cardiol 1997; 79:115–119.

52. Leor J, Reicher-Reiss H, Goldbourt U, Boyko V, Gottlieb S, Battler A, Behar S. Aspirin and mortality in patients treated with angiotensin-converting enzyme inhibitors. J Am Coll Cardiol 1999; 33:1920–1925.

53. Anti-Platelet Trialists Collaboration. Collaborative overview of randomized trials of antiplatelet treatment. Part I: Prevention of vascular death, myocardial infarction and stroke by prolonged antiplatelet therapy in different categories of patients. Br Med J 1994; 308:81–106.

54. ACE Inhibitor Myocardial Infarction Collaborative Group. Indications for ACE inhibitors in the early treatment of acute myocardial infarction. Systematic overview of individual data from 100,000 patients in randomized trials. Circulation 1998; 97: 2202–2212.

9
Detection of Peripheral Arterial Occlusion in the Vascular Laboratory

Marie Gerhard-Herman
*Brigham and Women's Hospital and Harvard Medical School,
Boston, Massachusetts*

Symptomatic arterial occlusive disease generally occurs when the artery lumen is reduced to half normal. Atherosclerosis is by far the most common cause of peripheral arterial occlusive disease (1). Other etiologies must be considered in individuals who do not have risk factors for atherosclerosis or in those who have an unusual distribution of arterial occlusive disease. These etiologies include Takayasu arteritis and giant cell arteritis. Both of these arteritides may result in stenosis of any extremity vessel, visceral vessels, or the aorta. Other forms of vasculitis also result in symptomatic arterial occlusive disease. Thromboangiitis obliterans should be suspected if the distal arteries of the upper and lower extremities are involved, particularly in those who smoke cigarettes (2). Acute arterial occlusion occurs as a consequence of embolism or thrombosis in situ. Thrombosis can develop acutely in atherosclerotic arteries or it can occur in locations such as the renal arteries in the presence of antithrombin-III deficiency.

Symptomatic lower extremity atherosclerosis is reported in 3% of those individuals over age 50 (3). In individuals greater than 70, over 25% have evidence of peripheral arterial occlusive disease by noninvasive testing. The prevalence of peripheral arterial disease is threefold greater when determined by noninvasive testing for arterial stenosis rather than by questionnaires regarding symptoms, consistent with the observation that two-thirds of affected individuals are asymptomatic by traditional history. Yet, in a recent community screening program, these asymptomatic individuals had lower functional capacity than those without peripheral arterial disease, as well as an increased risk of cardiovascular death. These findings corroborate an earlier observation linking noninvasive

161

detection of peripheral arterial disease to decreased functional capacity (4). In the clearly symptomatic patients, it is estimated that 10% have arterial stenoses limited to the aorta and iliac arteries, and the other 90% have diffuse disease extending to the femoral and tibioperoneal vessels.

I. IDENTIFICATION OF ARTERIAL OCCLUSIVE DISEASE

Noninvasive testing for lower extremity arterial occlusive disease provides objective information that, together with the history and physical examination, is used to make decisions regarding further evaluation and treatment (5). These tests can be used for screening, for physiological assessment of hemodynamically significant stenosis, and to follow-up after revascularization procedures. The most simple and widely used noninvasive test of extremity arterial occlusive disease is measurement of systolic pressure using a sphygmomanometric cuff and a Doppler device to detect arterial flow. Duplex scanning extends the capabilities of noninvasive testing by identifying anatomical and physiological information at the sites of arterial stenoses.

Three-dimensional arterial reconstruction using magnetic resonance imaging (MRI) arteriography (Fig. 1) and spiral CT arteriography can provide noninvasive assessment of the distal aorta and iliac vessels, but presently with less clarity than is available with invasive arteriography. Contrast arteriography is necessary to completely evaluate the anatomical extent of disease in the distal aorta and lower extremity arteries. It is generally performed only in order to determine the optimal revascularization procedure because of its invasive nature and risk (6). The functional significance of the arterial occlusive disease can be confirmed by invasive pressure measurements proximal and distal to the stenosis, and can be determined before and after administration of a vasodilator.

II. LOWER EXTREMITY ARTERIAL OCCLUSIVE DISEASE

A. Segmental Pressure Measurements

The initial confirmation of peripheral atherosclerotic disease can be acquired by determining the systolic blood pressure in the ankle and comparing it to the systolic blood pressure in the arm (7). Ankle pressure is greater or equal to arm pressure in the absence of arterial occlusive disease. The ankle pressure is less than the highest brachial pressure in the presence of peripheral atherosclerosis, with an ankle brachial ratio of ≤0.90 considered abnormal. The ankle brachial systolic pressure ratio is referred to as the ankle brachial index. Multiple epidemiological studies have shown the ankle brachial index to be a strong independent

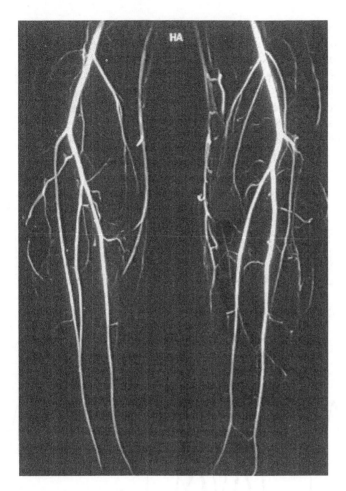

Figure 1 Magnetic resonance angiography. Three vessel runoff can be appreciated on this magnetic resonance angiogram.

risk factor not only for peripheral atherosclerotic disease, but also for risk of myocardial infarction and stroke.

More information about the location of limb arterial occlusive disease is obtained through segmental systolic blood pressure measurements. Blood pressure cuffs are placed on the proximal thigh, distal thigh, proximal calf, and above the ankle. A Doppler probe placed over a distal artery is used to determine systolic blood pressures at these cuff locations. The vascular laboratory staff determines the systolic pressure at each level by listening for the onset of flow as each cuff is inflated to suprasystolic pressures and then deflated. A pressure drop of 20 mmHg indicates the presence of significant stenosis between the two adjacent levels. Doppler waveforms are also recorded at each level by either pulse volume recording (Fig. 2) or pulse-wave Doppler using duplex ultrasound. The normal waveform has a rapid upstroke and is triphasic. When stenosis is present, there is a triphasic waveform proximal to the stenosis to a biphasic or monophasic pattern beyond the stenosis. When pulse-wave Doppler waveforms are determined along the length of the artery, an increase in the peak systolic velocity is

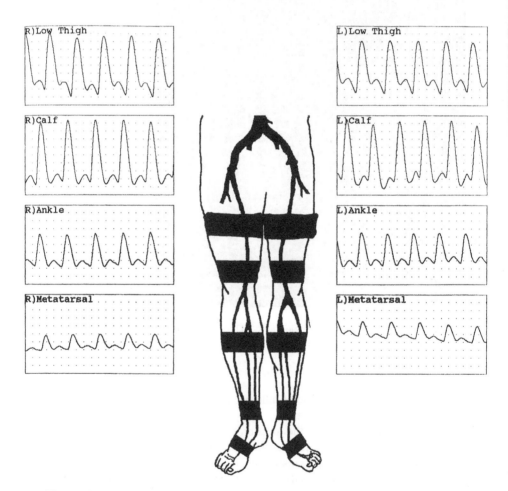

Figure 2 Normal segmental pulse volume recordings. Normal waveforms are seen throughout both lower extremities.

seen at the site of stenosis. With aortoiliac disease, thigh pressures will be less than arm pressures and the femoral waveforms are generally biphasic or monophasic (Fig. 3).

The segmental pressure measurements may be normal at rest and should be repeated following exercise if the clinical suspicion of peripheral arterial disease is high. If hemodynamically significant arterial occlusive disease is present, there will be a sustained drop in the ankle pressures after exercise.

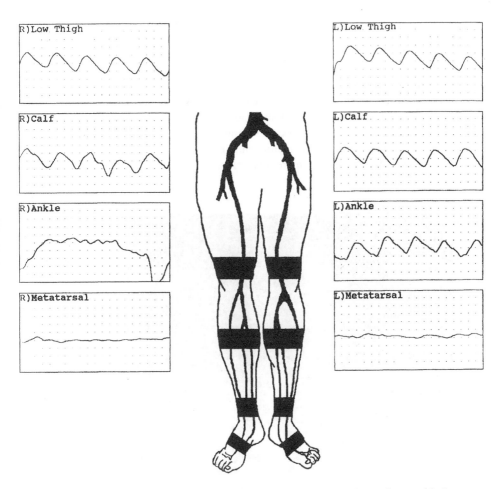

Figure 3 Abnormal segmental pulse volume recordings. Blunted waveforms with slow upstroke and delayed downstroke are seen throughout both lower extremities. This suggests distal aortic stenosis and/or bilateral iliac stenoses.

B. Peripheral Arterial Duplex Ultrasonography

The combination of B-mode ultrasound scanning and pulsed Doppler interrogation allows noninvasive assessment of the anatomy and hemodynamic abnormalities in the arterial segments from the distal aorta to the popliteal trifurcation (8). For example, soft plaque and thrombi may have similar acoustic properties to blood and, therefore, may not be detected by B-mode imaging, but they will result in a flow disturbance that can be detected by Doppler evaluation. Equipment for peripheral arterial testing includes a linear array transducer, operating at a gray-scale frequency of 4 to 10 MHz, and capable of providing frequencies above 3 MHz for Doppler signal analysis. Gray-scale imaging is used to examine the arteries and the presence of detectable atherosclerotic plaque or thrombus. The pulsed Doppler spectral analysis is used to document the presence of blood flow and to determine blood flow velocity. Normal Doppler waveforms in the lower extremity will be triphasic (Fig. 4), with a peak velocity less than 120 cm/s. Color Doppler flow mapping allows for a rapid survey of the arteries in order to identify those sites where more labor-intensive and precise Doppler spectral analysis is needed (Fig. 5). Still, full evaluation of the lower extremity arteries takes from 1 to 2 h.

The basic principle for detecting and grading stenotic lesions is the identification and measurement of increased velocity seen at the site of stenosis. At

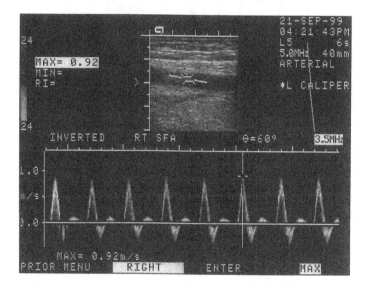

Figure 4 Duplex arterial examination. The inset demonstrates the gray-scale image of the vessel. The Doppler waveform is triphasic with a peak systolic velocity of 92 cm/s and indicative of normal peripheral arterial flow.

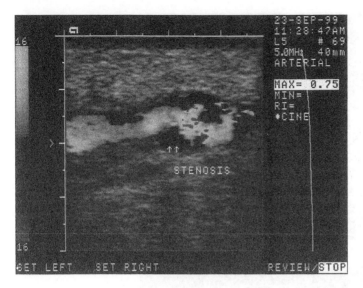

Figure 5 Color Doppler arterial mapping. The mixed color signals in the area of stenosis indicates turbulent flow that merits further pulsed Doppler evaluation.

the site of stenosis, the velocity of moving blood is uniformly increased. The measured Doppler frequency shift is proportional to the percent stenosis and inversely proportional to the residual lumen. A ratio of two or more for the peak systolic velocity at the site of stenosis compared to the more proximal velocity is used to identify stenoses resulting in a 50% or greater reduction in the lumen diameter (Fig. 6). A number of studies have shown that a 50% or greater reduction in arterial diameter is equivalent to a 75% reduction in cross-sectional area, resulting in a fall in distal arterial pressure and blood flow.

The duplex criteria for recognizing a 50% arterial reduction include a loss of reverse flow with forward flow seen throughout the cardiac cycle, extensive spectral broadening, and a doubling in peak systolic velocity (PSV) (9). When comparing the PSV within the stenosis to that in the nearest proximal disease-free segment, a ratio is created that is independent of individual variations in cardiac function, blood pressure, and vascular compliance. These criteria appear to discriminate the presence of significant stenoses adequately, even in situations with multilevel stenoses (10).

The arterial segments commonly evaluated (iliac, common femoral, superificial femoral, and popliteal) were prospectively studied using these criteria and compared to angiography. The duplex examination was found to have a sensitivity of 77%, specificity of 98%, a positive predictive value of 94%, a negative

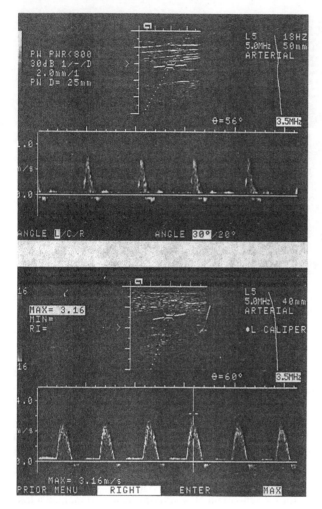

Figure 6 Pulsed Doppler evaluation. (top) Normal waveform is seen proximal to the arterial stenosis with PSV 82 cm/s^{-1}. (bottom) Biphasic waveform with increased velocity (PSV 316 cm/s) is seen at the site of the arterial stenosis.

predictive value of 92% in the presence of greater than 50% stenosis. These results are consistent with and comparable to the interobserver variability in estimating the degree of stenosis in conventional angiograms (6). The accuracy and noninvasive nature of duplex scanning make it ideal for detailed, serial, long-term evaluation in symptomatic and asymptomatic patients. In intermittent claudication, flow characteristics change with the increased inflow demand of exercise. Duplex examination can be combined with exercise testing to detect disproportionate velocity increases with exercise and therefore identify the lesions responsible for a patient's symptoms. The duplex scan is potentially superior to angiography in the evaluation of iliac artery, and in determining the hemodynamic status of ostial lesions in the profunda and superficial femoral arteries. Peripheral artery bypass grafts can be followed serially with duplex ultrasonography (11). The first month after surgery and every 1 to 2 years following surgery are key times to identify early changes consistent with stenosis within the graft. The criteria for discrete stenosis in bypass grafts is similar to that in native vessels. In addition, a peak systolic velocity that is decreased to 45 cm/s indicates a dramatically increased likelihood of graft failure and provides a rationale for early intervention. In addition, duplex evaluation is likely to be similarly useful in the follow-up of peripheral arteries following percutaneous revascularization.

A new advance in ultrasound imaging relies on pulse-length compression and allows direct visualization of blood echoes. This B-flow extends the wideband (multiple frequency) resolution and high-frame-rate possibilities of B-mode-to-image flowing blood and tissues simultaneously. Both blood echo strength and increased velocities result in increased brightness of the signal (Fig. 7). This technique will delineate the pattern of red cells flowing through a stenosis without obscuring the arterial wall. It provides a clear view of the vessel lumen.

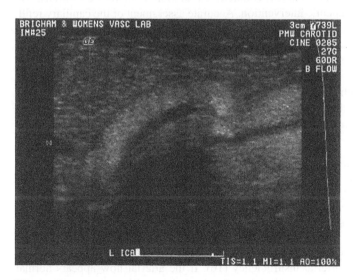

Figure 7 B-flow imaging of arterial segment. The bright regions indicate increased number of red blood cells in that region.

In contrast, color Doppler information tends to bleed into the surrounding gray-scale image and obscure the vascular pathology. Similarly, color artifact occurs with any movements of the transducer or nearby tissue and obscures the gray-scale image. Improvements such as B-flow imaging will be useful for those cases with severe stenoses, and to distinguish subtotal from total occlusion. This technology promises to extend the limited advance in this area made with power Doppler (12). This methodology will obviate the need for contrast agents in vascular ultrasound.

C. Acute Arterial Occlusion

Acute arterial occlusion requires quick and careful assessment in order to preserve the limb. The role of noninvasive testing in acute arterial occlusion is often one of follow-up. Arteriography is initially indicated for evaluation as revascularization is necessary for limb preservation. Sudden arterial occlusion may occur by embolism or by thrombosis. Embolism is the major cause and the primary source is the heart. Once emboli lodge in an artery, there may be further extension by thrombosis. Sudden arterial occlusion can occur in peripheral atherosclerosis patients when thrombosis occurs at the site of atherosclerotic plaque. Arterial thrombosis can occur in normal arteries exposed to hypercoagulable states. The presentation is often described as that of the six ps: pain, pallor, polar (cold), pulselessness, parasthesias, and paralysis. Outcome of acute arterial occlusion depends on the vessel occluded, collateral circulation, comorbid conditions, and the timing of therapeutic intervention. Accurate assessment of the capillary refill, muscle weakness, sensory loss, and Doppler signals from the vessels can establish the clinical grade of acute limb ischemia. For limbs that are viable or threatened but not irreversibly ischemic, reestablishing patency of the occluded vessel is achieved through thrombolytic therapy, embolectomy, or bypass surgery (13,14). If the patient with a viable or threatened limb cannot undergo surgery or thrombolysis, heparin should be administered and the extremity should be kept warm and in a dependent position.

D. Digital Arterial Occlusion

The isolated cold, blue digit requires further evaluation of the arterial supply to the digit. Arterial tests for the digits include systolic pressure measurements, digital plethysmography, skin temperature, laser Doppler flow, and Doppler flow (15). If abnormal arterial flow is seen, the study can be repeated with warming (Fig. 8). A prominent component of vasospasm may contribute to the clinical finding of severe arterial insufficiency (16). If the arterial flow appears normal after warming, vasospasm rather than fixed arterial occlusion is present. Additional testing can include the Allen test of ulnar artery patency. The radial artery

A. Before Warming   B. After Warming

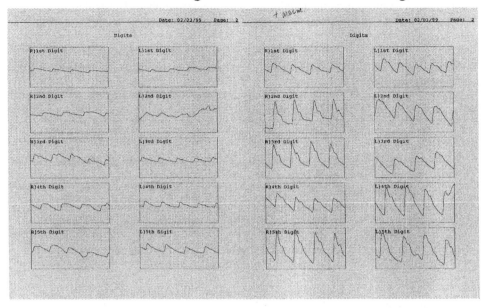

Figure 8 Finger pulse volume recordings in a patient with digital ischemia. The waveforms are abnormal at baseline. The normalization after warming suggests that vasospasm is playing a prominent role in the arterial occlusion.

at the wrist is occluded with manual pressure, and the patient exercises the hand until pallor develops in the palm. The examiner then observes the palm for a quick return of pink color to the palm to confirm arterial patency. This test can also be used to confirm radial artery patency. Arteriography is indicated only if an obstructive lesion requiring revascularization is sought.

III. CONCLUSION

There are a multitude of tests available in the vascular laboratory that vary in their precision for describing the extent of peripheral arterial disease (PAD). At one end of the spectrum is the ankle brachial index, identifying the presence or absence of PAD. At the other end of the spectrum is duplex scanning, with its ability to define the hemodynamic significance of individual stenoses. The limitation of duplex scanning has been in the ability to differentiate subtotal from total occlusion. Eventually, ultrasound will be able to make this differentiation reliably with B-mode imaging of flowing blood and tissues simultaneously. The study of digital ischemia can be made with an even greater number of tests that assess the hemodynamic significance of arterial disease in response to physiological changes.

REFERENCES

1. Weitz I, Byrne J, Clagett GP, et al. Diagnosis and treatment of chronic arterial insufficiency of the lower extremities: a critical review. Circulation 1996; 94(11):3026–3049.
2. Olin JW, Young JR, Graor RA, Ruschhaupt WF, Bartholomew JR. The changing clinical spectrum of thromboangiitis obliterans (Buerger's disease). Circulation 1990; 82(5 suppl):IV3–8.
3. Criqui MH, Denenberg JO, Langer RD, Fronek A. The epidemiology of peripheral arterial disease: importance of identifying the population at risk. Vasc Med 1997; 2(3):221–226.
4. McDermott MM, Liu K, Guralnik JM, et al. The ankle brachial index independently predicts walking velocity and walking endurance in peripheral arterial disease. J Am Geriatr Soc 1998; 46(11):1355–1362.
5. Gahtan V. The noninvasive vascular laboratory. Surg Clin North Am 1998; 78(4):507–518.
6. Moneta GL, Strandness DE, Jr. Peripheral arterial duplex scanning. J Clin Ultrasound 1987; 15(9):645–651.
7. Campbell WB, Wolfe JH. The role of non-invasive tests in arterial disease. Br J Surg 1987; 74(12):1075–1076.
8. Pemberton M, London NJ. Colour flow duplex imaging of occlusive arterial disease of the lower limb [see comments]. Br J Surg 1997; 84(7):912–919.
9. Jager KA, Phillips DJ, Martin RL, et al. Noninvasive mapping of lower limb arterial lesions. Ultrasound Med Biol 1985; 11(3):515–521.
10. Allard L, Cloutier G, Guo Z, Durand LG. Review of the assessment of single level and multilevel arterial occlusive disease in lower limbs by duplex ultrasound. Ultrasound Med Biol 1999; 25(4):495–502.
11. Roth SM, Bandyk DF. Duplex imaging of lower extremity bypasses, angioplasties, and stents. Semin Vasc Surg 1999; 12(4):275–284.
12. Allard L, Cloutier G. Power Doppler ultrasound scan imaging of the level of red blood cell aggregation: an in vitro study. J Vasc Surg 1999; 30(1):157–168.
13. Ouriel K, Shortell CK, Azodo MV, Guiterrez OH, Marder VJ. Acute peripheral arterial occlusion: predictors of success in catheter-directed thrombolytic therapy. Radiology 1994; 193(2):561–566.
14. Neuzil DF, Edwards WH, Jr., Mulherin JL, et al. Limb ischemia: surgical therapy in acute arterial occlusion. Am Surg 1997; 63(3):270–274.
15. Herrick AL, Clark S. Quantifying digital vascular disease in patients with primary Raynaud's phenomenon and systemic sclerosis. Ann Rheum Dis 1998; 57(2):70–78.
16. Wigley FM. Raynaud's phenomenon. Curr Opin Rheumatol 1993; 5(6):773–784.

10

Antithrombotic Therapy During Coronary Intervention

Jeffrey J. Popma
*Brigham and Women's Hospital and Harvard Medical School,
Boston, Massachusetts*

Arman T. Askari
The Cleveland Clinic Foundation, Cleveland, Ohio

Percutaneous coronary intervention (PCI) will be performed in more than 700,000 patients in the United States this year, exceeding the number of coronary artery bypass graft (CABG) surgeries. PCI will be primarily undertaken for the relief of ischemia in patients with atherosclerotic coronary artery disease. A number of methods are currently used for PCI, including balloon angioplasty, rotational and directional atherectomy, and coronary stenting. Coronary stenting is most commonly (60 to 80%) used and is the preferred form of therapy in patients with native vessels or saphenous vein grafts (SVG) more than 2.75 mm in diameter.

The safety of PCI has improved with the routine use of oral antiplatelet agents (e.g., aspirin, ticlopidine, and clopidogrel) and intravenous glycoprotein IIb-IIIa (GP IIb-IIIa) inhibitors. Antithrombin therapy with intravenous unfractionated heparin or low-molecular-weight heparin and novel thrombin inhibitors (e.g., hirudin, hirulog, argatroban) have also been used to prevent ischemic complications during PCI. The purposes of this review are to discuss contemporary strategies of anticoagulation to improve early clinical outcomes after PCI and review the current trials that have used antithrombotic agents for the prevention of late restenosis.

I. ANTIPLATELET THERAPY

A. Oral Antiplatelet Therapy

Aspirin reduces the frequency of ischemic complications [e.g., Q-wave myocardial infarction (MI), emergency CABG, and reocclusion] after PCI by 64 to 77% (1,2). The minimum effective aspirin dosage for PCI is not known, but doses ranging from 80 to 325 mg given $\geq$2 h before PCI have generally proven effective. Dipyridamole is no longer used after PCI, as it provides no incremental value over aspirin alone (3). Ticlopidine, 500 mg loading and 250 mg twice daily, has been used as an alternative antiplatelet agent among aspirin-intolerant patients (2). Another thienopyridine, clopidogrel, 300 mg loading followed by 75 mg daily, can also be used. Both these agents should be given for >24 h prior to elective PCI to achieve maximum platelet inhibition (4).

Two randomized studies have shown that as an adjunct to aspirin ticlopidine reduces the frequency of 30-day clinical events in patients undergoing stent implantation, including the occurrence of subacute thrombosis (5,6). A clinical trial of 517 patients at high risk for stent thrombosis after Palmaz–Schatz stenting were randomly assigned to treatment with aspirin + ticlopidine or aspirin + intravenous heparin + phenprocoumon. Those treated with aspirin + ticlopidine experienced a 75% reduction in early complications compared with those who received conventional antithrombotic therapy (5). Those patients who received antiplatelet therapy also had an 82% lower risk of MI and a 78% lower need for repeat balloon angioplasty compared with patients receiving anticoagulation therapy (5). It was also shown in this study that bleeding complications were lower in patients treated with antiplatelet therapy (5). The STent Anti-thrombotic Regimen Study (STARS) evaluated the effect of aspirin alone, aspirin + ticlopidine, and aspirin + warfarin on the occurrence of 30-day ischemic endpoints in 1653 low-risk patients undergoing successful Palmaz–Schatz stent placement (6). There was an 85% reduction in clinical events, including subacute thrombosis, in patients treated with aspirin + ticlopidine (6).

Ticlopidine has a number of side effects that limit its clinical use, including gastrointestinal distress (20%), cutaneous rashes (4.8 to 15%), and liver function test abnormalities. Neutropenia that is severe but generally reversible and aplastic anemia occur in $\leq$1% of patients. Rare fatal thrombotic thrombocytopenic purpura has been reported with ticlopidine (7). Shorter durations (10 to 14 days) of ticlopidine therapy may reduce the risk of these side effects (8,9).

Clopidogrel is an alternative thienopyridine derivative and inhibitor of adenosine diphosphate–induced platelet aggregation that has been used as an increasingly popular alternative to ticlopidine in patients undergoing stent placement (10,11). The CLASSICS trial showed no difference in clinical efficacy between clopidogrel and ticlopidine, with fewer side effects in patients treated with clopidogrel (12). Based on this randomized study and single center registries that do not shown a difference in outcomes using these two agents (13), clopidogrel, 300 mg loading followed by 75 mg daily for 14 to 30 days, may be used as an alternative to ticlopidine therapy in patients undergoing stent implantation. Some have advocated pretreatment with clopidogrel for several days before PCI, but this strategy may be associated with more bleeding complications should urgent CABG be needed. Longer durations (6 to 12 months) of clopidogrel therapy may provide an added benefit to aspirin as secondary prevention in patients with ischemic coronary disease. This strategy is currently being evaluated in the CREDO Trial. Longer durations (6 to 12 months) of clopidogrel may also be needed in patients treated with radiation therapy for in-stent restenosis or primary PCI. Although rare cases of thrombotic thrombocytopenic purpura have also been reported with clopidogrel (14), its side-effect profile is more benign than ticlopidine for patients undergoing stent implantation.

B. Glycoprotein IIb-IIIa Inhibitors

Early ischemic events may still develop in 3.0 to 12.8% of aspirin-treated patients undergoing PCI, as aspirin inhibits only cyclo-oxygenase-mediated platelet activation (15–17). Aspirin provides insufficient inhibition of platelet activation and adhesion stimulated by adenosine diphosphate (ADP), collagen, serotonin, or thrombin (18). GP IIb-IIIa receptor activation serves as the "final common pathway" of platelet aggregation, allowing binding of fibrinogen and other adhesive proteins that bridge one platelet to another (19). A number of intravenous and oral inhibitors of the GP IIb-IIIa receptor have been developed for clinical use.

The Evaluation of 7E3 for the Prevention of Ischemic Complications (EPIC) trial was the first to evaluation the safety and efficacy of abciximab in high-risk patients for acute ischemic complications (20) (Table 1). High-risk criteria included patients with acute MI, refractory unstable angina, and high-risk clinical and angiographic features. The study included 2099 patients who received 325 mg aspirin and a 10,000 to 12,000 IU bolus of non-weight-adjusted heparin, and randomly assigned to treatment with placebo, a 0.25 mg/kg bolus of abciximab, or the same bolus of abciximab followed by a 12-h abciximab infusion of 10 µg/min. A 35% reduction in the frequency of the composite of death, nonfatal MI, repeat revascularization, or procedural failure was found in patients treated with bolus and infusion abciximab (8.3 vs. 12.8% in placebo-treated patients; $p = 0.008$) (20).

The benefit of abciximab in the EPIC trial was highest in patients with unstable clinical syndromes (acute MI and refractory unstable angina) (21). In a subsequent randomized clinical trial of 429 patients with acute MI, pretreatment with abciximab resulted in a significant reduction ($p = 0.03$) in the incidence of

Table 1 Early and Late Outcome in Randomized Trials of GP IIb-IIIa Inhibitors

| | EPIC (20) | | | EPILOG (27) | | | EPISTENT (29) | | | IMPACT-II (29) | | | RESTORE (30) | |
	Placebo	Abciximab Bolus	Bolus + Inf	Placebo +SD Heparin	Abciximab +SD Heparin	+LD Heparin	Placebo +Stent	Abciximab +Stent	+PTCA	Placebo	Eptifibatide Low Dose	High Dose	Placebo	Tirofiban
Lesion type	High risk			Low risk			Low risk			Low and high risk			High risk	
Years of entry	11/91–11/92			2/95–12/95			7/96–9/97			11/93–11/94			1/95–12/95	
Number of patients	697	695	708	939	918	935	809	794	796	1328	1349	1333	1070	1071
Baseline factors														
Mean Age, years	61	60	62	60	60	60	59	59	60	60	62	60	59	59
Women, %	27	28	29	28	27	29	25.5	25	25	25	27	24	28	28
Diabetes mellitus	26	23	23	24	22	23	21.4	20.4	19.6	22	23	23	20	20
Unstable angina, %	NA	NA	NA	50	46	46	60.4	56.4	54.8	38	38	38	68	67
Stent use (%)	0.6	1.7	0.6	NR	NR	NR	96.0	97.3	19.3	4.5	3.6	4.1	NA	NA
Composite 1° endpoint	12.8	11.4	8.3****	11.7	5.4****	5.2****	10.8	5.3****	6.9***	11.4	9.2	9.9	12.2	10.3
Early complications														
Death (%)	1.7	1.3	1.7	0.8	0.4	0.3	0.6	0.3	0.8	1.1	0.5	0.8	0.7	0.8
Q-wave infarction, (%)	2.3	1.0	3.0	0.8	0.5	0.4	1.4	0.9	1.5	1.6	0.9	1.1	5.7	4.2
Emergency CABG (%)	3.6	2.3	2.4	1.7	0.9	0.4	1.1	0.8	0.6	2.8	1.6	2.0	2.2	1.9
Emergency PTCA (%)	4.5	3.6	0.8***	3.8	1.5***	1.2****	1.2	0.6	1.3	2.8	2.6	2.9	5.4	4.2
Major bleeding	7	11****	14****	3.1	3.5	2.0	2.2	1.5	1.4	4.8	5.1	5.2	3.7	5.3
Follow-up time	3 years			6 month			6 month			6 month			6 month	
Late clinical outcome	47.2	47.4	41.1	25.8	22.3	22.8	18.3	13.0	15.5	11.6	10.5	10.1	27.1	24.1
Death (%)	8.6	8.1	6.8	1.7	1.4	1.1	1.2	0.5	1.8	NR	NR	NR	1.4	1.8
Q-wave MI	13.6	12.2	10.7	1.6	1.4	1.3	1.5	1.3	2.1	NR	NR	NR	7.6	6.3
Revascularization (%)	40.1	38.6	34.8	19.4	18.4	19.0	10.6	8.7	15.4	NR	NR	NR	17.1	15.7
Repeat PTCA	NR	NR	NR	NR	NR	NR	NR	NR	NR	NR	NR	NR	NR	NR
CABG	NR	NR	NR	NR	NR	NR	NR	NR	NR	NR	NR	NR	6.8	5.5

CABG = coronary artery bypass surgery; CVA = cerebrovascular accident; IH = In-hospital; MI = myocardial infarction; PCI = percutaneous coronary intervention; NR = not reported; TLR = target lesion revascularization.
* $p < 0.05$; ** $p < 0.01$; *** $p < 0.005$; **** $p < 0.001$.
Source: Adapted from Popma JJ, Kuntz RF. 6th ed. In: Braunwald, E, ed. Percutaneous Intervention in Heart Disease.

death, reinfarction, or urgent target vessel revascularization at 30 days in patients treated with abciximab (4.9%) versus placebo (10.3%) (22). There was no difference in 6-month restenosis between the two groups (22).

To evaluate the effect of abciximab in low-risk patients undergoing PCI, the Evaluation of PTCA to Improve Long-Term Outcome by abciximab GP IIb-IIIa blockade (EPILOG) trial randomly assigned 2792 patients who were treated with aspirin to standard-dose, weight-adjusted (100 U/kg bolus) heparin and placebo, standard-dose, weight-adjusted heparin and abciximab, or low-dose, weight-adjusted (70 U/kg bolus) heparin. The 30-day composite event rate was significantly lower ($p < 0.001$) in patients treated with abciximab and low-dose (5.2%) or standard-dose (5.4%) heparin than in patients treated with standard-dose heparin and placebo (11.7%) (23). Bleeding complications were lowest in patients treated with abciximab and low-dose, weight-adjusted heparin.

The effect of GPIIb-IIIa inhibitors has been more variable in patients undergoing saphenous vein graft intervention. While one study suggested a beneficial effect with abciximab in patients undergoing SVG angioplasty (24), a larger study failed to demonstrate a convincing reduction in these patients at high risk for microembolization (25). Bailout abciximab is often given during or just after PCI for the presence of residual dissection, thrombus, or suboptimal results (26), although its value has not been demonstrated in prospective studies.

The EPISTENT trial randomly assigned 2399 patients with ischemic CAD to stenting plus placebo, stenting plus abciximab, or balloon PTCA plus abciximab (27) and found that the primary 30-day endpoint, a combination of death, MI, or need for urgent revascularization, occurred in 10.8% of patients in the stent plus placebo group, 5.3% of patients in the stent plus abciximab group (hazard ratio 0.48; $p < 0.001$), and 6.9% of patients in the balloon plus abciximab group (0.63; $p = 0.007$) (27). The primary benefit of abciximab was in the reduction of death and large (CPK-MB $> 5 \times$ normal) MI, which occurred in 7.8% of patients in the placebo group versus 3.0% of patients assigned to stent plus abciximab group ($p < 0.001$) and 4.7% of patients treated with balloon PTCA plus abciximab ($p = 0.01$) (27). No differences in bleeding complications were found among the groups (27).

Other GP IIb-IIIa inhibitors have also been used in patients undergoing PCI. The IMPACT-II trial evaluated the effect of bolus and infusion eptifibatide on 30-day clinical events in patients undergoing PCI. A total of 4010 patients undergoing PCI were assigned to placebo, eptifibatide bolus (135 µg/kg) followed by a low-dose eptifibatide infusion (0.5 µg/kg/min for 20 to 24 h) or the same eptifibatide bolus and higher dose infusion (0.75 µg/kg/min for 20 to 24 h) (29). The primary endpoint, a 30-day composite occurrence of death, MI, unplanned CABG or repeat PCI, or coronary stenting for abrupt closure, occurred in 11.4% patients in the placebo group compared with 9.2% in the 135/0.5 eptifibatide group ($p = 0.063$) and 9.9% in the eptifibatide 135/0.75 group ($p =$

0.22) (29). Using a treatment-received analysis, the eptifibatide 135/0.5 regimen produced a significant reduction in the composite endpoint (9.1% vs. 11.6% in placebo-treated patients; $p = 0.035$), but the eptifibatide 135/0.75 regimen produced a less substantial reduction (10.0% vs. 11.6% in placebo-treated patients; $p = 0.18$). There were no differences in major bleeding or transfusion rates among the three groups.

It is now understood that the eptifibatide dose used in the IMPACT-II trial was insufficient to provide adequate platelet inhibition during PCI. The recently completed, randomized ESPRIT trial compared a 180-μg/kg double bolus given 10 min apart of eptifibatide followed by a 2.0-μg/kg/min infusion with placebo in lower risk patients undergoing stent implantation. Preliminary results from this trial show a substantial benefit of eptifibatide compared with placebo in patients undergoing stent implantation (J. Tcheng, personal communications).

Tirofiban is a nonpeptidyl, tyrosine derivative that was evaluated after PCI in the Randomized Efficacy Study of Tirofiban for Outcomes and REstenosis (RESTORE) trial, a randomized, double-blind, placebo-controlled study involving 2139 patients undergoing PCI who presented within 72 h of an acute coronary syndrome (30). After treatment with aspirin and heparin, patients were randomly assigned to tirofiban bolus (10 μg/kg over 3 min) + infusion (0.15 μg/kg/min), or to placebo bolus + infusion for 36 h after PCI. There was a 16% reduction in the primary 30-day composite endpoint rate associated with tirofiban treatment ($p = 0.160$), although there was a 38% relative reduction in the composite endpoint at 48 h ($p < 0.005$) and a 27% relative reduction at 7 days ($p = 0.022$) (30). A 24% reduction was found when only urgent or emergency balloon angioplasty or CABG was included in the composite endpoint (30-day event rate: 10.5% for the placebo group and 8.0% for the tirofiban group; $p = 0.052$). Although major bleeding tended to be higher in tirofiban-treated patients (5.3 vs. 3.7% in the placebo-treated patients; $p = 0.096$), there was no difference in bleeding events using the TIMI criteria (31) for major bleeding (30) in those treated with tirofiban.

C. Effect of Antiplatelet on the Prevention of Restenosis

Studies evaluating the effect of aspirin on restenosis have produced conflicting results, potentially attributable to the varied dosage and duration of aspirin therapy (1,32–34). Although the majority of these studies have shown little, if any, sustained effect of aspirin on restenosis prevention, long-term aspirin (>80 mg daily) is recommended after PCI for secondary prevention of cardiac events (35). Ketanserin, prostacyclin, platelet thromboxane A_2 and serotonin receptor antagonists, respectively, have also been tried without success (36–40).

As platelet aggregation during PCI may occur as a result of GP IIb-IIIa activation by a number of agonists, inhibition of a single agonist for the prevention of restenosis may be problematic. Final common pathway GP IIb-IIIa platelet receptor inhibitors provide potent ($>80\%$) blockade of platelet aggregation during PCI, regardless of the platelet agonist. Although the EPIC study showed a 23% reduction in cumulative 6-month clinical events with abciximab ($p = 0.001$) (41), these events were primarily related to the prevention of early (<30 day) periprocedural events (20). Other studies have not shown a consistent reduction in clinical or angiographic restenosis with GP IIb-IIIa inhibitors (42). The need for late revascularization was not significantly lower ($p = 0.22$) in patients receiving stenting plus abciximab (8.7%) compared with patients receiving stenting + placebo (10.6%) (28), although there was a significant reduction ($p = 0.02$) in revascularization in diabetic patients assigned to stenting plus abciximab (8.1%) compared with patients receiving stenting plus placebo (16.6%) (28). This effect has been attributed to the enhanced activity of $\alpha_v \beta_3$ receptor activity in diabetic patients undergoing stent implantation.

The intravenously administered GP IIb-IIIa inhibitors (e.g., abciximab, eptifibatide, and tirofiban) improve clinical outcomes within the first 30 days in patients undergoing PCI. These agents as a class reduce ischemic complications after PCI, including non-Q-wave MI and recurrent ischemia. Oral GPIIb-IIIa inhibitors have not been effective in reducing early or late complications after PCI. It does not appear that GP IIb-IIIa inhibitors reduce the frequency of restenosis in nondiabetic patients; more study is needed to determine whether restenosis is reduced with abciximab in diabetic patients. These agents should be considered in all patients undergoing PCI, particularly in those patients with unstable angina, primary balloon PTCA or stent placement for acute MI, and in other patients at higher risk for ischemic complications after PCI.

II. ANTITHROMBIN THERAPY

Unfractionated heparin is used during PCI to prevent thrombus formation at the site of arterial injury and on the equipment used for PCI (44). Other antithrombin-III-dependent agents (i.e., low-molecular-weight heparins) and antithrombin-III-independent agents (i.e., hirudin, hirulog, and argatroban) have also been used during PCI, but have not yet achieved widespread use. Patients with acute coronary syndromes may also benefit from prolonged (>24-h) heparin therapy alone before PCI (45) or in combination with GP IIb-IIIa inhibitors (46–48).

A. Unfractionated Heparin

Activated partial thromboplastin times (aPTTs) are not useful for monitoring anticoagulation intensity during PCI, as large amounts of unfractionated heparin, greater than the aPTT assay can analyze, are required to prevent thrombus formation during arterial manipulations (49). Instead, near patient (also known as point of care) activated clotting time (ACT) monitoring is used to facilitate unfractionated heparin dose titration during PCI (50). ACT responses have shown marked variability in patients who received a non-weight-adjusted unfractionated heparin bolus. These differences have been attributed to patient-to-patient differences in heparin sensitivity and clearance, body weight, nitroglycerin use, and coexisting conditions that predispose to heparin resistance (e.g., heparin antibodies, oral contraceptive use, endocarditis, disseminated intravascular coagulation, and placement of an intra-aortic balloon pump). Patients with unstable angina and those with complex coronary lesions (irregular borders, overhanging edges, or filling defects) also have higher heparin dosing requirements (51). Heparin resistance may also be a marker of high-risk anatomy (52).

Two retrospective studies have related the ACT value to clinical outcome after PCI (53,54). In one study, patients who had complications after PCI had lower mean baseline ACT (Hemo Tec®) values after the initial heparin bolus and at the end of the procedure than those without complications (54). In another study, patients with abrupt closure had a lower mean ACT (Hemochron®) at the time of first balloon inflation than those without this complication (352 s vs. 388 s, respectively; $p < 0.002$) (53). An inverse relationship was shown between in-laboratory ACT values and the probability of abrupt closure ($p = 0.018$) (53). Higher ACT levels (55) and other markers of excess anticoagulation (56) also may serve as independent predictors of bleeding complications after PCI, although this relationship has not been confirmed. These studies have formed the empiric recommendations of target ACT levels during PCI.

With the availability of coronary stents, some recent studies show that lower dose heparin during PCI may also be safe and effective. In a series of 1375 consecutive patients undergoing PCI, low-dose bolus heparin (5000 IU) with early (<12 h) postprocedural sheath removal was associated with infrequent fatal complications (0.3%), emergency CABG (1.7%), MI (3.3%), or repeat angioplasty within 48 h (0.7%) (57). ACT levels were not available in this study. Lower dose unfractionated heparin may prevent excessive anticoagulation, but at this juncture monitoring a low-dose heparin strategy with ACTs seems prudent.

Although weight-adjusted heparin seems to lower bleeding complications compared with fixed-dose heparin in association with GP IIb-IIIa inhibitor use (23), the advantage of weight-adjusted heparin over fixed-dose heparin in one randomized trial of 400 patients that did not use GP IIb-IIIa inhibitors appeared to relate only to early sheath removal. Patients assigned to fixed-dose heparin (15,000 IU) or weight-adjusted heparin (100 IU/kg) had similar clinical outcomes (95% success rates) (58). Use of the weight-adjusted heparin did result in earlier sheath removal and more rapid transfer to a stepdown unit (58).

The following empiric recommendation can be made with respect to anticoagulation during PCI. Weight-adjusted heparin dosing regimens (70 to 100 IU/

kg) or gender-adjusted bolus heparin (7000 U for women and 8000 U for men) should be used in an attempt to avoid "overshooting" the ACT (35). Sufficient unfractionated heparin should be administered during PCI to achieve an ACT between 250 and 300 s using the HemoTec® monitor and between 300 and 350 s using the Hemochron® monitor (50). The ACT should be monitored frequently and additional, smaller heparin boluses of 2000 to 5000 IU should be given until the target ACT is achieved. Lower target ACT levels (>200 s) are adequate when GPIIb-IIIa inhibitors are used. A number of studies have now shown that routine use of intravenous heparin after PCI is no longer indicated (59,60). Early sheath removal is strongly encouraged when the ACT falls to less than 150 to 180 s.

B. Low-Molecular-Weight Heparin

Patients with unstable angina may now be treated with low-molecular-weight heparin (LMWH) and, on occasion, require PCI for ongoing symptoms (61). While it is difficult to monitor anticoagulation levels using LMWH during PCI, conventional dosages of unfractionated heparin are generally recommended. It is important to note that conventional monitoring methods, such as the ACT, may underestimate the true degree of periprocedural anticoagulation. One pilot randomized trial of 60 patients undergoing PCI, treated with unfractionated heparin or enoxaparin (1 mg/kg intravenously), showed no difference in safety between the two anticoagulants (62). Similar favorable results with the use of intravenous LMWH have been reported when this agent is used alone (NICE-1) or in combination with GPIIb-IIIa inhibitors (NICE-3 and NICE-4). Routine use of LMWH as the sole anticoagulant during PCI cannot be recommended at this time, pending the results of a large, multicenter trials evaluating the safety of LMWH compared with unfractionated heparin during PCI.

C. Direct Thrombin Inhibitors

Direct thrombin inhibitors have been evaluated during PCI as an alternative to heparin. In the Hirudin in a European Trial Versus Heparin in the Prevention of Restenosis after PTCA (HELVETICA) study (63), 1141 patients with unstable angina scheduled for PCI were treated with aspirin and then randomly assigned to bolus heparin (10,000 U) plus infusion (15 U/kg/h for 24 h), hirudin bolus (40 mg + intravenous infusion, 0.2 mg/kg/h for 24 h) or hirudin bolus (40 mg plus intravenous infusion, 0.2 mg/kg/h for 24 h), followed by subcutaneous injection (40 mg twice daily) for an additional 3 days. Hirudin use was associated with a 39% reduction in early cardiac events ($p = 0.023$), although clinical outcomes were similar 7 months later in the three groups. Recombinant hirudin (Lepirudin™) bolus (0.4 mg/kg) and infusion (0.15 mg/kg/h) and argatroban have now been approved for use in the United States in patients with heparin-induced thrombocytopenia.

The direct thrombin inhibitor argatroban, unlike hirudin, does not require downward dose adjustment for renal insufficiency. None of the direct thrombin inhibitors have antidotes for bleeding.

Another direct thrombin inhibitor, bivalirudin (AngioMax™) was compared with unfractionated heparin in the Hirulog Angioplasty study, a randomized trial of 4098 patients with postinfarction or unstable angina undergoing PCI. After pretreatment with aspirin, patients were then assigned to heparin bolus (175 U/kg bolus and 15 U/kg/h infusion for 18 to 24 h) or bivalirudin bolus (1.0 mg/kg bolus and 2.5 mg/kg/h infusion for 4 h followed by 0.2 mg/kg/h for 14 to 20 h) (64). Bivalirudin did not reduce the likelihood of in-hospital death, Q-wave or non-Q-wave MI, or emergency CABG, although it did reduce the likelihood of bleeding complications (OR = 0.4; $p < 0.001$) (64). In a prospectively stratified cohort of 704 patients with post-MI angina, bivalirudin therapy did result in lower rates of major ischemic complications (9.1% vs. 14.2% in heparin-treated patients; $p = 0.04$), and lower rates of bleeding (3.0% vs. 11.1% in heparin-treated patients; $p < 0.001$). Bivalirudin has been approved by the Food and Drug Administration for use as an alternative to unfractionated heparin in patients undergoing PCI in the United States.

D. Antithrombin Therapy for the Prevention of Restenosis After PCI

Neither intravenous heparin (59) subcutaneous (65) unfractionated heparin, nor low-molecular-weight heparins, including enoxaparin, reviparin, nadroparin, and fraxiparin (66–68), prevent restenosis after PCI. Antithrombin-III-independent thrombin inhibitors, such as bivalirudin (69), hirudin (63), and long-term warfarin (70), also have had little effect on the prevention of restenosis.

The safety of PCI has advanced substantially over the past several years, owing to both improvements in the techniques of coronary revascularization (e.g., coronary stents) and the availability of novel adjunct pharmacology (e.g., GP IIb-IIIa inhibitors). This review has focused on the advances that have been achieved with antithrombotic agents during PCI. The most dramatic advances have been with the GP IIb-IIIa inhibitors, which as a class have achieved a 30 to 50% reduction in 30-day clinical events, and with the use of clopidogrel, which has reduced the occurrence of subacute stent thrombosis to <1% in most centers. There has also been a steady advance in our understanding of the use of unfractionated heparin during PCI. Near-patient monitoring has allowed the titration of unfractionated heparin, avoiding excessive anticoagulation, which may result in bleeding complications, and empiric guidelines have been established. Newer antithrombins, including LMWH, have been evaluated during PCI, but only the antithrombin III-independent bivalirudin has been approved for clinical use as an alternative to unfractionated heparin. No antithrombotic agent has been shown thus far to reduce restenosis, although abciximab may lower the restenosis rates in diabetic patients undergoing stent implantation. During the next few years, we will witness continued rapid evolution of the pharmacological regimens during PCI.

REFERENCES

1. Schwartz L, Bourassa M, Lesperance J, Aldridge H, Kazim F, Salvatori V, et al. Aspirin and dipyridamole in the prevention of restenosis after percutaneous transluminal coronary angioplasty. N Engl J Med 1988; 318:1714–1719.
2. White C, Chaitman B, Lassar T, Marcus M, Chisholm R, Knudson M, et al. Antiplatelet agents are effective in reducing the immediate complications of PTCA. Results of the ticlopidine multicenter trial (abstr). Circulation 1987; 76:IV–400.
3. Lembo NJ, Black, AJ, Roubin GS, Wilentz JR, Mufson LH, Douglas JS, Jr., et al. Effect of pretreatment with aspirin versus aspirin plus dipyridamole on frequency and type of acute complications of percutaneous transluminal coronary angioplasty. Am J Cardiol 1990; 65:422–426.
4. Gregorini L, Marco J, Fajadet J, Bernies M, Cassagneau B, Brunel P, et al. Ticlopidine and aspirin pretreatment reduces coagulation and platelet activation during coronary dilation procedures. J Am Coll Cardiol 1997; 29:13–20.
5. Schomig A, Neumann FJ, Kastrati A, Schuhlen H, Blasini R, Hadamitzky M, et al. A randomized comparison of antiplatelet and anticoagulant therapy after the placement of coronary-artery stents. N Engl J Med 1996; 334:1084–1089.
6. Leon M, Baim D, Popma J, Gordon P, Cutlip D, Ho K, et al. A clinical trial comparing three antithrombotic-drug regimens after coronary-artery stenting. N Engl J Med 1998; 339:1665–1671.
7. Bennett C, Weinberg P, Rozenberg-Ben-Dror K, et al. Thrombocytopenic purpura associated with ticlopidine. Ann Intern Med 1998; 128:541–544.
8. Szto G, Linnemeier T, Lewis S. Safety of 10 days of ticlopidine after coronary stenting—A randomized comparison with 30 days: Strategic ALternatives with Ticlopidine in Stenting Study (SALTS) (abstr). J Am Coll Cardiol 1998; 31:352A.
9. Berger P, Grill D, Melby S, et al. Can ticlopidine be safely discontinued two weeks after coronary stent placement (abstr). J Am Coll Cardiol 1998; 31:458A.
10. Coukell AJ, Markham A. Clopidogrel. Drugs 1997; 54:745–750.
11. The CAPRIE Committee. A randomised, blind, trial of clopidogrel versus aspirin in patients at risk of ischemic events (CAPRIE). Lancet 1996; 348:1239–1339.
12. Bertrand M. CLASSICS Study. Circulation 2000, in press.
13. Moussa I, Oetgen M, Roubin G, Colombo A, Wang X, Iyer S, et al. Effectiveness of clopidogrel and aspirin versus ticlopidine and aspirin in preventing stent thrombosis after coronary stent implantation. Circulation 1999; 99:2364–2366.
14. Bennett C, Connors J, Carwile J. Thrombotic thrombocytopenic purpura associated with clopidogrel. N Engl J Med 2000; 342:1773–1777.

15. de Feyter P, van den Brand M, Jaarman G, van Domburg R, Serruys P, Suryapranata H. Acute coronary artery occlusion during and after percutaneous transluminal coronary angioplasty: Frequency, prediction, clinical course, management and follow-up. Circulation 1991; 83:927–936.

16. Myler RK, Shaw RE, Stertzer SH, Hecht HS, Ryan C, Rosenblum J, et al. Lesion morphology and coronary angioplasty: current experience and analysis. J Am Coll Cardiol 1992; 19:1641–1652.

17. Lincoff AM, Popma JJ, Ellis SG, Hacker JA, Topol EJ. Abrupt vessel closure complicating coronary angioplasty: clinical, angiographic and therapeutic profile. J Am Coll Cardiol 1992; 19:926–935.

18. Ruggeri Z. Receptor-specific antiplatelet therapy. Circulation 1989; 80:1920–1922.

19. Phillips D, Charo I, Parise L, Fitzgerald L. The platelet membrane glycoprotein IIb-IIIa complex. Blood 1988; 71:831–843.

20. The EPIC Investigators. Use of a monoclonal antibody directed against the platelet glycoprotein IIb/IIIa receptor in high-risk coronary angioplasty. The EPIC Investigation. N Engl J Med 1994; 330:956–961.

21. Lincoff AM, Califf RM, Anderson KM, Weisman HF, Aguirre FV, Kleiman NS, et al. Evidence for prevention of death and myocardial infarction with platelet membrane glycoprotein IIb/IIIa receptor blockade by abciximab (c7E3 Fab) among patients with unstable angina undergoing percutaneous coronary revascularization. EPIC Investigators. Evaluation of 7E3 in Preventing Ischemic Complications. J Am Coll Cardiol 1997; 30:149–156.

22. Brener SJ, Barr LA, Burchenal JE, Katz S, George BS, Jones AA, et al. Randomized, placebo-controlled trial of platelet glycoprotein IIb/IIIa blockade with primary angioplasty for acute myocardial infarction. ReoPro and Primary PTCA Organization and Randomized Trial (RAPPORT) Investigators. Circulation 1998; 98:734–741.

23. The EPILOG Investigators. Platelet glycoprotein IIb/IIIa receptor blockade and low-dose heparin during percutaneous coronary revascularization. The EPILOG Investigators [see comments]. N Engl J Med 1997; 336:1689–1696.

24. Mak KH, Challapalli R, Eisenberg MJ, Anderson KM, Califf RM, Topol EJ. Effect of platelet glycoprotein IIb/IIIa receptor inhibition on distal embolization during percutaneous revascularization of aortocoronary saphenous vein grafts. EPIC Investigators. Evaluation of IIb/IIIa platelet receptor antagonist 7E3 in preventing ischemic complications. Am J Cardiol 1997; 80:985–988.

25. Mathew V, Grill D, Scott C, Grantham J, Ting H, Garratt K, et al. The influence of abciximab use on clinical outcome after aortocoronary vein graft interventions. J Am Coll Cardiol 1999; 34:1163–1169.

26. Muhlestein JB, Karagounis LA, Treehan S, Anderson JL. "Rescue" utilization of abciximab for the dissolution of coronary thrombus developing as a complication of coronary angioplasty. J Am Coll Cardiol 1997; 30:1729–1734.

27. The EPISTENT Investigators. Randomised placebo-controlled and balloon-angioplasty-controlled trial to assess safety of coronary stenting with use of platelet glycoprotein-IIb/IIIa blockade. The EPISTENT Investigators. Evaluation of Platelet IIb/IIIa Inhibitor for Stenting. Lancet 1998; 352:87–92.

28. Lincoff A, Califf R, Moliterno D, Ellis S, Ducas J, Kramer J, et al. Complementary

clinical benefits of coronary artery stenting and blockade of platelet glycoprotein IIb/IIIa receptors. N Engl J Med 1999; 341:319–327.

29. The IMPACT-II Investigators. Randomised placebo-controlled trial of effect of eptifibatide on complications of percutaneous coronary intervention: IMPACT-II. Integrilin to Minimise Platelet Aggregation and Coronary Thrombosis-II. Lancet 1997; 349:1422–1428.

30. The RESTORE Investigators. Effects of platelet glycoprotein IIb/IIIa blockade with tirofiban on adverse cardiac events in patients with unstable angina or acute myocardial infarction undergoing coronary angioplasty. The RESTORE Investigators. Randomized Efficacy Study of Tirofiban for Outcomes and REstenosis. Circulation 1997; 96:1445–1453.

31. Rao T, Pratt C, Berke A, Jaffe A, Ockene I, Schreiber T, et al. Thrombolysis in Myocardial Infarction (TIMI) trial, phase I: hemorrhagic manifestations and changes in fibrinogen and the fibrinolytic system in patients treated with recombinant tissue plasminogen activator and streptokinase. J Am Coll Cardiol 1988; 11:1–11.

32. Thornton M, Gruentzig A, Hollman J, King SI, Douglas J. Coumadin and aspirin in prevention of recurrence after transluminal coronary angioplasty: A randomized study. Circulation 1984; 69:721–727.

33. Taylor R, Gibbons F, Cope G, Cumpston G, Mews G, Luke P. Effects of low-dose aspirin on restenosis after coronary angioplasty. Am J Cardiol 1991; 68:874–878.

34. Schwartz L, Lesperance J, Bourassa MG, Eastwood C, Kazim F, Arafah M, et al. The role of antiplatelet agents in modifying the extent of restenosis following percutaneous transluminal coronary angioplasty. Am Heart J 1990; 119:232–236.

35. Popma JJ, Weitz J, Bittl JA, Ohman EM, Kuntz RE, Lansky AJ, et al. Antithrombotic therapy in patients undergoing coronary angioplasty. Chest 1998; 114:728S–741S.

36. Serruys PW, Rutsch W, Heyndrickx GR, Danchin N, Mast EG, Wijns W, et al. Prevention of restenosis after percutaneous transluminal coronary angioplasty with thromboxane A2-receptor blockade. A randomized, double-blind, placebo-controlled trial. Coronary Artery Restenosis Prevention on Repeated Thromboxane-Antagonism Study (CARPORT). Circulation 1991; 84:1568–1580.

37. Savage M, Goldberg S, Macdonald R, Bass T, Margolis J, Whitworth H, et al. Multihospital Eastern Atlantic restenosis trial II: A placebo-controlled trial of thromboxane blockade in the prevention of restenosis following coronary angioplasty. Am Heart J 1991; 122:1239–1244.

38. Serruys PW, Klein W, Tijssen JP, Rutsch W, Heyndrickx GR, Emanuelsson H, et al. Evaluation of ketanserin in the prevention of restenosis after percutaneous transluminal coronary angioplasty. A multicenter randomized double-blind placebo-controlled trial. Circulation 1993; 88:1588–601.

39. Knudtson ML, Flintoft VF, Roth DL, Hansen JL, Duff HJ. Effect of short-term prostacyclin administration on restenosis after percutaneous transluminal coronary angioplasty. J Am Coll Cardiol 1990; 15:691–697.

40. Raizner A, Hollman J, Abukhalil J, Demke D. Ciprostene for restenosis revisited: Quantitative analysis of angiograms (abstr). J Am Coll Cardiol 1993; 21:321A.

41. Topol EJ, Califf RM, Weisman HF, Ellis SG, Tcheng JE, Worley S, et al. Randomised trial of coronary intervention with antibody against platelet IIb/IIIa integrin for

reduction of clinical restenosis: results at six months. The EPIC Investigators. Lancet 1994; 343:881–886.

42. Gibson CM, Goel M, Cohen DJ, Piana RN, Deckelbaum LI, Harris KE, et al. Six-month angiographic and clinical follow-up of patients prospectively randomized to receive either tirofiban or placebo during angioplasty in the RESTORE trial. Randomized Efficacy Study of Tirofiban for Outcomes and Restenosis. J Am Coll Cardiol 1998; 32:28–34.

43. Marso S, Bhatt D, Tanguay J-F, Hammoud T, Sapp S, Robbins M, et al. Synergy of stenting plus abciximabl in diabetic patients: Persistence through 1-year follow-up from EPISTENT (abstr). Circulation 1999; 100:I–365.

44. Grayburn P, Willard J, Brincker M, Eichhorn E. In vivo thrombus formation on a guidewire during intravascular ultrasound imaging: Evidence for inadequate heparinization. Cathet Cardiovasc Diagn 1991; 23:141–143.

45. Laskey MA, Deutsch E, Barnathan E, Laskey WK. Influence of heparin therapy on percutaneous transluminal coronary angioplasty outcome in unstable angina pectoris. Am J Cardiol 1990; 65:1425–1429.

46. The CAPTURE Investigators. Randomised placebo-controlled trial of abciximab before and during coronary intervention in refractory unstable angina: the CAPTURE Study. Lancet 1997; 349:1429–1435.

47. The PRISM PLUS Investigators. Inhibition of the platelet glycoprotein IIb/IIIa receptor with tirofiban in unstable angina and non-Q-wave myocardial infarction. Platelet Receptor Inhibition in Ischemic Syndrome Management in Patients Limited by Unstable Signs and Symptoms (PRISM-PLUS) Study Investigators. N Engl J Med 1998; 338:1488–1497.

48. The PURSUIT Investigators. Inhibition of platelet glycoprotein IIb/IIIa with eptifibatide in patients with acute coronary syndromes. The PURSUIT Trial Investigators. Platelet Glycoprotein IIb/IIIa in Unstable Angina: Receptor Suppression Using Integrilin Therapy. N Engl J Med 1998; 339:436–443.

49. Dougherty K, Gaos C, Bush H, Leachman D, Ferguson J. Activated clotting times and activated partial thromboplastin times in patients undergoing coronary angioplasty who receive bolus doses of heparin. Cathet Cardiovasc Diagn 1992; 26:260–263.

50. Bowers J, Ferguson J. The use of activated clotting times to monitor heparin therapy during and after interventional procedures. Clin Cardiol 1994; 17:357–361.

51. Marmur J, Merlini P, Sharma S, Khaghan N, Torre S, Israel D, et al. Thrombin generation in human coronary arteries after percutaneous transluminal balloon angioplasty. J Am Coll Cardiol 1994; 24:1484–1491.

52. Marmur J, Sharma S, Kantrowitz N, Gupta V, Cocke T, Duvvuri S, et al. Angiographically complex lesions are associated with increased levels of thrombin generation and activity following PTCA (abstr). J Am Coll Cardiol 1995; 25:155A.

53. Narins CR, Hillegass WB, Jr., Nelson CL, Tcheng JE, Harrington RA, Phillips HR, et al. Relation between activated clotting time during angioplasty and abrupt closure. Circulation 1996; 93:667–671.

54. Ferguson J, Dougherty K, Gaos C, Bush H, Marsh K, Leachman D. Relation between procedural activated clotting time and outcome after percutaneous transluminal coronary angioplasty. J Am Coll Cardiol 1994; 23:1061–1065.

55. Hillegass W, Narins C, Brott B, Haura E, Phillips H, Stack R, et al. Activated clotting time predicts bleeding complications from angioplasty (abstr). J Am Coll Cardiol 1994:184A.

56. Popma JJ, Satler LF, Pichard AD, Kent KM, Campbell A, Chuang YC, et al. Vascular complications after balloon and new device angioplasty. Circulation 1993; 88: 1569–1578.

57. Koch KT, Piek JJ, de Winter RJ, Mulder K, David GK, Lie KI. Early ambulation after coronary angioplasty and stenting with six French guiding catheters and low-dose heparin. Am J Cardiol 1997; 80:1084–1086.

58. Boccara A, Benamer H, Juliard J, et al. A randomized trial of a fixed high dose versus a low weight adjusted low dose of intravenous heparin during coronary angioplasty. Eur Heart J 1997; 18:631–635.

59. Ellis S, Roubin G, Wilentz J, Douglas J, King S. Effect of 18- to 24-hour heparin administration for prevention of restenosis after uncomplicated coronary angioplasty. Am Heart J 1989; 117:777–782.

60. Friedman HZ, Cragg DR, Glazier SM, Gangadharan V, Marsalese DL, Schreiber TL, et al. Randomized prospective evaluation of prolonged versus abbreviated intravenous heparin therapy after coronary angioplasty. J Am Coll Cardiol 1994; 24: 1214–1219.

61. Cohen M, Demers C, Gurfinkel E, al e. A comparison of low-molecular-weight heparin with unfractionated heparin for unstable coronary artery disease. N Engl J Med 1997; 1997:447–452.

62. Grines C. Anticoagulation requirements for coronary interventions and the role of low molecular weight heparins. J Invas Cardiol 1999; 11:7A–12A.

63. Serruys PW, Herrman JP, Simon R, Rutsch W, Bode C, Laarman GJ, et al. A comparison of hirudin with heparin in the prevention of restenosis after coronary angioplasty. Helvetica Investigators. N Engl J Med 1995; 333:757–763.

64. Bittl JA, Strony J, Brinker JA, Ahmed WH, Meckel CR, Chaitman BR, et al. Treatment with bivalirudin (Hirulog) as compared with heparin during coronary angioplasty for unstable or postinfarction angina. Hirulog Angioplasty Study Investigators. N Engl J Med 1995; 333:764–769.

65. Brack MJ, Ray S, Chauhan A, Fox J, Hubner PJ, Schofield P, et al. The Subcutaneous Heparin and Angioplasty Restenosis Prevention (SHARP) trial. Results of a multicenter randomized trial investigating the effects of high dose unfractionated heparin on angiographic restenosis and clinical outcome. J Am Coll Cardiol 1995; 26:947–954.

66. Faxon DP, Spiro TE, Minor S, Cote G, Douglas J, Gottlieb R, et al. Low molecular weight heparin in prevention of restenosis after angioplasty. Results of Enoxaparin Restenosis (ERA) Trial. Circulation 1994; 90:908–914.

67. Karsch KR, Preisack MB, Baildon R, Eschenfelder V, Foley D, Garcia EJ, et al. Low molecular weight heparin (reviparin) in percutaneous transluminal coronary angioplasty. Results of a randomized, double-blind, unfractionated heparin and placebo-controlled, multicenter trial (REDUCE trial). Reduction of Restenosis After PTCA, Early Administration of Reviparin in a Double-Blind Unfractionated Heparin and Placebo-Controlled Evaluation. J Am Coll Cardiol 1996; 28:1437–1443.

68. Lablanche JM, McFadden EP, Meneveau N, Lusson JR, Bertrand B, Metzger JP,

et al. Effect of nadroparin, a low-molecular-weight heparin, on clinical and angiographic restenosis after coronary balloon angioplasty: the FACT study. Fraxiparine Angioplastie Coronaire Transluminale. Circulation 1997; 96:3396–3402.

69. Burchenal JE, Marks DS, Tift Mann J, Schweiger MJ, Rothman MT, Ganz P, et al. Effect of direct thrombin inhibition with Bivalirudin (Hirulog) on restenosis after coronary angioplasty. Am J Cardiol 1998; 82:511–515.

70. Urban P, Buller N, Fox K, Shapiro L, Bayliss J, Rickards A. Lack of effect of warfarin on the restenosis rate or on clinical outcome after balloon coronary angioplasty. Br Heart J 1988; 60:485–488.

11

Percutaneous Interventions for Obstructive Atherosclerotic Peripheral Arterial Disease

Joseph M. Garasic
*Massachusetts General Hospital and Harvard Medical School,
Boston, Massachusetts*

Andrew C. Eisenhauer
*Brigham and Women's Hospital and Harvard Medical School,
Boston, Massachusetts*

The increasing recognition of the clinical importance of atherosclerotic peripheral vascular disease and widespread availability of noninvasive diagnostic modalities have brought increased attention to therapeutic options. While surgery has historically been the mainstay of therapy for peripheral vascular disease, catheter-based therapies have advanced significantly in recent years. Percutaneous vascular intervention now provides patients with a less invasive, efficacious modality for the treatment of atheromatous disease over a wide spectrum of anatomical and clinical situations. Catheter-based intervention can provide symptomatic relief of claudication and has proved useful for definitive therapy in the renal, brachiocephalic, and carotid vessels.

I. LOWER EXTREMITY OBSTRUCTIVE DISEASE

Intermittent claudication involving the lower extremities is commonly caused by stenosis or occlusion of the iliofemoral or crural vessels. While first-line therapy has included aggressive risk-factor modification and exercise training, progressive symptomatic claudication and rest symptoms often dictate more aggressive investigation and therapy. The goals of therapy for lower extremity claudication are symptomatic relief and, in more extreme cases, limb salvage. While surgical therapy has historically been reserved for patients with limb-threatening ischemia and rest pain, the availability of endovascular therapies has lowered the threshold for intervention. As most percutaneous interventions are associated with low procedural risk, patients with lifestyle-limiting claudication are now being considered for angiographic investigation and intervention. In addition, percutaneous treatment usually preserves the surgical option should it be needed. An increasingly aware patient population will, given the choice, often opt for less invasive therapies, accepting results that may be less durable or even less efficacious than those with a more invasive approach such as surgery. For the clinician treating patients with lower extremity vascular disease, both patient satisfaction and long-term results are important in weighing potential treatments.

In some instances, lower extremity arterial occlusive disease has been considered merely an outpatient problem and a nuisance. However, the United States National Institutes of Health suggest that this disease results in over 60,000 hospitalizations annually, with an average length of stay greater than 11 days (1). It has been estimated that 1% of men and 2% of women aged 45–69 have clinical evidence of intermittent claudication (2). However, with advancing age, the incidence of lower extremity claudication rises. Among 2415 initial cardiovascular events in the Framingham study, 9.6% of the events in men were intermittent claudication. Using the subset of patients aged 65 to 74 years, 11.6% of men and 9.4% of women had intermittent claudication (3). Well-described risk factors for lower extremity disease include: tobacco use, diabetes mellitus, hyperlipidemia, and systolic hypertension. Smoking appears to be the greatest modifiable risk factor and one of the most deleterious. Of 343 patients with intermittent claudication, 16% of patients who continued to smoke developed rest pain within 1 year, while none of the former smokers were similarly afflicted (4). Though progression of claudication to limb-threatening ischemia has been said to occur in less than 10% of claudicants, the diabetic patient is at particularly high risk. One study showed that over 6 years of follow-up, examining a cohort of diabetic and nondiabetic patients with claudication, 40% of diabetics and 18% of nondiabetics progressed to ischemic rest pain or gangrene.

While noninvasive modalities such as segmental Doppler pressures and pulse-volume recordings are helpful in localizing the level of obstructive disease and characterizing its severity, patient symptoms drive further investigation, especially diagnostic angiography. The broad indications for lower extremity angiography include symptomatic arterial occlusive disease unresponsive to conservative measures, rest claudication, and critical limb-threatening ischemia. The goals of revascularization include relief of symptoms, aid in wound healing, and limb salvage. In cases where percutaneous therapy is entertained, one must consider whether these goals can be accomplished percutaneously and with what durability. The likelihood of clinical success, the durability, and the technical approach vary according to anatomical site. These aspects are best considered separately for aortoiliac, femoropopliteal, and infrapopliteal segments.

A. Aortoiliac Obstruction

While many patients with iliac artery disease have concomitant femoral and crural obstructive disease, initial treatment of iliac obstruction is often undertaken first. In some cases, symptomatic improvement may be accomplished through increasing the proximal pressure head, and thus collateral blood flow to the distal extremity. Bilateral claudication resulting from distal abdominal aortic disease, or unilateral symptoms from iliac artery disease, can be treated percutaneously with good short- and long-term success. In a randomized study, Wilson et al. saw no significant difference in 3-year patency rates between iliac stenoses treated with balloon angioplasty versus surgery (5). Though the ease of stent placement has bolstered its popularity, there is insufficient evidence to advocate primary stent placement as uniformly superior to PTA alone for iliac disease. A comparison of 279 patients with claudication, randomized to primary stent placement or primary angioplasty with stent placement for iliac lesions, showed no substantial difference between treatment groups. When similar angiographic and hemodynamic results were obtained, patency rates were similar (about 70% at 2 years), as were clinical success rates (about 78%) (6). However, the restenosis rate for iliac artery lesions treated with stent placement appears quite low, with 6-month angiographic follow-up showing a rate of 0.5%, and 86% target vessel patency at 4 years. Moreover, stented segments that did restenose were successfully treated with repeat angioplasty in most cases (7). Examples of the types of complex aortic and iliac disease that can now be treated percutaneously are shown in Figures 1 and 2.

While there is good evidence to support the endovascular therapy of iliac artery stenoses, total occlusions have been a more difficult problem. Though early studies demonstrated poor results with unacceptably high complication rates, the advent of hydrophilic guidewires and technical advances have allowed the recanalization of occluded iliac segments with an estimated 88% rate of primary success independent of location (external, internal, or common iliac artery) (8,9). The secondary patency rate at 6 years in the same series was 77%. The most common serious complication associated with recanalization of iliac occlusions remains distal embolism, with rates ranging from 4 to 7% (10). Thrombolytic therapy combined with balloon dilatation in an attempt to avoid embolic complications has been proposed, but requires further investigation. In addition, covered stents are now being used for iliac artery lesions with associated aneurysm or anatomical complexities and may increase the applicability of percutaneous therapy. At present, iliac PTA and stenting, when performed for obstructive iliac disease, are excellent first-line therapies and, when successful, have a durability similar to that of surgical reconstruction.

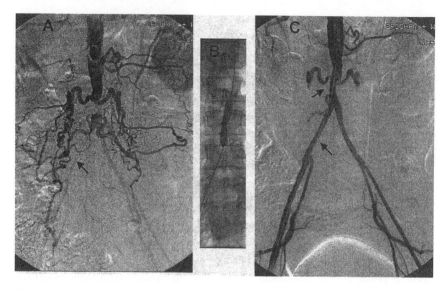

Figure 1 Percutaneous treatment of chronic aortic occlusion. A middle-aged woman with a history of tobacco use presented with chronic claudication and diminished femoral pulses. Angiography via the brachial approach (panel A) showed a distal aortic occlusion bridged by extensive lumbar collaterals faintly reconstituting the iliacs. In addition, there was an intrinsic stenosis of the right common iliac (arrow). The occlusion was pierced from above using a hydrophilic guidewire. The guidewire was snared via the common femoral on the right, exteriorized, and the aorta and right common iliac dilated (panel B) and stented. Care was taken not to overexpand the stented segment at the initial recanalization to minimize the possibility of rupture. The final result is shown in panel C.

B. Femoropopliteal Obstruction

The superficial femoral artery, particularly within the adductor canal of the thigh, is a frequent site of infrainguinal atherosclerotic disease. While procedural success in the relief of femoropopliteal stenoses and the recanalization of superficial femoral occlusions has been reasonable, concerns regarding high restenosis rates persist. Henry et al. report an 11% restenosis rate in SFA lesions and 20% for popliteal lesions at 6-month angiographic follow-up (7). All lesions were treated with stent placement. The 4-year patency rates among the same cohort were 65% for SFA lesions and 50% for popliteal lesions. While Matsi et al. reported high rates of procedural success for patients with SFA stenosis and recanalized total occlusions, clinical follow-up via ankle-brachial indices and reported symptoms demonstrated primary patency of less than 50% at 1 to 3 years (11). Excimer laser angioplasty, rotational atherectomy, and hydrophilic guidewires have all been employed to aid in the technical approach to totally occluded femoropopli-

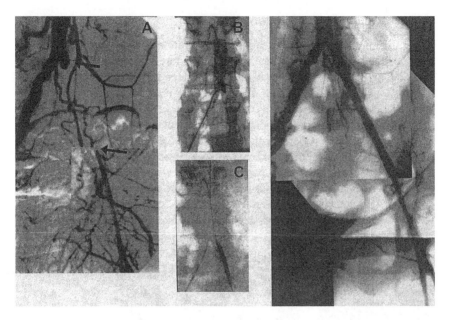

Figure 2 Percutaneous treatment of chronic iliac occlusion. A middle-aged man who was a former smoker presented with left leg claudication. Angiography was accomplished via the right common femoral approach. Composite frames of digital subtraction pelvic angiography are shown in panel A. There is a nubbin of the common iliac (upper arrow) and late reconstitution of the external iliac (lower arrow). The area of total occlusion was instrumented (panel B) from the contralateral approach using both antegrade and retrograde technique; the total occlusion was eventually pierced; and the guidewire was free in the aorta. Balloon recanalization was accomplished followed by stenting. The final result is shown in panel D. Note the absence of the left internal iliac. Generally, when this vessel is a retrograde collateral pathway, it can be covered without consequence in this setting.

teal vessels. However, once recanalized, there is little evidence to support the superiority of endovascular stents in this anatomical locale. Furthermore, the optimal role of thrombolytic therapy in the management of SFA occlusions, acute and subacute, remains to be elucidated. Given the moderate rates of procedural success with femoropopliteal intervention, percutaneous treatment may be considered in patients at high risk for surgical therapy, in attempts at improved wound healing, and for symptomatic relief despite concerns over aggressive restenosis in this anatomical locale. A potential advantage of endovascular therapy in this area is that restenosis or occlusion of previously successfully treated limbs seldom results in incremental deterioration. In contrast, occlusion of surgical bypasses has been associated with overall worsening of ischemia.

C. Infrapopliteal Obstruction

While the infrapopliteal vessels are a common site of arterial occlusive disease, single or multiple stenoses of one crural vessel rarely provoke lower extremity claudication. Rather, significant disease of all three infrapopliteal arteries (anterior tibial, peroneal, and posterior tibial) is usually required to provoke symptomatic calf ischemia in the absence of more proximal flow-limiting disease. While some operators may limit the indications for percutaneous revascularization below the knee to those patients with rest claudication, threatened limbs, or symptoms at low levels of exertion, patients with more moderate symptoms have been the subject of many studies. In particular, catheter-based techniques have been employed in patients at high risk for bypass graft surgery, those patients who had a greater saphenous vein unusable for bypass surgery, and in patients with more proximal interventions with the hope of maintaining adequate distal runoff (12). Superior long-term patency rates after proximal interventions and saphenous

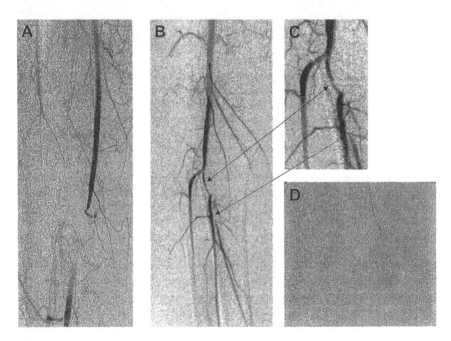

Figure 3 Percutaneous treatment of femoral and tibial disease. Short-segment stenoses and occlusions of the superficial femoral artery are readily approached. This 46-year-old diabetic smoker developed severe unilateral claudication. The initial angiogram showed a short-segment total occlusion of the SFA (panel A), severe obstruction of the tibioperoneal trunk and origin of the posterior tibial (panel B; magnified in panel C), and very sluggish single-vessel supply to the foot via the posterior tibial (panel D).

vein bypasses have been reported in circumstances with improved distal runoff, further supporting the utility of such a strategy (13). Short-term results with modern equipment have been promising, with primary success rates as high as 96% and a cumulative patency rate of 75.3% after 2 years (14). While there have been particular concerns regarding small-vessel interventions in diabetic patients, there is evidence that balloon angioplasty of the crural vessels can salvage ischemic limbs in the diabetic population (15). Overall infrapopliteal interventions are characterized with high rates of technical success and the potential to achieve improved distal arterial runoff, symptomatic improvement, and even limb salvage, despite the specter of high rates of late restenosis and reocclusion. Figures 3–5 demonstrate both the potential for success and the unresolved issues of femoral and tibial intervention.

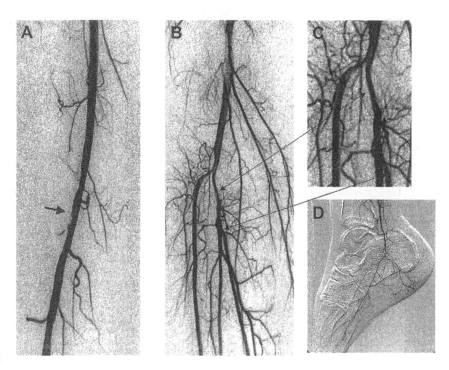

Figure 4 Following PTA, blood flow in the limb of the patient shown in Figure 3 has improved markedly. The prior total occlusion is resolved (panel A, arrow) and the stenoses in the tibioperoneal trunk and the posterior tibial origin are markedly improved (panel B; magnified in panel C). Perfusion to the foot (using the same contrast injection and filming technique as in Fig. 3) is now vigorous (panel D) though small-vessel disease remains. The patient's symptoms resolved completely after this procedure.

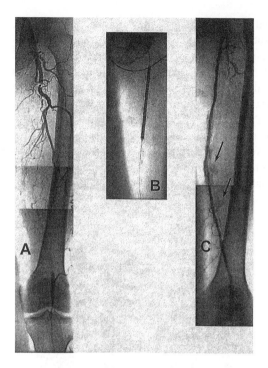

Figure 5 Chronic long-segment total occlusions of the superficial femoral artery remain difficult to treat. Panel A shows a composite view of a left leg angiogram in a patient with a chronic, long total occlusion of the SFA. Note the distal reconstitution at the popliteal. These lesions can often be pierced (panel B) and dilated. However, as shown in panel C, the results are irregular with contrast ''extravasation'' into arteriovenous communications with the femoral vein (arrows). These results can be improved angiographically with the use of self-expanding stents. Unfortunately, regardless of technique, reocclusion remains common.

D. Summary

Patients with lower extremity arterial occlusive disease and associated symptoms, but without limb-threatening ischemia, should be considered for percutaneous endovascular treatment. The physician must provide a frank discussion of the risk, potential symptomatic benefit, and durability of such intervention. There is little to suggest that the natural history of lower extremity occlusive disease is altered by an early and aggressive mechanical approach and thus treatment directed to early symptom management should be guided by the patient's symptoms and his or her wishes. On the other hand, limb-threatening ischemia is often best treated by the modality that will provide the most complete and durable revascularization. Often in isolated iliac occlusive disease, endovascular treatment is equivalent hemodynamically and may be preferable to surgery. Infrainguinal disease is often diffuse, and extensive long-segment femoral obstructive disease is often best addressed by saphenous vein bypass (see Fig. 5). However, given the diffuse nature of atherosclerosis and the widespread coexistence of coronary disease with peripheral vascular disease, a less invasive endovascular approach may be a preferable first step. For more urgently required revascularization, surgery is usually the preferred approach, especially for infrainguinal disease. As medical comorbidities increase, however, the more likely one is to turn to an initial percutaneous approach.

II. RENAL ARTERY OBSTRUCTIVE DISEASE

Renovascular disease is an important and often unrecognized contributor to renal insufficiency and difficult-to-manage hypertension. However, because not all patients with angiographic evidence of renovascular disease are hypertensive or have renal failure, patient selection for more invasive therapy is very important. Additionally, since the clinical syndrome associated with this anatomical diagnosis can be reminiscent of more common clinical diagnoses, such as isolated essential hypertension, a renovascular cause may not be entertained. The onset of diastolic hypertension after the age of 55, refractory or malignant hypertension, resistant hypertension in a previously well-controlled patient, and/or an increasing serum creatinine level, should alert the clinician and prompt further diagnostic testing. Unfortunately, modalities such as converting enzyme inhibitor–induced venous plasma renin sampling and intravenous urography lack the sensitivity and specificity necessary for a valuable screening and diagnostic tool (16,17). While converting enzyme inhibitor–induced renal scintigraphy has high levels of sensitivity and specificity in some patient subsets, its utility is limited by loss of sensitivity and specificity in patients with bilateral disease or abnormal renal function (18). Duplex renal artery ultrasound (19), spiral computerized tomography (20), and, more recently, magnetic resonance angiography (19) have all been used in the noninvasive assessment of the renal vasculature with high degrees of accuracy. While these modalities vary in their sensitivity and specificity, ultimately one's clinical conviction regarding the diagnosis must weigh heavily in the decision to pursue angiographic evaluation, as none of the techniques allows assessment of the functional significance of a renovascular lesion. Furthermore, even the "gold standard" of angiography is itself associated with significant intra- and inter-observer variability (21,22). Determining the functional significance of an anatomical finding remains one of the greatest unresolved dilemmas of renal intervention.

Once the anatomical diagnosis of renal artery stenosis is secure, one must consider what management is most appropriate. The goals of treatment, both surgical and percutaneous, for renal artery stenosis include preservation of renal function, improved control of hypertension, and forestalling hemodialysis. Fibromuscular dysplasia is the prototypical human condition upon which our notions about the relevance of renovascular obstruction are based. Therapy here is generally aimed at the amelioration of refractory hypertension and, in this case, balloon dilatation has been proven a successful modality (23).

The natural history of atherosclerotic renovascular disease differs somewhat and, while potentially a contributor in patients with difficult-to-control hypertension, concomitant essential hypertension often coexists. Preservation of renal function may be considered the primary goal of therapy, as improvement in blood pressure control and reduction in the number of antihypertensive medications is common, and complete resolution of hypertension is unusual (24–27). As deteriorating renal function has been associated with severe renal artery obstruction, the identification of functionally significant renal artery stenosis and its appropriate therapy could provide great benefit (28). The major question remaining is whether percutaneous renal revascularization can slow, delay, or prevent this deterioration in renal function and subsequent hemodialysis.

Data from the surgical literature support treatment of patients with both unilateral and bilateral renal artery stenosis. Among a cohort of 152 patients treated mechanically for the above anatomy, 90% had an improvement in blood pressure control, while 15% had ''cure'' of their hypertension (29). In another study of 51 patients with chronic renal insufficiency (serum creatinine >2 mg/dL) and bilateral renal artery lesions greater than 75%, surgical therapy was followed by improvement in renal function in 67% of patients, and stabilization in 27% of patients (30).

While anatomical revascularization may allow improved antihypertensive management and preserve renal parenchymal function, how does percutaneous therapy compare to surgery? This question is of particular importance given the advanced age of many patients with atherosclerotic disease, and the significant perioperative morbidity and operative mortality rates (up to 6%) associated with surgical therapy (29,31,32). One randomized, controlled study has compared surgical therapy versus balloon angioplasty for unilateral atherosclerotic renal artery stenosis (33). The authors reported slightly lower primary patency rates in the balloon angioplasty group, as one might expect in the prestent era. However, secondary patency was 90% in the PTA group and 97% in the surgical group, with comparable improvement in blood pressure and similar likelihood of improvement or stabilization in renal function after intervention (83% for PTA/72% for surgery).

Improved blood pressure has been reported in 60 to 75% of patients treated with stenting for renovascular disease, and is often associated with a reduction in the number of antihypertensive medications (24–27). In a metanalysis of 20 published series of balloon angioplasty for atherosclerotic renal artery disease, 54% of patients experienced improvement in hypertension, with 9% normalization of blood pressure. One problem in assessing the efficacy of renal artery intervention is that the anatomical presence of arterial stenosis does not guarantee causation. Patients with renovascular disease are also commonly afflicted by other nephrotoxic conditions: diabetes, essential hypertension, atheroemboli, and medicine-related insults. Thus, the outcome of intervention in patients with isolated renovascular disease differs from that in candidates with additional causes of renal parenchymal disease. How, then, can one determine if revascularizing one of two kidneys will achieve the targeted goals?

A recent study from the Dutch Renal Artery Stenosis Intervention Cooperative Study Group prospectively studied 106 patients with difficult-to-control hypertension, unilateral atherosclerotic renal artery stenosis (>50% decrease in luminal diameter), and a serum creatinine of less than 2.3 mg/dL to PTA versus continued medical therapy (34). This study reported little advantage of angioplasty over medical therapy in the management of hypertension. However, the inclusion of patients with moderate renal artery stenoses, the failure to utilize vascular stents, and the authors' isolated investigation of the effects of therapy on blood pressure control

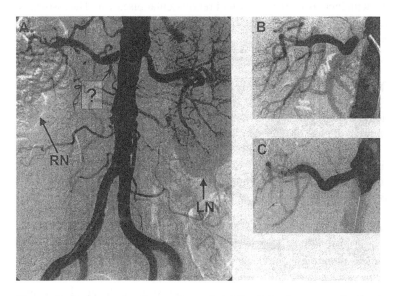

Figure 6 Renovascular disease. Several pitfalls of simple aortography for the detection of anatomical renal artery obstruction are illustrated in panel A. In this aortogram, performed with slight right anterior oblique angulation in an elderly man with the sudden exacerbation of previously mild hypertension, there appears to be no defined stenosis of the origin of the right renal artery. Though no other vessel obscures the origin of this vessel, one should be suspicious because right nephrogram (RN) is delayed in comparison to the left (LN) and the renal branch vessels are less well opacified. A selective angiogram (panel B) clearly shows a severe eccentric stenosis that was amenable to stenting (panel C).

all limit the utility of this investigation. Harden et al. studied patients with both bilateral and unilateral renal artery stenosis and were able to suggest a slowing of renal impairment after stenting (35). Additionally, we have recently completed a study of the effects of renal artery stenting showing that in patients with severe (>75%) bilateral disease, or unilateral disease with a lone kidney, such intervention improves or stabilizes renal function and preserves kidney size (36).

Percutaneous treatment of renovascular disease, then, offers a safe and efficacious therapy that is now widely considered preferable to vascular surgery for this indication. Current techniques (Fig. 6) permit the accurate demonstration of aortorenal anatomy and renal revascularization in the same procedural setting. Renal artery stenting has been shown to improve or stabilize renal function, and potentially forestall hemodialysis. Improved hypertensive control and a reduction in the number of antihypertensive medications necessary to achieve that control have both been associated with percutaneous renal artery revascularization. With the advent of distal protection devices to limit atheroembolic complications, operators may hope for even greater safety and renal parenchymal preservation. Meanwhile, with increasing recognition of renovascular disease and its associated morbidity, even more rigorous examination of such therapy and its efficacy can take place.

III. BRACHIOCEPHALIC OBSTRUCTIVE DISEASE

While brachiocephalic and subclavian artery obstructions are generally considered uncommon, the use of internal mammary conduits for coronary bypass surgery over the last decade has brought increasing attention to atherosclerotic disease in this locale. Subclavian steal syndrome arises because of reversal of flow in the vertebral artery as blood is shunted into the brachial circulation (37–39). Symptoms of dizziness, syncope, and vertigo are most common, while upper extremity claudication in the ipsilateral limb is another presenting feature (22,40). In coronary-subclavian steal, there is reversal of flow within the left internal mammary artery because of proximal subclavian stenosis. These patients often come to clinical attention with myocardial ischemia (41–43). While some clinical improvement may be seen with conservative therapy, relief of the anatomical obstruction is usually necessary (44,45). Although surgical therapy has historically been the ''first-choice'' treatment for symptomatic brachiocephalic and subclavian obstructive disease, balloon angioplasty has shown patency rates comparable to surgery, but with a low rate of complication and infrequent mortality.

We recently reviewed and compared experiences in surgical revascularization and stenting as reported in the literature (46). Review of nearly 2000 surgical patients over 25 years revealed an initial technical success rate of 96%, with a 3% initial stroke rate and 2% mortality. The overall complication rate was estimated as 16%, including such complications as stroke, hemorrhage, infection, Horner's syndrome, graft thrombosis, and anesthetic-related problems. Overall, open-chest procedures had a higher morbidity and mortality than extrathoracic bypasses. Review of the published series of patients treated with endovascular stenting was quite revealing. Adverse events were reported in 6% of cases, though the incidence of specific postprocedure complications is unknown. Technical success was achieved in 97% of nearly 100 patients. Target vessel occlusion or in-stent restenosis was reported in 6% of cases. The recent reports of vascular stenting suggest that periprocedural strokes are uncommon. Al-Mubarak et al. reported no strokes in a series of 38 patients (47), while Henry et al. reported stroke in 0.9% of patients in their series of subclavian procedures (48). Primary patency in the Al-Mubarak patients was 94% at 20 months and 75% at 8 years.

No direct comparison of surgical and endovascular therapy has been undertaken for patients with brachiocephalic and subclavian disease, and such a trial is unlikely in the near future. The involvement of the internal mammary and vertebral artery distributions is increasingly recognized and endovascular techniques, as shown in Figure 7, are available to address these clinical situations.

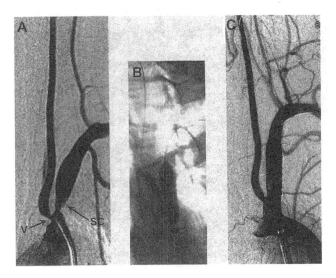

Figure 7   Complex atherosclerotic disease at the origin of the left subclavian involving the vertebral origin. Such lesions are becoming recognized more frequently as clinicians follow more patients in the years after internal mammary coronary bypass. The initial angiogram (panel A) illustrates the stenosis of the subclavian (SC) also involving the vertebral artery (V). These lesions were successfully treated with initial low-pressure stent deployment in the subclavian followed by instrumentation of the vertebral and "kissing" balloon dilatation (panel B). The final result is shown in panel C.

At present, examination of published series supports the consideration of a percutaneous approach in most patients with symptomatic obstructive disease.

IV. EXTRACRANIAL CEREBROVASCULAR OBSTRUCTIVE DISEASE

For patients, stroke and its associated debilitation is one of the most dreaded threats to health. As a result, clinical data in support of surgical therapy for significant carotid stenosis were embraced by the medical community. Carotid endarterectomy has become one of the most performed procedures by vascular surgeons in an effort to alter the natural history of cerebrovascular disease. Now, developing technology has permitted the expansion of endovascular treatment to atherosclerotic cerebrovascular disease and is one of the most exciting and controversial areas of investigation. As illustrated in Figure 8, carotid stenting can produce excellent anatomical results and is not associated with the inconve-

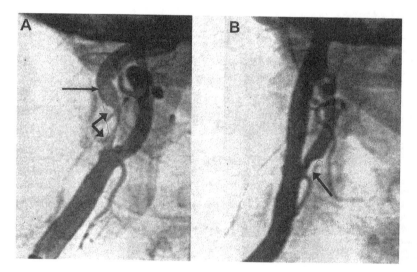

Figure 8 Carotid stenting. A 70-year-old gentleman presented with multiple hemispheric transient ischemic attacks (TIA). The angiogram demonstrated a severe origin stenosis of the internal carotid (panel A, thick arrows). Downstream, there were mobile filling defects consistent with thrombus (thin arrow). After heparinization and the use of a platelet IIb/IIIa receptor antagonist, this lesion was successfully treated with a single self-expanding stent. The final result is shown in panel B: stenoses of the external carotid caused by plaque shift (arrow) are inconsequential and should not be treated.

nience and discomfort of a cervical incision. However, though catheter-based therapy may offer a less invasive option to carotid endarterectomy, controversy still exists regarding where and when the endovascular treatment of cerebrovascular disease should be applied.

Before consideration of therapy for cerebrovascular disease, the clinician must first consider the potential goals of such treatment. The ultimate goal of treating cerebrovascular disease, and carotid artery disease in particular, is to reduce or eliminate disabling stroke and prolong life if possible. All potential therapies should be judged on their ability to achieve these endpoints—other surrogate endpoints are unimportant to the patient and clinician. In planning mechanical treatment for cerebrovascular disease, knowledge of the natural history of the problem is essential.

The natural history of symptomatic and asymptomatic carotid stenoses has been examined and is the impetus for aggressive treatment strategies. Among 3000 patients with a history of recent TIA in the Dutch TIA trial, entrants were randomized to treatment with low- or moderate-dose aspirin (49). After 36 months, the risk of nonfatal stroke was 5.7% in the low-dose group and 6.9% in the high-dose group.

Given the natural history of cerebrovascular disease and the unknown effects of carotid endarterectomy, several randomized trials were organized to determine whether endarterectomy had benefits over medical therapy for both symptomatic and asymptomatic disease. In the early 1990s, the European Medical Research Council, European Carotid Endarterectomy Surgery Trialists (ECST) (50) enrolled patients with 70 to 99% carotid stenosis and ipsilateral TIA within 180 days. Patients were randomized to medical versus surgical therapy, yielding a 21.9% risk of stroke at 36 months for the medically treated group, and a 12.3% risk in the surgically treated group. The death rate over the same period did not differ between treatment groups, although most were related to cardiovascular causes.

The North American Symptomatic Carotid Endarterectomy Trial (NAS-CET) randomized patients with 70 to 99% stenosis and ipsilateral TIA symptoms within 120 days of randomization to medical or surgical therapy (51). The 30-day follow-up showed a benefit of medical therapy with a 5.8% rate of all stroke and death in the surgical group, and a 3.6% risk in the medical group. As with the ECST data, the 36-month death rate did not differ significantly between groups in the NASCET study (9.9% surgical vs. 12.7% surgical). Again, the majority of these deaths were cardiovascular. However, by 36-month follow-up, the total stroke rate (9 vs. 26%) and major stroke rate (2.5 vs. 13.1%, surgical vs. medical) was less in the surgical group. The results of this study have served as the ''gold standard'' in the field, and clearly suggest that surgical endarterectomy stabilizes the treated lesion and effectively eliminates it as a cause of patient morbidity for at least 3 years. Similar data have been developed for severe asymptomatic stenoses (52). The data, however, are less powerful and the number of patients that must be treated to defer one stroke is in excess of that for symptomatic disease.

While these randomized trials suggest that high-quality carotid endarterectomy, despite procedural risk, decreases long-term risk of ipsilateral stroke in patients with severe carotid stenoses, endarterectomy has not been shown to prolong life. In addition, a significant number of surgical complications were reported with carotid endarterectomy in the NASCET trial, including a 7.6% rate of cranial nerve palsy, a 5.5% rate of neck hematomas, and a 3.4% rate of wound infections (51). While cardiac complications were uncommon in the NASCET group, 0.9% did suffer a periprocedural myocardial infarction. To understand these data fully, however, one must first explore which medical institutions and patients participated in the study. To participate, institutions were required to demonstrate acceptably low rates of complication and stroke in their surgically treated patients. In addition, beyond meeting the angiographic and symptomatic criteria, selected patients needed to be surgical candidates *and* consent to randomization. Many patients with significant comorbidities were excluded—such as those with atrial fibrillation, severe symptomatic coronary disease, recent myocardial infarction, past ipsilateral carotid endarterectomy, ipsilateral disabling stroke, age >79 years, or life expectancy <5 years. Clearly, it is difficult to generalize the NASCET data because patients were low risk in comparison to those often encountered in clinical practice. Furthermore, in an analysis of the variation in carotid endarterectomy mortality among the Medicare populations, hospitals that participated in the NASCET or ACAS trials presented a 1.44% 30-day mortality; there was a 1.77% rate in nonparticipating hospitals (53). Both values were greater than the 0.6% mortality reported by the same institutions in the NASCET. Furthermore, the majority of endarterectomies done nationwide are performed in low-volume hospitals and by surgeons who do less than 20 cases per year. Such low-volume hospitals have reported mortality rates as high as 2.5% (54).

Thus, while an effective strategy for reducing the incidence of ipsilateral stroke, carotid endarterectomy is not without associated problems. Is it possible less invasive approaches to plaque stabilization could prove similarly beneficial? Like other interventions in other territories, endovascular stenting has achieved excellent hemodynamic results. However, critics of carotid stenting have suggested that early data report a high rate of procedural complication. Roubin et al. reported their complication rates in a series of patients treated with carotid stenting (55,56). While a 6% rate of all strokes was reported by 30 days postprocedure, this rate compares favorably with the 5.8% overall stroke and death rate reported for the NASCET surgical group. Additionally, there appears to be a steep learning curve associated with carotid stenting procedures (55). While the earliest group of patients from the University of Alabama/Lenox Hill Hospital (UAB-LHH) cohort suffered a 7 to 8% procedural rate of minor stroke, this rate fell to 4.5%, and subsequently to 2.3% in the more recent groups. To allow comparison of the surgical risk of carotid endarterectomy and the current best estimate of morbidity and mortality from carotid stenting, one can compare the NASCET data to the overall 30-day follow-up data from the UAB-LHH cohort (55,57). The overall surgical stroke rate of 5.5% appears comparable to the 6% stroke rate reported for stenting. Also, the major stroke and death rates of 2.1 and 2.8% (surgery vs. stenting) are nearly numerically identical. The most common procedural morbidity for the group treated endovascularly is minor stroke, with a 5.2% rate. By definition, the sequelae of these events resolved entirely within 7 days and did not produce long-term morbidity. Again, recent data from UAB-LHH reports a 30-day minor stroke rate of 0% among 88 patients. Certainly, the short-term outcomes for endovascular carotid intervention are encouraging.

While this evidence supports potential equivalence of surgical and catheter-based therapies in the immediate periprocedural period, it is in the 36-month period after intervention that the real benefits of surgical therapy became evident in the NASCET group. How, then, do stent patients fare after more extended follow-up? Up to 13-month follow-up is available on 225 patients and 266 vessels treated percutaneously in the UAB-LHH group. No patients suffered a major stroke. The minor stroke rate was 1.7%, and one patient died of a noncerebrovascular cause. Although comparison of these data to the NASCET group is difficult, some interesting points can be made. By subtracting the 30-day NASCET events from the overall 36-month events, a 4.5% late stroke rate is obtained, considerably higher than the endovascular rate. These data are from admittedly different patient groups, although one may wonder whether the stented group is at higher baseline risk.

The International Society for Carotid Artery Treatment (ISCAT) has compiled registry data of ongoing endovascular carotid procedures (57,58). These data support the concept of a learning curve where the highest rates of major stroke and death occur in centers that have performed less than 50 procedures. However, taking into account all involved centers, the reported rate of TIA and minor stroke is still less than 3%, major stroke 1.35%, and death <1%. These data clearly support the notion that carotid stenting, while a developing technology subject to developing experience, offers an exciting and less invasive modality with benefits comparable to surgical endarterectomy. With increasing operator experience, and future use of distal embolization protection devices and antiplatelet therapy, endovascular techniques will undoubtedly advance rapidly. Only with randomized controlled trials can the question of which modality is "better" come to a reasonably convincing conclusion. For the present, carotid endarterectomy is the "gold standard" for extracranial cervical carotid revascularization.

Clearly, though no randomized comparative data exist, the results available thus far suggest that the "order of magnitude" of the outcomes with endovascular carotid stenting is close to that of surgery. Unless and until definitive studies are reported, it remains reasonable to offer carefully screened and informed patients an endovascular alternative to surgical or medical therapy. These procedures should be performed in centers that collect, analyze, and review their results carefully and participate in clinical research and investigation.

V. CONCLUSION

Although the specific tools and techniques vary, the theme of endovascular intervention is similar across many vascular territories. In general, vascular stenting has become the mainstay of percutaneous revascularization for relief of symptoms. The challenge for the future will be to improve the long-term durability of endovascular therapy and explore its potential for preventing the complications of progressive atherosclerosis.

REFERENCES

1. National Institutes of Health (USDHHS). Chartbook on cardiovascular, lung and blood diseases. Bethesda, MD: National Institutes of Health, 1994.
2. Hughson W, Mann J, Garrod A. Intermittent claudication: prevalence and risk factors. Br Med J 1978; 1:1379–1381.
3. Kannel W. The demographics of claudication and the aging of the American population. Vasc Med 1996; 1:60–64.
4. Jonason T, Bergstrom R. Cessation of smoking in patients with intermittent claudication. Effects on the risk of peripheral vascular complications, myocardial infarction and mortality. Acta Med Scand 1987; 221:253–260.
5. Wilson SE, Wolf GL, Cross AP. Percutaneous transluminal angioplasty versus operation for peripheral arteriosclerosis. Report of a prospective randomized trial in a selected group of patients. J Vasc Surg 1989; 9:1–9.
6. Tetteroo E, van der Graaf Y, Bosch JL, et al. Randomised comparison of primary stent placement versus primary angioplasty followed by selective stent placement in patients with iliac artery occlusive disease. Dutch iliac stent trial study group. Lancet 1998; 351:1153–1159.
7. Henry M, Amor M, Ethevenot G, et al. Palmaz stent placement in iliac and femoropopliteal arteries: primary and secondary patency in 310 patients with 2–4 year follow-up. Radiology 1995; 197:167–174.
8. Colapinto RF, Stronell RD, Johnston WK. Transluminal angioplasty of complete iliac obstructions. Am J Roentgenol 1986; 146:859–862.
9. Ring EJ, Freiman DB, McLean GK, Schwarz W. Percutaneous recanalization of common iliac artery occlusions: an unacceptable complication rate? Am J Roentgenol 1982; 139:587–589.
10. Henry M, Amor M, Ethevenot G, Henry I, Mentre B, Tzvetanov K. Percutaneous endoluminal treatment of iliac occlusions: long-term follow-up of 105 patients. J Endovasc Surg 1998; 5:228–235.

11. Matsi PJ, Manninen HI, Vanninen RL, et al. Femoropopliteal angioplasty in patients with claudication: primary and secondary patency in 140 limbs with 1–3 year follow-up. Radiology 1994; 191:727–733.

12. Greenfield AJ. Femoral, popliteal, and tibial arteries: percutaneous transluminal angioplasty. Am J Roentgenol. 1980; 135:927–935.

13. Darling RC, Linton RR. Durability of femoropopliteal reconstructions. Endarterectomy versus vein bypass grafts. Am J Surg 1972; 123:472–479.

14. Horvath W, Oertl M, Haidinger D. Percutaneous transluminal angioplasty of crural arteries. Radiology 1990; 177:565–569.

15. Hanna GP, Fujise K, Kjellgren O, et al. Infrapopliteal transcatheter interventions for limb salvage in diabetic patients: importance of aggressive interventional approach and role of transcutaneous oximetry. J Am Coll Cardiol 1997; 30:664–669.

16. Bookstein JJ, Abrams H, Buenger R, et al. Radiologic aspects of renovascular hypertension. Part 2: the role of intravenous urography in unilateral renovascular disease. JAMA 1972; 220:1225–1230.

17. Lenz T, Kia T, Rupprecht G, Schulte KL, Geiger H. Captopril test: time over? J Hum Hypertens 1999; 13:431–435.

18. Olin JW, Novick AC. Renovascular disease. In: Young JR, et al., eds. Peripheral Vascular Diseases, 2nd ed. St. Louis: C.V. Mosby, 1996:321–342.

19. Leung DA, Hoffman U, Pfammatter T, et al. Magnetic resonance angiography versus duplex sonography for diagnosis renovascular disease. Hypertension 1999; 33:726–731.

20. Johnson PT, Halpern EJ, Kuszyk BS, et al. Renal artery stenosis: CT angiography-comparison of real-time volume-rendering and maximal intensity projection algorithms. Radiology 1999; 211:337–343.

21. vanJaarsveld BC, Pieterman H, vanDijk LC, et al. Inter-observer variability in the angiographic assessment of renal artery stenosis. J Hypertens 1999; 17:1731–1736.

22. Schreij G, deHaan MW, Oei TK, Koster D, deLeeuw PW. Interpretation of renal angiography by radiologists. J Hypertens 1999; 17:1737–1741.

23. Ramsay LR, Waller PC. Blood pressure response to percutaneous transluminal angioplasty for renovascular hypertension: an overview of published series. BMJ 1990; 300:569–572.

24. Losino F, Zuccala A, Busato F, Zucchelli P. Renal artery angioplasty for renovascular hypertension and preservation of renal function: long-term angiographic and clinical follow-up. Am J Roentgenol 1994; 162:853–857.

25. Jensen G, Zachrisson B-F, Denlin K, Volkmann R, Aurell M. Treatment of renovascular hypertension: one year results of renal angioplasty. Kidney Int 1995; 48:1936–1945.

26. Rundback JH, Jacobs JM. Percutaneous renal artery stent placement for hypertension and azotemia: pilot study. Am J Kidney Dis 1996; 28:214–219.

27. Gross CM, Jochen K, Waigand J, et al. Ostial renal artery stent placement for atherosclerotic renal artery stenosis in patients with coronary artery disease. Cathet Cardiovasc Diag 1998; 45:1–8.

28. Caps MT, Zierler RE, Polissar ML, et al. Risk of atrophy in kidneys with atherosclerotic renal artery stenosis. Kidney Int 1998; 53:735–742.

29. Hansen KJ, Starr SM, Sands RE, Burkhart JM, Plonk GWJ, Dean RH. Contemporary surgical management of renovascular disease. J Vasc Surg 1992; 16:319–330.

30. Novick AC, Pohl MA, Schreiber M, Gifford RWJ, Vidt DG. Revascularization for preservation of renal function in patients with atherosclerotic renovascular disease. J Urol 1983; 129:907–912.

31. Cambria RP, Brewster DC, L'Italien GJ, et al. The durability of different reconstructive techniques for atherosclerotic renal artery disease. J Vasc Surg 1994; 20: 76–87.

32. Novick AC, Ziegelbaum M, Vidt DT, Gifford RW, Pohl MA, Goormastic M. Trends in surgical revascularization for renal artery disease. JAMA 1987; 257:498–501.

33. Weibull H, Bergquist P, Bergentz SE, Jonsson K, Hulthen L, Manhem P. Percutaneous transluminal renal angioplasty versus surgical reconstruction of atherosclerotic renal artery stenosis: a prospective randomized study. J Vasc Surg 1993:841–852.

34. vanJaarsveld BC, Krijnen P, Pieterman H, et al. The effect of balloon angioplasty on hypertension in atherosclerotic renal artery stenosis. N Engl J Med 2000; 342: 1007–1014.

35. Harden PN, Macleod MJ, Rodger RSC, et al. Effect of renal artery stenting on progression of renovascular renal failure. Lancet 1997; 349:1133–1136.

36. Watson PS, Hadjipetrou P, Cox SV, Piemonte TC, Eisenhauer AC. Effect of renal artery stenting on renal function and size in patients with atherosclerotic renovascular disease. Circulation; in press.

37. Tyras DH, Barner HB. Coronary-subclavian steal. Arch Surg 1977; 112:1125–1127.

38. Editorial. A new vascular syndrome: "The subclavian steal." N Engl J Med 1961; 265:912.

39. Reivich M, Holling HE, Roberts B, et al. Reversal of blood flow through vertebral artery and its effects on cerebral circulation. N Engl J Med 1961; 265:878–885.

40. Smith JM, Koury HI, Hafner CD, et al. Subclavian steal syndrome—a review of 59 consecutive cases. J Cardiovasc Surg 1994; 35:11–14.

41. Breall JA, Kim D, Baim DS, Skillman JJ, Grossman W. Coronary-subclavian steal: an unusual cause of angina pectoris after successful internal mammary-coronary artery bypass grafting. Cathet Cardiovasc Diagn 1991; 24:274–276.

42. Granke K, Van Meter CH, Jr., White CJ, Ochsner JL, Hollier LH. Myocardial ischemia caused by postoperative malfunction of an internal mammary coronary artery graft. J Vasc Surgery 1990; 11:659–664.

43. Olsen CO, Dunton RF, Maggs PR, Lahey SJ. Review of coronary-subclavian steal following internal mammary artery—coronary artery bypass surgery. Ann Thorac Surg 1988; 46:675–678.

44. Ackermann H, Diener HC, Seboldt H, Huth C. Ultrasonographic follow-up of subclavian stenosis and occlusion: natural history and surgical treatment. Stroke 1988; 19:431–435.

45. Moran KT, Zide RS, Persson AV, et al. Natural history of subclavian steal syndrome. Am Surg 1988; 54:643–644.

46. Hadjipetrou P, Cox S, Piemonte T, Eisenhauer A. Percutaneous revascularization of atherosclerotic obstruction of aortic arch vessels [see comments]. J Am Coll Cardiol 1999; 33:1238–1245.

47. Al-Mubarak N, Liu MW, Dean LS, et al. Immediate and late outcomes of subclavian artery stenting. Cathet Cardiovasc Intervent 1999; 46:169–172.
48. Henry M, Amor M, Henry I, Ethevenot G, Tzvetanov K, Chati Z. Percutaneous transluminal angioplasty of the subclavian arteries. J Endovasc Surg 1999; 6:33–41.
49. Group TDTTS. A comparison of two doses of aspirin (30 mg vs. 283 mg a day) in patients after a transient ischemic attack or minor stroke. N Engl J Med 1991; 325:1261–1266.
50. Group ECST. Randomised trial of endarterectomy for recently symptomatic carotid stenosis: final results of the MRC European Carotid Surgery Trial (ECST). Lancet 1998; 351:1379–1387.
51. Collaborators NASCET. Beneficial effect of carotid endarterectomy in symptomatic patients with high-grade carotid stenosis. N Engl J Med 1991; 325:445–453.
52. Study ECftACA. Endarterectomy for asymptomatic carotid artery stenosis. J Am Med Assoc 1995; 273:1421–1428.
53. Wennberg DE, Lucas FL, Birkmeyer JD, et al. Variation in carotid endarterectomy mortality in the Medicare Population. Trial hospitals, volume and patient characteristics. J Am Med Assoc 1998; 279:1278–1281.
54. Cebul RD, Snow JS, Pine R, et al. Indications, outcomes, and provider volumes for carotid endarterectomy. J Am Med Assoc 1998; 279:1282–1287.
55. Roubin GS, Iyer SS, Vitek J. Carotid artery stenting: rationale, indications, technique. In: Heuser R, ed. Peripheral Vascular Stenting for Cardiologists. City: Martin Dunitz, 1999:67–117.
56. Yadav JS, Roubin GS, Iyer S, et al. Elective stenting of the extracranial carotid arteries. Circulation 1997; 95:376–381.
57. Wholey MH. Global carotid artery stent registry: updated results. Carotid Interven 1999; 1:94–96.
58. Wholey MH, Wholey M, Bergeron P, et al. Current global status of carotid artery stent placement. Cathet Cardiovasc Diagn 1998; 44:1–6.

12

Venous Thromboembolism: Clinical Impact and Multifactorial Etiology

Samuel Z. Goldhaber
*Brigham and Women's Hospital and Harvard Medical School,
Boston, Massachusetts*

Venous thromboembolism (VTE), which encompasses deep venous thrombosis (DVT) and pulmonary embolism (PE), is a major cardiovascular illness with an incidence in western countries of at least 1 per 1000 annually in adults.

I. INCIDENCE

In the Brest District of western France, with a defined population of 342,000 inhabitants, the incidence of VTE was 1.8 per 1000 per year (1). DVT without PE had an incidence of 1.2 per 1000 per year, whereas PE with or without DVT had an incidence of 0.6 per 1000 per year. VTE incidence increased markedly with increasing age for both men and women. For those over age 75 years, the incidence was 1 per 100 per year. VTE occurred at home in 63% of the population. Of those, 16% had been hospitalized within the previous 3 months.

In Olmsted County, a retrospective review of a population-based cohort showed an incidence of 1.2 per 10,000 per year (2). The incidence rose markedly with increasing age. The risk factors for VTE are attracting increasing attention (3) because of our improved understanding of the interaction among genetic, environmental, and medical factors that contribute to this condition.

II. CLINICAL IMPACT

PE is potentially fatal, with a high mortality rate when patients are assessed prospectively (4,5). The International CoOperative Pulmonary Embolism Registry (ICOPER) enrolled 2454 consecutive patients from 52 hospitals in 7 countries and is the largest prospective PE registry that has ever been published. In ICOPER, the mortality rate was 15% during the first 3 months after diagnosis; most deaths occurred during the first 2 weeks after diagnosis. Importantly, most patients who died had succumbed to PE, not to other comorbidities such as cancer. Age greater than 70 years increased the likelihood of death by 60%. Six other risk factors independently increased the likelihood of mortality by a factor of two- to threefold: cancer, clinical congestive heart failure, chronic obstructive pulmonary disease, systemic arterial hypotension with a systolic blood pressure of <90 mmHg, tachypnea (defined as >20 breaths per minute), and right ventricular hypokinesis on echocardiogram, an especially useful sign to identify high-risk patients who might be suitable for aggressive interventions such as thrombolysis or embolectomy. Nonfatal recurrent PE occurred in 4% of patients.

The Bounameaux Risk Score was developed using data from 296 PE patients (6). It predicts the risk of major adverse outcomes such as death, recurrent PE, and major bleeding. Six prognostic variables are considered: cancer, heart failure, prior DVT, hypotension, hypoxemia, and DVT on ultrasound. Patients receive a point score for each variable and an estimate of the likelihood of an adverse outcome (Table 1).

When PE is not fatal, it can cause chronic pulmonary hypertension with disabling fatigue and breathlessness. Especially troubling among survivors is the high rate of recurrent VTE after anticoagulation is discontinued. With long-term follow-up, as many as 30% of patients suffer recurrence (7) (Fig. 1). Risk factors for recurrence include idiopathic (as opposed to postoperative) DVT (8) as well as cancer and cardiopulmonary disease (9).

Table 1   (A) The Bounameaux
PE Risk Score

Variable	Point score
Cancer	+2
Heart failure	+1
Prior DVT	+1
Hypotension	+2
Hypoxemia	+1
DVT on ultrasound	+1

Table 1 (B) The Bounameaux PE Risk Score

Number of points	Number of patients	Cumulative (%)	Percent of patients with adverse outcome (n)
0	52	19.4	0 (0)
1	79	48.9	2.5 (2)
2	49	67.2	4.1 (2)
3	56	88.1	17.8 (10)
4	22	96.3	27.3 (6)
5	7	98.9	57.1 (4)
6	3	100	100 (3)

DVT often impairs quality of life by causing limb discomfort, especially calf swelling, tenderness, and aching. The post-thrombotic syndrome, also known as chronic venous insufficiency, occasionally causes skin discoloration and ulceration over the medial malleolus. In Olmsted County, the cumulative incidence of venous insufficiency was 14% over the first 5 years following acute VTE and 20% after 10 years (10). Among those patients less than 40 years of age, chronic venous insufficiency was three times more likely to develop if the clot involved the proximal leg veins rather than only the calf veins. The economic impact of

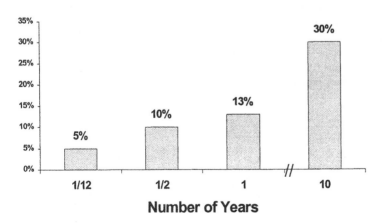

Figure 1 Rate of recurrent venous thromboembolism with long-term follow-up in Olmsted County. (Adapted with permission from Ref. 7.)

chronic venous insufficiency is considerable. The additional long-term health-care cost of the post-thrombotic syndrome is about 75% of the cost of initial management of acute DVT (11).

VTE also extracts a high psychological toll from patients stricken with this illness. They are often angered by delay in diagnosis and live with great uncertainty as to whether they will at some point suffer a recurrent event. They are concerned about the welfare of their children and siblings and, in the back of their minds, they often wonder about the possibility of an occult cancer that is lurking but as yet undetected (12).

III. MULTIFACTORIAL ETIOLOGY

Our paradigm for discerning the etiology of VTE has become more sophisticated as we recognize that those individuals predisposed to VTE may emerge with clinical disease when multiple risk factors are superimposed (Table 2). For exam-

Table 2   Major Risk Factors for VTE

Genetic
Factor V Leiden
Prothrombin gene mutation
Antithrombin-III deficiency
Protein C deficiency
Protein S deficiency
Mutations of cystathionine beta-synthase or methylene tetrahydrofo-
    late reductase (MTHFR)
Thrombophilic
Anticardiolipin antibodies (including lupus anticoagulant)
Hyperhomocysteinemia (usually due to folate deficiency)
High concentrations of Factor VIII and XI
Environmental
Obesity
Cigarette smoking
Immobility (including airline travel)
Medical Comorbidities
Increasing age
Pregnancy, oral contraceptives, and hormone replacement therapy
Cancer
Operation, especially neurosurgery
Trauma
Hypertension

ple, the risk of fatal PE increases in postoperative patients who are morbidly obese compared with other postoperative patients (13).

It appears that minor events—such as short periods of immobilization during travel, brief illness, or minor surgery or trauma—increase the risk of VTE by about threefold (14). Those who have minor events plus thrombophilia with genetic mutations such as factor V Leiden have an increased risk that is estimated at 17-fold. Asian Americans have about one-fifth the risk of VTE as black, Hispanic, or white Americans, based upon a study of more than 128,000 members of Kaiser-Permanente in Northern California (15). One of the main reasons is that Asian Americans as a group rarely carry the factor V Leiden or prothrombin gene mutation.

Environmental factors that predispose to VTE include obesity and cigarette smoking (16). Medical factors include systemic arterial hypertension, cancer, and surgery. Recently, a sevenfold increase in VTE has been found with exposure to conventional antipsychotic drugs. Risk seems most pronounced during the first 3 months of exposure. Ironically, VTE risk was higher for low-potency drugs such as chlorpromazine and thioridazine than for high-potency drugs such as haloperidol (17).

A. Thrombophilia

Whether to screen for genetic factors that predispose to VTE is controversial (18). The factor V Leiden (19) and prothrombin gene (20) mutations are autosomal dominant. They are associated with a severalfold increased risk of VTE. However, there may be a paradox with factor V Leiden (21). Those with this mutation and VTE may have less extensive thrombosis.

Well-designed studies have found conflicting results regarding the controversial issue of whether factor V Leiden predisposes to recurrent VTE after anticoagulation is discontinued (22,23). The prothrombin gene mutation is associated with an increased risk of recurrent VTE, especially in patients who have coinherited the factor V Leiden mutation (24–26).

High plasma levels of coagulation factors VIII and XI (27) are also risk factors for VTE. Recurrent VTE occurs more often in the presence of a high factor VIII plasma level (28).

Traditionally, patients with VTE were screened for deficiencies of antithrombin III, protein C, and protein S. However, this strategy is low-yield, with positive findings in fewer than 5% of patients. Furthermore, it may result in the diagnosis of spurious deficiencies. For example, heparin decreases the antithrombin-III level. Warfarin, pregnancy, and oral contraceptives decrease the protein C and S levels. Therefore, to assay for protein C and S, patients must not take warfarin for at least 3 to 4 weeks.

Screening for thrombophilia remains controversial. Nevertheless, in pa-

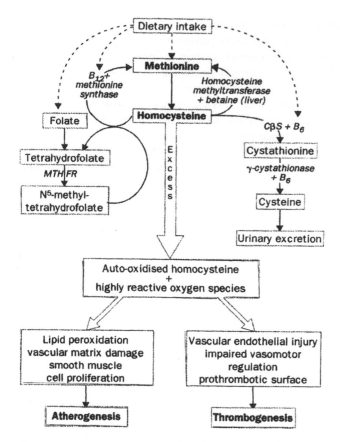

Figure 2 Homocysteine metabolism and possible mechanism of atherothrombotic disease. (Reprinted with permission from Ref. 30.)

tients with newly diagnosed VTE, I usually screen for factor V Leiden and the prothrombin gene mutation, which are more common than other inherited thrombophilias (29), as well as acquired hyperhomocysteinemia (Fig. 2) and anticardiolipin antibodies. Elevated levels of homocysteine are usually easily treated with folate (30,31), and the presence of anticardiolipin antibodies suggests the possible need for prolonged and intensive anticoagulation (32,33).

B. Cancer

Data from the Danish National Registry of Patients were used to investigate the risk of a diagnosis of cancer following the detection of VTE not associated with

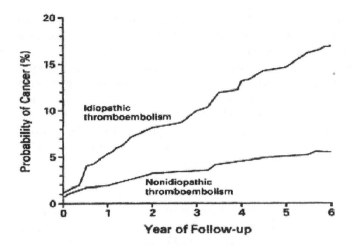

Figure 3 Cumulative probability of newly diagnosed cancer after a first VTE episode, according to whether the VTE was idiopathic or nonidiopathic. (Reprinted with permission from Ref. 35.)

surgery, known cancer, or pregnancy (34). There was a 30% increased risk of a diagnosis of cancer among those with newly detected VTE. The risk was substantially elevated only during the first 6 months of follow-up and declined rapidly thereafter. Of those diagnosed with cancer within 1 year after the initial VTE hospitalization, 40% had distant metastases at the time of the cancer diagnosis. The association between cancer and VTE was most pronounced for cancers of the pancreas, ovary, liver (primary hepatic cancer), and brain.

In the Swedish Cancer Registry, the risk of diagnosed cancer after a first episode of VTE was elevated during at least the following 2 years (35). The standardized incidence ratio for newly diagnosed cancer was 3.4 during the first year after VTE and remained between 1.3 and 2.2 for the following 5 years. Of the 854 patients with VTE, 534 had idiopathic VTE occurring in the absence of surgery, trauma, temporary immobilization, or oral contraceptive use. These were the patients in whom the association between VTE and the subsequent diagnosis of cancer was apparent (Fig. 3).

IV. WOMEN'S HEALTH

A. Generations of Oral Contraceptives

First-generation oral contraceptives contained more than 50 µg of estrogen and were associated with an alarming increase in the frequency of VTE, especially massive PE. Second-generation oral contraceptives contain less than 50 μg and were introduced in the United States in 1967. Eventually, in 1989, first-generation pills were withdrawn from the market.

Third-generation oral contraceptives utilize the new progestogens, desogestrel or gestodene. They cause acne and hirsutism less often and have a more favorable effect on carbohydrate metabolism and lipid profiles than second-generation pills. Ironically, they are associated with a doubling or tripling of the VTE rate compared with second-generation oral contraceptives (36,37). The explanation for this surprising finding is that third-generation oral contraceptives lead to acquired resistance to activated protein C, thus creating an effect similar to the factor V Leiden mutation (38).

Despite the high relative risk of VTE from oral contraceptives, the absolute risk is low. A New Zealand study of oral contraceptives and fatal PE estimated the absolute risk of death from PE in current users as 1 per 10.5 million woman-years. In this study, the risk of fatal PE was double among those taking third-generation pills (39).

B. Oral Contraceptives and Thrombophilia

Oral contraceptives and thrombophilia appear to interact synergistically to increase the risk of VTE. In a case-control study at Leiden University, women with the factor V Leiden mutation who used oral contraceptives were at a 35-fold greater risk of VTE than controls (40). In a subsequent analysis from the Leiden Thrombophilia Study, which included cases with factor V Leiden, protein C or S deficiency, the prothrombin gene 20210 A mutation, and antithrombin-III deficiency, the overall risk of developing DVT during the first 6 months of oral contraceptive use was increased 19-fold in thrombophilic women compared with controls (41).

Whether women with a family history of VTE but no personal past history of VTE should be screened prior to oral contraceptive use is controversial. For women with known thrombophilia but no prior VTE, the safest policy is to use alternative forms of contraception. However, no definitive ban on using oral contraceptives can be justified in this setting because the absolute risk of VTE remains very low.

C. Pregnancy

PE is the leading cause of maternal death in the United Kingdom. Beginning in the 1980s, the number of fatal PEs began to increase, especially following vaginal delivery. In the mid-1990s, about two-thirds of the fatal PEs classified as maternal deaths occurred postpartum, with cesarean section accounting for approximately half of these catastrophic events (42).

Two-thirds of DVT occur during pregnancy, and the remainder occur post-partum. The risk of DVT is present throughout pregnancy and increases during the third trimester. Of all antepartum DVT, about one-fifth occur during the first trimester, one-third during the second trimester, and almost one-half during the third trimester (43). After delivery, two of the most important risk factors for VTE are increased maternal age and cesarean section. Emergency cesarean section increases the VTE risk by about 50% compared with elective cesarean section.

Thrombophilia increases the risk of VTE during pregnancy and the puerperium. In a control study, the prevalence of factor V Leiden was 44% among women with a history of VTE during pregnancy or the puerperium, and the prevalence of the prothrombin gene mutation was 17%. Compared with controls, the Leiden mutation increased the risk of VTE ninefold, and the prothrombin gene mutation increased the risk by a factor of 15. The combination of the Leiden and prothrombin gene mutations virtually multiplied the risk, estimated to be 107 times greater than control. Fortunately, the absolute risk of VTE among carriers of each mutation was low: 0.2% for Leiden and 0.5% for the prothrombin gene. However, among those few women with both thrombophilic mutations, the absolute risk soared to 4.6% (44). Regardless of factor V Leiden, pregnancy itself causes hypercoagulability because it induces a relative state of activated protein C resistance.

Thrombophilia has also been implicated in otherwise unexplained recurrent pregnancy loss. The factor V Leiden mutation appears to double the risk of fetal loss, possibly because of an increased frequency of placental vein thrombosis (45,46). In addition to fetal demise, genetic thrombophilia appears to be associated with obstetrical complications, such as preeclampsia, abruptio placentae, fetal growth retardation, and stillbirth (47).

It has been common practice to prophylax with heparin those pregnant women who suffered a prior VTE. In a prospective study of 125 pregnant women with a single prior VTE, antepartum heparin was withheld but postpartum anticoagulation was administered for 4 to 6 weeks (48). Only 3 of the 125 women (2.4%) developed antepartum VTE. Thus, VTE during pregnancy may be less common in this population than had been previously thought.

D. Hormone Replacement Therapy

The traditional teaching used to be that hormone replacement therapy (HRT) does not predispose to VTE. In 1996, this assumption was challenged when three separate large data sets implicated HRT as doubling, tripling, or even quadrupling the risk of VTE (49–51). As with oral contraceptives, the risk of VTE was highest during the first year of HRT.

The Heart and Estrogen/progestin Replacement Study was a randomized trial of 2763 postmenopausal women who had a history of coronary heart disease but no previous VTE. They were allocated to conjugated equine estrogens, 0.625

mg, plus medroxyprogesterone acetate, 2.5 mg, versus placebo. In results that surprised the medical community, HRT did not reduce the rate of new coronary events (52). Furthermore, the rate of VTE tripled among those women receiving HRT (53). Certain subgroups were at especially high risk of increased VTE, including women with lower extremity fractures (18-fold increase), cancer (4-fold increase), postoperative state (5-fold increase), or nonsurgical hospitalization (6-fold increase). Women with factor V Leiden seem to be at especially high risk of VTE if they take HRT (54).

E. Selective Estrogen Receptor Modulators

An alternative to HRT is raloxifene, a selective estrogen receptor modulator that has estrogenic effects on bone, lipid metabolites, and blood clotting but an estrogen antagonist effect on breast tissue. In a randomized controlled trial of 7705 osteoporotic postmenopausal women, raloxifene decreased the risk of breast cancer by 75% and decreased the rate of vertebral fractures, as had been hoped, but it tripled the rate of VTE (55).

Tamoxifen, another selective estrogen receptor modulator, also acts as an estrogen agonist on bone and an estrogen antagonist on breast tissue. In the British Cancer Prevention Trial of women at high risk of breast cancer, 55 months of treatment with tamoxifen 20 mg daily halved the rate of breast cancer. However, the DVT rate increased by 60%, and the PE rate tripled (56).

V. CONCLUSIONS

In summary, VTE has enormous clinical impact. PE has a high mortality rate despite advances in therapy, and VTE has a high recurrence rate after anticoagulation is discontinued. DVT is often characterized by leg discomfort and postthrombotic venous insufficiency that adversely impacts the quality of life. Patients with VTE often feel like they have a sword dangling over them because this disease may be latent for many years and then recur. The etiologies of VTE are multifactorial, and we have arrived at an exciting juncture where we can identify with increasing sophistication predisposing genetic, environmental, and hormonal factors that contribute to the risk of this illness.

REFERENCES

1.   Oger E. Incidence of venous thromboembolism: a community-based study in Western France. EPI-GETBP Study Group. Groupe d'Etude de la Thrombose de Bretagne Occidentale. Thromb Haemost 2000; 83:657–660.

2. Silverstein MD, Heit JA, Mohr DN, Petterson TM, O'Fallon WM, Melton LJ, III. Trends in the incidence of deep vein thrombosis and pulmonary embolism: a 25-year population-based study. Arch Intern Med 1998; 158:585–593.

3. Heit JA, Silverstein MD, Mohr DN, Petterson TM, O'Fallon WM, Melton LJ, III. Risk factors for deep vein thrombosis and pulmonary embolism: a population-based case-control study. Arch Intern Med 2000; 160:809–815.

4. Goldhaber SZ, Visani L, De Rosa M, for ICOPER. Acute pulmonary embolism: Clinical outcomes in the International Cooperative Pulmonary Embolism Registry (ICOPER). Lancet 1999; 353:1386–1389.

5. Heit JA, Silverstein MD, Mohr DN, Petterson TM, O'Fallon WM, Melton LJ, III. Predictors of survival after deep vein thrombosis and pulmonary embolism: a population-based, cohort study. Arch Intern Med 1999; 159:445–453.

6. Wicki J, Perrier A, Perneger TV, Bounameaux H, Junod AF. Predicting adverse outcome in patients with acute pulmonary embolism: a risk score. Thromb Haemost 2000; 84:548–552.

7. Heit JA, Mohr DN, Silverstein MD, Petterson TM, O'Fallon WM, Melton LJ, III. Predictors of recurrence after deep vein thrombosis and pulmonary embolism: a population-based cohort study. Arch Intern Med 2000; 160:761–768.

8. Hansson PO, Sorbo J, Eriksson H. Recurrent venous thromboembolism after deep vein thrombosis: incidence and risk factors. Arch Intern Med 2000; 160:769–774.

9. Douketis JD, Foster GA, Crowther MA, Prins MH, Ginsberg JS. Clinical risk factors and timing of recurrent venous thromboembolism during the initial 3 months of anticoagulant therapy. Arch Intern Med 2000; 160:3431–3436.

10. Mohr DN, Silverstein MD, Heit JA, Petterson TM, O'Fallon WM, Melton LJ. The venous stasis syndrome after deep venous thrombosis or pulmonary embolism: a population-based study. Mayo Clin Proc 2000; 75:1249–1256.

11. Bergqvist D, Jendteg S, Johansen L, Persson U, Odegaard K. Cost of long-term complications of deep venous thrombosis of the lower extremities: an analysis of a defined patient population in Sweden. Ann Intern Med 1997; 126:454–457.

12. Walrath K, Berkovitz P, Morrison R, Goldhaber SZ. Frequently asked questions of the Venous Thromboembolism Support Group. Brigham and Women's Hospital. 1999. Available at: *http://web.mit.edu/karen/www/faq.html*)

13. Blaszyk H, Bjornsson J. Factor V Ieiden and morbid obesity in fatal postoperative pulmonary embolism. Arch Surg 2000; 135:1410–1413.

14. Eekhoff EM, Rosendaal FR, Vandenbroucke JP. Minor events and the risk of deep venous thrombosis. Thromb Haemost 2000; 83:408–411.

15. Klatsky AL, Armstrong MA, Poggi J. Risk of pulmonary embolism and/or deep venous thrombosis in Asian-Americans. Am J Cardiol 2000; 85:1334–1337.

16. Goldhaber SZ, Grodstein F, Stampfer MJ, Manson JE, Colditz GA, Speizer FE et al. A prospective study of risk factors for pulmonary embolism in women. JAMA 1997; 277:642–645.

17. Zornberg GL, Jick H. Antipsychotic drug use and risk of first-time idiopathic venous thromboembolism: a case-control study. Lancet 2000; 356:1219–1223.

18. Guidelines on diagnosis and management of acute pulmonary embolism. Task Force on Pulmonary Embolism, European Society of Cardiology. Eur Heart J 2000; 21:1301–1336.

19. Price DT, Ridker PM. Factor V Leiden mutation and the risks for thromboembolic disease: A clinical perspective. Ann Intern Med 1997; 127:895–903.
20. Nguyen A. Prothrombin G20210A polymorphism and thrombophilia. Mayo Clin Proc 2000; 75:595–604.
21. Bounameaux H. Factor V Leiden paradox: risk of deep-vein thrombosis but not of pulmonary embolism. Lancet 2000; 356:182–183.
22. Ridker PM, Miletich JP, Stampfer MJ, Goldhaber SZ, Lindpaintner K, Hennekens CH. Factor V Leiden and risks of recurrent idiopathic venous thromboembolism. Circulation 1995; 92:2800–2802.
23. Simioni P, Prandoni P, Lensing AWA, Scudeller A, Sardella C, Prins MH, Villalta S, Dazzi F, Girolami A. The risk of recurrent venous thromboembolism in patients with an Arg^{506}® Gln mutation in the gene for factor V (factor V Leiden). N Engl J Med 1997; 336:399–403.
24. Margaglione M, D'Andrea G, Colaizzo D, Cappucci G, del Popolo A, Brancaccio V et al. Coexistence of factor V Leiden and Factor II A20210 mutations and recurrent venous thromboembolism. Thromb Haemost 1999; 82:1583–1587.
25. De S, V, Martinelli I, Mannucci PM, Paciaroni K, Chiusolo P, Casorelli I et al. The risk of recurrent deep venous thrombosis among heterozygous carriers of both factor V Leiden and the G20210A prothrombin mutation. N Engl J Med 1999; 341:801–806.
26. Miles JS, Miletich JP, Goldhaber SZ, Hennekens CH, Ridker PM. G20210A Mutation in the prothrombin gene and the risk of recurrent venous thromboembolism. JACC 2001; 37:1–4.
27. Meijers JC, Tekelenburg WL, Bouma BN, Bertina RM, Rosendaal FR. High levels of coagulation factor XI as a risk factor for venous thrombosis. N Engl J Med 2000; 342:696–701.
28. Kyrle PA, Minar E, Hirschl M, Bialonczyk C, Stain M, Schneider B et al. High plasma levels of factor VIII and the risk of recurrent venous thromboembolism. N Engl J Med 2000; 343:457–462.
29. Rosendaal FR. Venous thrombosis: a multicausal disease. Lancet 1999; 353:1167–1173.
30. Hankey GJ, Eikelboom JW. Homocysteine and vascular disease. Lancet 1999; 354:407–413.
31. Langman LJ, Ray JG, Evrovski J, Yeo E, Cole DE. Hyperhomocyst(e)inemia and the increased risk of venous thromboembolism: more evidence from a case-control study. Arch Intern Med 2000; 160:961–964.
32. Greaves M. Antiphospholipid antibodies and thrombosis. Lancet 1999; 353:1348–1353.
33. Schulman S, Svenungsson E, Granqvist S. Anticardiolipin antibodies predict early recurrence of thromboembolism and death among patients with venous thromboembolism following anticoagulant therapy. Duration of Anticoagulation Study Group. Am J Med 1998; 104:332–338.
34. Sorensen HT, Mellemkjaer L, Steffensen FH, Olsen JH, Nielsen GL. The risk of a diagnosis of cancer after primary deep venous thrombosis or pulmonary embolism. N Engl J Med 1998; 338:1169–1173.
35. Schulman S, Lindmarker P. Incidence of cancer after prophylaxis with warfarin

against recurrent venous thromboembolism. Duration of Anticoagulation Trial. N Engl J Med 2000; 342:1953–1958.

36. Chasan-Taber L, Stampfer MJ. Epidemiology of oral contraceptives and cardiovascular disease. Ann Intern Med 1998; 128: 467–477.

37. Jick H, Kaye JA, Vasilakis-Scaramozza C, Jick SS. Risk of venous thromboembolism among users of third generation oral contraceptives compared with users of oral contraceptives with levonorgestrel before and after 1995: cohort and case-control analysis. BMJ 2000; 321:1190–1195.

38. Rosing J, Middeldorp S, Curvers J, Thomassen MCLGD, Nicolaes GAF, Meijers JCM, Bouma BN, Büller HR, Prins MH, Tans G. Low-dose oral contraceptives and acquired resistance to activated protein C: A randomized cross-over study. Lancet 1999; 354:2036–2040.

39. Parkin L, Skegg DCG, Wilson M, Herbison GP, Paul C. Oral contraceptives and fatal pulmonary embolism. Lancet 2000; 355:2133–2134.

40. Vandenbroucke JP, Koster T, Briët E, Reitsma PH, Bertina RM, Rosendaal FR. Increased risk of venous thrombosis in oral-contraceptive users who are carriers of factor V Leiden mutation. Lancet 1994; 344:1453–1457.

41. Bloemenkamp KWM, Rosendaal FR, Helmerhorst FM, Vandenbroucke JP. Higher risk of venous thrombosis during early use of oral contraceptives in women with inherited clotting defects. Arch Intern Med 2000; 160:49–52.

42. Greer IA. Thrombosis in pregnancy: maternal and fetal issues. Lancet 1999; 353: 1258–1265.

43. Ray JG, Chan WS. Deep vein thrombosis during pregnancy and the puerperium: A meta-analysis of the period of risk and the leg of presentation. Obstet Gynecol Surv 1999; 54:265–271.

44. Gerhardt A, Scharf RE, Beckmann MW, Struve S, Bender HG, Pillny M, Sandmann W, Zotz RB. Prothrombin and factor V mutations in women with a history of thrombosis during pregnancy and the puerperium. N Engl J Med 2000; 342:374–380.

45. Ridker PM, Miletich JP, Buring JE, Ariyo AA, Price DT, Manson JE, Hill JA. Factor V Leiden mutation as a risk factor for recurrent pregnancy loss. Ann Intern Med 1998; 128:1000–1003.

46. Meinardi JR, Middeldorp S, de Kam PJ, Koopman MMW, van Pampus ECM, Hamulyák K, Prins MH, Büller HR, van der Meer J. Increased risk for fetal loss in carriers of the factor V Leiden mutation. Ann Intern Med 1999; 130:736–739.

47. Kupferminc MJ, Eldor A, Steinman N, Many A, Bar-Am A, Jaffa A, Fait G, Lessing JB. Increased frequency of genetic thrombophilia in women with complications of pregnancy. N Engl J Med 1999; 340:9–13.

48. Brill-Edwards P, Ginsberg JS, Gent M, Hirsh J, Burrows R, Kearon C et al. Safety of withholding heparin in pregnant women with a history of venous thromboembolism. N Engl J Med 2000; 343:1439–1444.

49. Daly E, Vessey MP, Hawkins MM, Carson JL, Gough P, Marsh S. Risk of venous thromboembolism in users of hormone replacement therapy. Lancet 1996; 348:977–980.

50. Jick H, Derby LE, Myers MW, Vasilakis C, Newton KM. Risk of hospital admission for idiopathic venous thromboembolism among users of postmenopausal oestrogens. Lancet 1996; 348:981–983.

51. Grodstein F, Stampfer MJ, Goldhaber SZ, Manson JE, Colditz GA, Speizer FE, Willett WC, Hennekens CH. Prospective study of exogenous hormones and risk of pulmonary embolism in women. Lancet 1996; 348:983–987.

52. Hulley C, Grady D, Bush T, et al. Randomized trial of estrogen plus progestin for secondary prevention of coronary heart disease in postmenopausal women. Heart and Estrogen/progestin Replacement Study (HERS) Research Group. JAMA 1998; 280:605–613.

53. Grady D, Wenger NK, Herrington D, Khan S, Furberg C, Hunninghake D, Vittingh-off E, Hulley S, for the Heart and Estrogen/progestin Replacement Study Research Group. Postmenopausal hormone therapy increases risk for venous thromboembolic disease. The Heart and Estrogen/progestin Replacement Study. Ann Intern Med 2000; 132:689–696.

54. Lowe G, Woodward M, Vessey M, et al. Thrombotic variables and risk of idiopathic venous thromboembolism in women aged 45–64 years. Relationships to hormone replacement therapy. Thromb Haemost 2000; 83:530–535.

55. Cummings SR, Eckert S, Krueger KA, Grady D, Powles TJ, Cauley JA, Norton L, Nickelsen T, Bjarnason NH, Morrow M, Lippman ME, Black D, Glusman JE, Costa A, Jordan VC. The effect of raloxifene on risk of breast cancer in postmenopausal women: results from the MORE randomized trial. Multiple Outcomes of Raloxifene Evaluation. JAMA 1999; 281:2189–2197.

56. Fisher B, Costantino JP, Wickerham L, et al. Tamoxifen for the prevention of breast cancer: report of the National Surgical Adjuvant Breast and Bowel Project P-1 Study. J Natl Cancer Inst 1998; 90:1371–1388.

13

Integrated Diagnostic Approach to Venous Thromboembolism

Henri Bounameaux
University Hospital of Geneva and Geneva School of Medicine, Geneva, Switzerland

Diagnosis of deep vein thrombosis (DVT) depends mainly upon three clinical tools: venous compression ultrasonography (US), assessment of prior clinical probability (PCP), and measurement of fibrin D-Dimer (DD). In suspected pulmonary embolism (PE), the same tools can be applied, in addition to ventilation/perfusion lung scan (V/Q scan). In a few patients, venography (suspected DVT) or pulmonary angiography (suspected PE) may also be required.

I. BRIEF DESCRIPTION OF THE DIAGNOSTIC TOOLS

Today venous compression ultrasonography (US) is the key diagnostic tool in patients with a first episode of clinically suspected DVT. The sensitivity and specificity exceed 90% for proximal DVT (1). The corresponding values are definitely less (50% or less) for isolated distal DVT. Although these results may be superior in experienced hands, they clearly highlight the need for integrating the US result in a comprehensive approach.

A crucial issue in this regard is clinical assessment, which can be made either by means of a standardized Wells score (2) or in an empirical way (3). These two means have been compared in the case of suspected DVT (4). Both the Wells score and the empirical evaluation can triage patients into a low, intermediate, or high clinical probability category. However, the empirical method performed slightly better in categorizing patients in the high-probability class, while the Wells score categorized more patients in the low-probability class.

Because of the very high sensitivity of some DD tests to the presence of DVT and PE, they can be used alone or in combination with other findings (US or clinical probability) to exclude venous thrombosis with a high negative predictive value (5). The rapid tests that have been validated in large patient populations include a rapid ELISA (VIDAS DD from bioMerieux), an automated turbidimetric method (LIA test from Diagnostica STAGO), and the whole blood latex test SimpliRED (from AGEN). Table 1 gives a summary of the performances of these commercial tests. Other rapid tests (Turbiquant, Tinaquant, MDA D-Dimer) are currently undergoing intensive clinical investigation.

Ventilation/perfusion lung scanning has been investigated in the large PIOPED study (6), which defined clear interpretation categories. Briefly, while a normal/near-normal perfusion scan virtually rules out PE, a high-probability ventilation/perfusion pattern allows one to diagnose PE. Low-probability and intermediate-probability categories were also defined, but are considered in most centers as nondiagnostic patterns.

In recent years, interest has developed in using spiral computed tomography (CT) for PE diagnosis. Two systematic reviews have independently and simultaneously concluded that this new technique has not been adequately evaluated (7,8) and that additional research is required to establish its place in clinical practice. In particular, sensitivity of spiral CT to the presence of PE appears to be lower than anticipated from the initial studies, especially if the embolus is located in subsegmental vessels.

Gold standards for DVT and PE diagnosis are ascending venography and pulmonary angiography, respectively. Both exams are invasive, costly, and not devoid of risk. Moreover, their interpretation may be equivocal, as interobserver agreement is far from optimal. The aim of any diagnostic strategy is to reduce the number of invasive exams without increasing the number of false diagnoses.

Table 1 Comparison of Three Rapid DD Tests for Diagnosing DVT and/or PE

DD test	Patients with DVT and/or PE (n)	Sensitivity (%, 95% CI)	Specificity (%, 95% CI)
VIDAS DD	1311, 305	98.7 (96.7–99.6)	39.6 (36.5–42.6)
LIA test	971, 310	99.4 (97.7–99.9)	39.6 (35.9–43.4)
SimpliRED	2393, 489	90.2 (87.2–92.7)	68.5 (66.5–70.6)

DD, D-dimer, DVT, deep vein thrombosis; PE, pulmonary embolism; 95% CI, 95% confidence interval.

II. BACKGROUND OF DIAGNOSTIC STRATEGIES IN SUSPECTED DVT AND PE

Contemporary diagnostic strategies have been formulated according to two main observations. First, while more than 50% of suspected patients had confirmed DVT or PE in the early 1980s, this figure has decreased to 35% in the early 1990s and 20% in the late 1990s. This decrease in diagnostic yield most likely reflects heightened clinical awareness of practitioners to the presence and danger of venous thromboembolism. On the other hand, this trend means that the majority of patients referred to a diagnostic center for evaluation will have the disorder excluded rather than confirmed. Second, because DVT and PE are now recognized as two clinical manifestations of a single disease, treatment algorithms and diagnostic protocols have been streamlined.

As a consequence of these two observations, the first diagnostic step should ideally be highly sensitive in order to detect the disease in a substantial proportion of suspected patients. On the other hand, diagnosing DVT in a patient suspected of PE suffices to rule in venous thromboembolism and to indicate anticoagulant treatment.

The evaluation of a diagnostic tool or strategy culminates in management trials or outcome studies in which the overall clinical strategy is applied. The outcome at 3 or 6 months of follow-up is subsequently surveyed to determine thromboembolic events that might have occurred in patients in whom anticoagulant treatment had been withheld on the basis of a negative diagnostic workup (9).

III. DIAGNOSTIC STRATEGIES IN SUSPECTED DVT

Table 2 compares four recently proposed management strategies (2,3,10,11). One Italian study relies on serial US (10) (i.e., repetition of compression US after 1 week in all patients with no DVT on the initial exam). A second Italian study relies on serial US restricted to patients with a normal initial US and an abnormal DD result (rapid latex test) (11). In the third strategy, serial US was restricted to patients with a non-low-prior clinical probability (PCP) (2). In the fourth algorithm, a single US was performed in patients with a DD result above the critical cutoff (rapid ELISA method) (3), with PCP allowing the identification of patients requiring venography (those with a high PCP, a positive DD, and a negative US).

These four strategies were assessed in management trials with long-term (at least 3-month) follow-up. In the three trials in which DD (11), PCP (2), or both (3) were added to the initial US exam, the proportion of patients requiring a repeat US exam at 1 week was reduced from 76% in the study relying on US

Table 2 Comparison of Four Validated Diagnostic Strategies in Patients Clinically Suspected of DVT

Tool/strategy	Cogo et al. (10) RUS	Bernardi et al. (11) RUS + DD	Wells et al. (2) RUS + PCP	Perrier et al. (3) US + DD + PCP
Patients (n)	1702	946	593	474
DVT prevalence	24%	28%	16%	24%
PCP assessment	—	—	score	empirical
DD test	—	Instant-IA	—	Vidas DD
Patients with US (n, %)	1702 (100%)	946 (100%)	593 (100%)	346 (73%)
Patients with RUS (n, %)	1302 (76%)	88 (9%)	166 (28%)	0
Yield of RUS	0.9%	5.7%	1.8%	—
Venography (n, %)	0	0	33 (6%)	2 (0.4%)
3-month VTE risk [% (95% CI)]	0.7% (0.3–1.2)	0.4% (0–0.9)	0.6% (0.1–1.8)	2.6% (0.2–4.9)

VTE, venous thromboembolism; DVT, deep vein thrombosis; FU, follow-up; US, compression ultrasonography; RUS, repeat US. (Instant-IA and Vidas DD are D-dimer tests marketed by Stago, Asnières, France, and bioMérieux, Lyon, France, respectively.)

alone (10) to 9% when adding DD latex test (11), 28% when adding PCP (2), or 0% when adding DD ELISA test and PCP assessment (3) (Table 2).

Compression venous US appears to be the key diagnostic tool in outpatients clinically suspected of DVT. However, because the prevalence of DVT in the suspected population is quite low (approximately 20%), using a highly sensitive DD (ELISA) test as an initial screening would reduce the number of initial US exams by one-fourth to one-third. Alternatively, PCP or DD may be used to diminish the number of repeat US. However, the principle of repeat US after 1 week to pick up undiagnosed distal DVT that would have extended proximally, albeit very attractive at a first glance, has a low yield and is not cost effective (12). Last, the 3-month thromboembolic risk in these four studies (13) (Table 2) was low and comparable to the 1.9% (95% CI; 0.4–5.4%) observed in clinically suspected patients followed up after a negative venogram (14). Of note, these results were obtained by means of a compression US technique limited to the examination of the common and superficial femoral and popliteal veins. This at least questions the affirmation by some investigators that a complete, more time-consuming venous US examination (from the calf to the inferior vena cava) should be performed in all patients clinically suspected of DVT (15).

IV. DIAGNOSTIC STRATEGIES IN SUSPECTED PE

Recently, two sequential, mainly noninvasive strategies were applied in large cohorts of patients with suspected PE (3,16). They are based on PCP, assessed empirically (3) or by means of a clinical model (16); on a rapid DD ELISA test (3); on venous compression US (3,16); on a V/Q lung scan (3,16); and, in some cases, on pulmonary angiography. These strategies are depicted in Figures 1 and

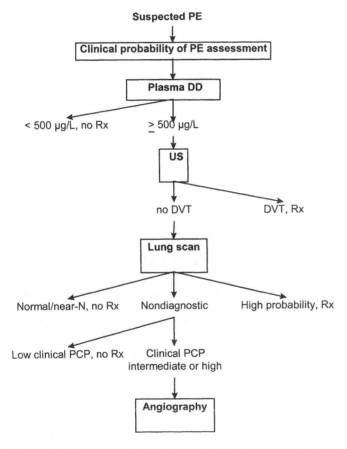

Figure 1 Diagnostic algorithm for suspected pulmonary embolism. PE, pulmonary embolism; US, lower limb venous ultrasonography; DVT, deep vein thrombosis; PCP, prior clinical probability; near-N, near-normal; Rx, treatment; no Rx, no treatment. (From Ref. 3.)

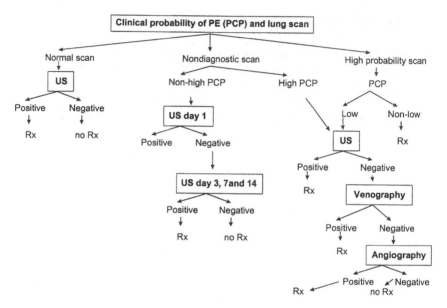

Figure 2 Diagnostic algorithm for suspected pulmonary embolism. PE, pulmonary embolism; US, lower limb venous ultrasonography; DVT, deep vein thrombosis; PCP, prior clinical probability; near-N, near-normal; Rx, treatment; no Rx, no treatment. (From Ref. 16.)

2. The 3-month thromboembolic risks that were associated with these algorithms were 0.9% (95% CI; 0.2–2.7%) (3) or 0.5% (95% CI; 0.1–1.3%) (16), respectively. Pulmonary angiography had to be performed in 11% (3) or 4% (16) of patients. These strategies allow the management of the majority of patients with widely available, noninvasive diagnostic tools. In a third, smaller Dutch study, a sequential strategy of ventilation/perfusion lung scan, rapid whole-blood DD test SimpliRED, US, and pulmonary angiography was used. The 3-month thromboembolic risk was 2.5% (95% CI; 0.5–7.1%) in the 121 patients in whom anticoagulant treatment had been withheld on the basis of a normal perfusion or a nondiagnostic lung scan pattern associated with a negative SimpliRED DD test. (17).

Finally, in a secondary analysis of a database of 1034 consecutive patients referred to a diagnostic center with clinically suspected PE, the diagnosis could be ruled out by the combination of a low clinical probability and a nondiagnostic lung scan (i.e., abnormal but non-high-probability pattern), provided no proximal DVT had been detected on US exam. This combination was present in 175 patients of the cohort (22%), and was safe to rule out PE since the 3-month thromboembolic risk was only 1.7% (95% CI; 0.4–4.9%) (18).

Because these strategies have a similar efficacy, the less resource-intensive strategy depicted in Figure 2 (3) is likely to be the most cost-effective one. However, formal cost-effectiveness studies comparing them are not yet available.

V. SCOPE AND LIMITATIONS OF THE PROPOSED INTEGRATED APPROACH

The strategies described above can be combined in a single, integrated algorithm (Fig. 3) that is, however, suitable for patients with clinical symptoms and/or signs of venous thromboembolism who are referred to an outpatient clinic or an emergency ward for ruling in/out the disease. It is not suited for patients who are hospitalized in medical or surgical wards for longer periods of time, nor is

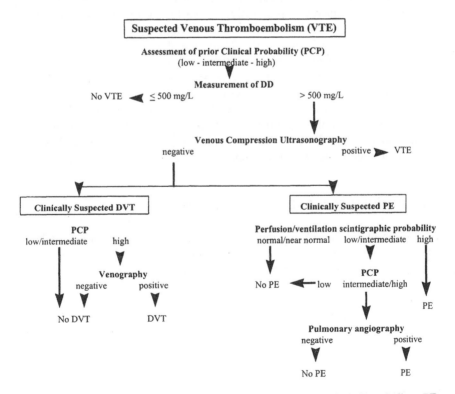

Figure 3   Integrated diagnostic algorithm for suspected venous thromboembolism. PE, pulmonary embolism; US, lower limb venous ultrasonography; DVT, deep vein thrombosis; PCP, prior clinical probability. (From Ref. 3.)

it suitable for patients who present with hemodynamic instability. In the latter case, the problem is therapeutic rather than diagnostic; moreover, emergency treatment (e.g., thrombolysis or embolectomy) must be considered in these patients without delay. Thus, echocardiography and/or spiral CT may be first-line diagnostic tools, because in this situation signs of right heart dysfunction or presence of proximal emboli are very likely to be present.

On the other hand, patients who are hospitalized in medical or surgical wards for more than 24 h are unlikely to present with DD concentrations below the critical cutoff due to comorbidities. Thus, in a diagnostic study of suspected PE in hospitalized patients, the yield of a negative DD result was very low (about 5%) (19), which at least questions its utility in this category of patients.

Last, age considerably influences the performance of all diagnostic tools (20). In an analysis of two large outcome studies that enrolled 1029 consecutive outpatients presenting in the emergency ward with clinically suspected pulmonary embolism (prevalence of pulmonary embolism 27%), the prevalence of pulmonary embolism increased progressively from 12% below age 40 to 44% above age 80. The positive predictive value of a high clinical probability of pulmonary embolism was higher in the elderly (71 to 78% above 60 vs. 40 to 64% below 60). Sensitivity of DD testing was 100% in all age subgroups, but specificity decreased markedly with age, from 67% below age 40 to 10% above age 80. The diagnostic yield of lower limb venous compression US was higher in the elderly [46% (95% CI; 26–67%) below 40 vs. 56% (95% CI; 44–68%) above 80]. The proportion of diagnostic (normal/near-normal or high probability) lung scans also decreased from 68% to 42% with increasing age. This variable should be kept in mind in the diagnostic approach of this disease.

VI. CONCLUSION AND PERSPECTIVES

Diagnosing DVT and PE has improved over the past 15 years primarily due to the development of venous compression ultrasound of the lower limbs and D-dimer measurement. If carefully applied, these strategies can reduce the need for venography and pulmonary angiography to less than 10% of patients evaluated and thus are likely to be cost effective. These newer diagnostic strategies should thus be implemented in daily practice, taking into account local facilities and expertise (21). In the near future, spiral CT might be included in the diagnostic approach of PE, but its exact place remains to be determined.

REFERENCES

1. Kearon C, Julian JA, Math M, Newman TE, Ginsberg JS. Noninvasive diagnosis of deep venous thrombosis. Ann Intern Med 1998; 128:663–677.

2. Wells PS, Anderson DR, Bormanis J, Guy F, Mitchell M, Gray L, Clement C, Robinson KS, Lewandowski B. Value of assessment of pretest probability of deep-vein thrombosis in clinical management. Lancet 1997; 350:1795–1798.

3. Perrier A, Desmarais S, Miron MJ, de Moerloose P, Lepage R, Slosman D, Didier D, Unger PF, Patenaude JV, Bounameaux H. Noninvasive diagnosis of venous thromboembolism in outpatients. Lancet 1999; 353:190–195.

4. Miron MJ, Perrier A, Bounameaux H. Clinical assessment of suspected deep vein thrombosis: comparison between a score and empirical assessment. J Intern Med 2000; 247:249–254.

5. Bounameaux H, de Moerloose P, Perrier A, Miron MJ. D-dimer testing in suspected venous thromboembolism: an update. Q J Med 1997; 90:437–442.

6. The PIOPED Investigators. Value of the ventilation/perfusion scan in acute pulmonary embolism. Results of the Prospective Investigation of Pulmonary Embolism Diagnosis (PIOPED). JAMA 1990; 263:2753–2759.

7. Rathbun SW, Raskob GE, Whitsett TL. Sensitivity and specificity of helical computed tomography in the diagnosis of pulmonary embolism: a systematic review. Ann Intern Med 2000; 132:227–232.

8. Mullins MD, Becker DM, Hagspiel KD, Philbrick JT. The role of spiral volumetric computed tomography in the diagnosis of pulmonary embolism. Arch Intern Med 2000; 160:293–298.

9. Büller HR, Lensing AWA, Hirsh J, tenCate JW. Deep vein thrombosis: new non-invasive diagnostic tests. Thromb Haemost 1991; 66:133–137.

10. Cogo A, Lensing AWA, Koopman MMW, Piovella F, Siragusa S, Wells PS, Villalta S, Büller HR, Turpie AGG, Prandoni P. Compression ultrasonography for diagnostic management of patients with clinically suspected deep vein thrombosis: prospective cohort study. BMJ 1998; 316:17–20.

11. Bernardi E, Prandoni P, Lensing AWA, Agnelli G, Guazzaloca G, Scannapieco G, Piovella F, Verlato F, Tomasi C, Moia M, Scarano L, Girolami A. D-dimer testing as an adjunct to ultrasonography in patients with clinically suspected deep vein thrombosis: prospective cohort study. BMJ 1998; 317:1037–1040.

12. Perone N, Bounameaux H, Perrier A. Comparison of four strategies for diagnosing deep vein thrombosis: a cost-effectiveness analysis. Am J Med 2001; 110:33–40.

13. Bounameaux H, Perrier A. Rapid diagnosis of deep vein thrombosis: a comparison between four strategies. Thromb Haemost 1999; 82:1360–1361.

14. Hull R, Hirsh J, Sackett DL, Taylor DW, Carter C, Turpie AGG, Powers P, Gent M. Clinical validity of a negative venogram in patients with clinically suspected venous thrombosis. Circulation 1981; 64:622–625.

15. Gena Frederick M, Hertzberg BS, Kliewer MA, Paulson EK, Bowie JD, Lalouche KJ, DeLong DM, Carroll BA. Can the US examination for lower extremity deep venous thrombosis be abbreviated? A prospective study of 755 examinations. Radiology 1996; 199:45–47.

16. Wells PS, Ginsberg JS, Anderson DR, Kearon C, Gent M, Turpie AGG, Bormanis J, Weitz J, Chamberlain M, Bowie D, Barnes D, Hirsh J. Use of a clinical model for safe management of patients with suspected pulmonary embolism. Ann Intern Med 1998; 129:997–1005.

17. de Groot MR, van Marwijk Kooy M, Pouwels JG, Engelage AH, Kuipers BF, Büller

HR. The use of a rapid D-dimer blood test in the diagnostic work-up for pulmonary embolism: a management study. Thromb Haemost 1999; 82:1588–1592.

18. Miron MJ, Perrier A, Bounameaux H, de Moerloose P, Slosman D, Didier D, Junod A. Contribution of noninvasive evaluation to the diagnosis of pulmonary embolism in hospitalized patients. Eur Resp J 1999; 13:1365–1370.

19. Perrier A, Miron MJ, Desmarais S, de Moerloose P, Slosman D, Didier D, Unger PF, Junod A, Patenaude JV, Bounameaux H. Using clinical evaluation and lung scan to rule out suspected pulmonary embolism: Is it a valid option in patients with normal results of lower-limb venous compression ultrasonography? Arch Intern Med 2000; 160:512–516.

20. Righini M, Goehring C, Bounameaux H, Perrier A. Influence of age on performances of common diagnostic tests in suspected pulmonary embolism. Am J Med 2000; 109:357–361.

21. Fennerty T. Pulmonary embolism. Hospitals should develop their own strategies for diagnosis and management. BMJ 1998; 317:791–792.

14

The Management of Massive Pulmonary Embolism

Jeremy P. Feldman
University of California at San Francisco, San Francisco, California

Samuel Z. Goldhaber
Brigham and Women's Hospital and Harvard Medical School, Boston, Massachusetts

Venous thromboembolism (VTE) remains a leading cause of cardiovascular morbidity and mortality. The disease encompasses a spectrum of disorders including distal calf vein thrombosis, proximal deep vein thrombosis, asymptomatic pulmonary embolism, hemodynamically stable symptomatic pulmonary embolism without right ventricular dysfunction, impending hemodynamically unstable pulmonary embolism with right ventricular dysfunction, and hemodynamically unstable massive pulmonary embolism. This chapter will focus on massive and submassive pulmonary embolism.

I. DEFINITION

Massive pulmonary embolism is accompanied by hemodynamic instability. Submassive disease is associated with moderate or severe right ventricular dysfunction on echocardiography.

II. PATHOGENESIS AND PATHOPHYSIOLOGY

Virchow described three factors involved in the genesis of VTE: stasis, endothelial injury, and hypercoagulability. These remain the major culprits. Progress has come in our understanding of the myriad genetic thrombophilias. Clots formed in the lower extremity veins (and occasionally the upper extremities) may propagate proximally and embolize to the pulmonary vasculature. In the lungs, platelets, vascular endothelium, and fibrin interact to increase pulmonary vascular resistance due to loss of cross-sectional area of the pulmonary vascular tree, atelectasis, and bronchoconstriction (1,2). Imbalances result in ventilation-perfusion mismatching, largely due to changes in regional perfusion that cause hypoxia, and potentially right ventricular pressure overload, right-to-left shunting, and hypotension. Right ventricular ischemia and bulging of the right ventricular septum into the left ventricle have also been shown in animal models to contribute to the hemodynamic effects of massive pulmonary embolism (3,4).

III. PROSPECTIVE REGISTRY

The International Cooperative Pulmonary Embolism Registry, a prospective study of 2454 consecutive patients from 52 centers in seven countries, found that 88.9% of patients are symptomatic and hemodynamically stable; 4.2% of patients presented in shock. Furthermore, of the patients undergoing echocardiography, 40% had right ventricular hypokinesis. The all-cause mortality rate of 11.4% at 2 weeks was highly correlated with more severe characteristics on presentation. Hemodynamically unstable patients had a 58.3% mortality rate compared with 15.1% for patients who were stable at presentation (5).

IV. CLINICAL PRESENTATION

The clinical presentation of massive and submassive pulmonary embolism is highly variable. In MAPPET (6), a multicenter registry that enrolled 1001 patients from 204 centers with massive or submassive pulmonary embolism, dyspnea was a near universal finding. Acute onset of symptoms and tachycardia were present in almost 70% of patients. One-third of patients presented with syncope. A variety of other findings may accompany massive pulmonary embolism (Table 1).

An important presentation in the emergency department is the patient with cardiopulmonary symptoms and an elevated troponin level. Although the majority of patients with markers of cardiac injury will have acute coronary syndromes, pulmonary embolism may also cause this abnormality (7). The mechanism is thought to be related to right ventricular ischemia due to acute dilatation (8). Additionally, patients with elevated troponin levels are more likely to have electrocardiographic findings suggestive of pulmonary embolism, including right-bundle branch block and precordial T-wave abnormalities (9).

Table 1 Physical Findings in
Massive Pulmonary Embolism

Finding
Tachycardia
Fever
Distended neck veins
Tricuspid regurgitation
Right-sided heave
Right-sided S3
S1Q3T3
Right bundle branch block
Anterior precordial T-wave inversion

V. DIFFERENTIAL DIAGNOSIS

Table 2 lists common diseases that must be distinguished from massive pulmonary embolism. Three diagnostic tests often are sufficient to distinguish pulmonary embolism from the other possibilities. All patients should have an immediate chest radiograph and an electrocardiogram, as well as blood pressures measured in both arms and a pulsus paradoxus checked. Results obtained from these simple and readily available tests should point the clinician toward pulmonary embolism as a possibility.

The best emergent bedside imaging test is echocardiography. Highly suggestive findings include: intracardiac thrombus, right ventricular septal bulging into the left ventricle, McConnell's sign (right ventricular hypokinesis with relative preservation of the apical region), pulmonary hypertension (estimated by the velocity of the tricuspid regurgitation jet), and dilation of the right ventricle and inferior vena cava (indicating elevated venous pressure) (10).

Table 2 Differential Diagnosis of Massive Pulmonary Embolism

Diagnosis	Comments
Myocardial infarction	Quality of pain, location, ECG
Cardiac tamponade	CXR, pulsus paradoxus, distant heart sounds, ECG
Tension pneumothorax	Lung exam, CXR, ECG
Aortic dissection	Quality of pain, pulse deficit, hypertension, CXR

d-Dimer, when measured using the ELISA method, is often helpful in the evaluation of suspected pulmonary embolism. A quantitative d-dimer of less than 500 mg/mL makes pulmonary embolism unlikely. The negative predictive value of the quantitative ELISA method exceeds 90%, and thus a negative result should strongly suggest an alternative diagnosis (11–13). The converse, however, is not true. An elevated d-dimer does not specifically point to pulmonary embolism.

Last, right heart catheterization may suggest the diagnosis. Elevated pulmonary pressures with a normal pulmonary capillary wedge pressure, with a difference between the mean pulmonary artery pressure and the pulmonary capillary wedge pressure of greater than 12 mmHg suggests the presence of pulmonary vascular disease. Often, in patients who are critically ill, hypoxemia and arterial hypotension are multifactorial, and assessment of the cardiac pressures may be useful in combination with evaluation for lower extremity thrombus and more conventional imaging modalities. Also, in patients receiving mechanical ventilation, increasing dead space may be attributable to pulmonary embolism.

VI. DIAGNOSTIC IMAGING STUDIES

Bedside echocardiography has several clear advantages in hemodynamically unstable patients. Myocardial infarction and pericardial tamponade can readily be identified and differentiated from pulmonary embolism. After the diagnosis of pulmonary embolism is established, assessing right ventricular function also provides prognostic information in the setting of submassive disease. Several studies have consistently shown that the presence of moderate or severe right ventricular hypokinesis is a marker for increased mortality (14,15).

Additional studies include spiral computed tomography (CT), magnetic resonance pulmonary angiography (MRPA), ventilation-perfusion (V/Q) scanning, and contrast pulmonary angiography (CPA). Each has advantages and disadvantages (Table 3). As more emergency departments acquire CT scanning capability, this modality is emerging as particularly useful, especially at times when echocardiography is not available. CT scanning is fast, provides high-quality images of the proximal pulmonary vasculature, and is noninvasive. It also provides information about the pericardial space and can be used (with a separate imaging acquisition protocol) to evaluate possible aortic dissection. However, in patients who are breathing very rapidly, image quality is compromised. Furthermore, the patient is exposed to intravenous contrast. In the hemodynamically unstable patient, chest CT scanning is the best diagnostic study of choice to exclude large proximal pulmonary emboli. Reported sensitivities range from 53 to 100%, and specificity ranges from 81 to 100% (16–19). However, a negative CT scan does not exclude peripheral emboli, and anticoagulation should not be withheld solely on the basis

Table 3 Diagnostic Imaging Tests

Test	Comments
Echocardiogram	Fast, portable, evaluates pericardium and left ventricle, risk stratifies submassive PE.
Chest CT scan	Readily available, can exclude massive disease, may reveal alternative diagnoses.
MRPA	Time-consuming, not widely available, not safe for an unstable patient.
V/Q lung scan	Widely available, no radiocontrast needed, often nondiagnostic.
CPA	Gold standard, invasive, limited availability.

MRPA, magnetic resonance pulmonary angiogram; CPA, contrast pulmonary angiogram.

of a negative spiral study (19,20). Although several studies have attempted to evaluate the safety of withholding anticoagulation after a negative spiral CT scan (21,22), none of these studies actually included consecutive patients who only were evaluated with spiral CT scanning. Rather, V/Q scanning and ultrasound were widely used in addition to clinical prior probability. Whereas a negative CT scan does not exclude peripheral pulmonary embolism, it does exclude proximal disease. Thus in a hypotensive patient with a negative CT scan, an alternative diagnosis must be sought.

Magnetic resonance pulmonary angiography (MRPA), although attractive in principle, has not gained wide acceptance. Interobserver variability remains high (23–25). Much as with CT angiography, proximal emboli are more easily visualized than distal ones. The specificity appears high, but the resolution is not as clear cut as with the most recent generation of chest CT scanners. In contrast to CT, MRPA requires a longer period of breath-holding. Also, monitoring unstable patients during MRPA is difficult. Settings where MRPA is particularly useful include patients with life-threatening reactions to intravenous contrast, or patients who refuse contrast pulmonary angiography. Currently, MRPA is not a suitable diagnostic modality for the evaluation of possible massive PE in an unstable patient.

In the more stable patient, V/Q scanning often provides enough information to make a diagnosis of pulmonary embolism. The two main disadvantages are a high frequency of nondiagnostic studies, especially in patients with coexisting lung disease, and the difficulty in monitoring unstable patients during the test. Spiral CT scanning of the chest may be at least as sensitive and specific. Furthermore, CT scanning has the advantage of identifying possible alternative diagnoses such as pneumonia, aortic dissection, or atelectasis. The primary advantage of V/Q lung scans is that no intravenous radiocontrast is required. Additionally, in the pregnant patient, V/Q scans are still preferred.

In contrast to the often nondiagnostic results from lung scanning, contrast pulmonary angiography (CPA) has long been considered the gold standard in the evaluation of pulmonary embolism. In addition to providing useful diagnostic information, catheter-directed therapy can be delivered once a diagnosis is established. The disadvantages of angiography are related to the morbidity and mortality of the procedure. It is an invasive procedure that also employs radiocontrast material. In experienced centers, however, the major morbidity rate is less than 1%. Zuckerman et al. reported no mortalities in a consecutive series of 547 patients (26).

VII. TREATMENT

The management of massive pulmonary embolism can be divided into two broad categories, supportive measures and clot removal or dissolution. Ensuring adequate oxygenation is paramount and may entail noninvasive positive pressure ventilation or even endotracheal intubation. (However, positive end expiratory pressure should be minimized as it imposes additional afterload to the right ventricle.) In patients with arterial hypotension, diagnostic evaluation must proceed in parallel with resuscitation.

Although data are sparse, several studies in animals suggest that fluid loading in massive PE may result in further hemodynamic deterioration. Two mechanisms have been set forth to explain this finding. The right and left ventricles share an interventricular septum. As the right ventricle dilates, the septum bulges into the left ventricle and limits diastolic volume and, thus, left ventricular stroke volume and cardiac output. A second mechanism involves right ventricular ischemia that may be exacerbated by increased wall stress associated with further increases in right ventricular end-diastolic volume caused by volume loading. Despite the data generated from animal studies, there are few prospective studies with humans. One study by Mercat et al. involving 13 patients did show that cardiac index improved in response to fluid loading (27). Given the paucity of data, a limited trial of fluids may be reasonable, but excessive volume resuscitation should be avoided.

Is there an ideal pressor agent in arterial hypotension due to pulmonary embolism? There have been no large prospective randomized controlled trials to address this question. The literature is replete with case reports and cases series describing the successful or unsuccessful use of a specific agent. Several small-scale studies, mostly in animals, have evaluated norepinephrine, dobutamine, dopamine, epinephrine, milrinone, neosynephrine, and even arteriolar dilating agents in cardiogenic shock from pulmonary embolism. The results in general are mixed. Although no single agent stands out as clearly superior, on balance, norepinephrine seems to have a beneficial effect on cardiac output and mean arterial pressure in the majority of the studies (28).

Systemic thrombolysis and catheter-directed lysis provide mechanical relief to the right ventricle by dissolving pulmonary emboli. In comparison to heparin, thrombolysis results in more rapid improvement in hemodynamic derangements, pulmonary perfusion, ventilation-perfusion matching, and oxygenation. However, there is not yet firm proof that survival is improved among unselected patients. In the National Institutes of Health-sponsored Urokinase in Pulmonary Embolism Trial (UPET), 160 patients with angiographically proven PE were randomized to urokinase followed by heparin or heparin alone. Mortality was not significantly different in the two groups (29).

Large randomized trials are lacking among patients presenting with hemodynamic collapse (30). Jerjes-Sanchez et al., in a study of eight patients who were randomly assigned to receive either streptokinase plus heparin or heparin alone, found 100% mortality in the heparin group and no deaths in the streptokinase group (31).

Patients presenting with submassive pulmonary embolism have been the subjects of several larger studies. In 1993, Goldhaber studied 101 patients with acute right heart dysfunction due to pulmonary embolism and found a trend toward reduced mortality in the thrombolysis group as compared to the heparin-treated group (32). In the Management Strategy and Prognosis of Pulmonary Embolism Registry, a multicenter registry, patients who were treated with thrombolytic therapy had a statistically significant reduced 30-day mortality compared to the heparin group (4.7% vs. 11.1%) (33).

Verstraete compared catheter-directed thrombolytic therapy delivered into the main pulmonary artery to systemic thrombolytic therapy (34). The results showed no significant differences between groups. In a small case series, intraembolic delivery of thrombolytic therapy was shown to be safe in patients with contraindications to systemic therapy. In theory, advantages to local or regional therapy include less systemic exposure to thrombolytic agents, and an ability to directly assess the angiographic results of therapy. On the other hand, this strategy requires pulmonary artery catheterization with its attendant risks.

Major hemorrhage is the most feared complication of thrombolysis. Although the precise definition varies slightly from study to study, it generally includes fatal hemorrhage, intracranial hemorrhage (ICH), and bleeding requiring a transfusion or a surgical procedure. In comparison to heparin therapy, thrombolysis causes significantly more episodes of major bleeding. The incidence of ICH is also significantly higher. In the International Cooperative Pulmonary Embolism Registry, patients receiving thrombolysis had a 3.0% rate of ICH (5).

Greenfield pioneered catheter embolectomy in the 1970s. Substantial improvements have been made to his original technique, which involved venotomy. Currently, there are a variety of techniques to assist with clot disruption and removal (Table 4). Experience at our institution has been disappointing in general, and we now have largely adopted surgical embolectomy in patients with massive PE and contraindications to systemic thrombolysis.

Surgical embolectomy is emerging as a promising treatment for massive pulmonary embolism associated with impending hemodynamic collapse. Improvements in operative technique have resulted in excellent outcomes. Patients most likely to benefit have centrally located thrombus. This can be assessed readily with spiral CT scan. The procedure involves cardiopulmonary bypass and pulmonary arteriotomy with manual clot extraction. At our institution, a vena caval filter is placed at the completion of the case. Patients are therapeutically anticoagulated on postoperative day 2, provided ongoing bleeding is not an issue.

Whereas there is significant controversy surrounding thrombolytic therapy and embolectomy, there is agreement on the need for anticoagulation. In patients not considered for lysis or embolectomy, rapid anticoagulation with unfractionated heparin with a goal of prolonging the partial thromboplastin time to 2.0 to 3.0 times baseline is the standard of care.

The role of low-molecular-weight heparin (LMWH) is evolving. Increasing data support its equivalence or superiority in the treatment of deep venous thrombosis of the leg veins. A few large studies in symptomatic pulmonary embolism have found it to be safe and effective. However, LMWH has not been specifically studied in massive pulmonary embolism. One of the main advantages of LMWH is more consistent dose response. Patients with large clot burden may require

Table 4 Catheter-Based Pulmonary
Thrombectomy and Embolectomy

Aspiration thrombectomy
  Greenfield technique
  Meyerovitz technique—8F sheath and 60
    mL suction syringe
Fragmentation thrombectomy
  Pulmonary artery catheter
  "Clot buster" Amplatz thrombectomy de-
    vice
  Pigtail rotational catheter
Rheolytic therapy
  Angioget rapid thrombectomy system
  Hydrolyster-Cordis thrombectomy catheter

large doses of UFH. Additionally, in patients with normal renal function and those not morbidly obese, there is no monitoring required for LMWH.

Inferior vena cava (IVC) interruption remains one of the least well-studied treatment modalities for VTE. Pioneered by Greenfield, inferior vena cava filters have been used in situations where anticoagulation was contraindicated. Typical applications include patients with ongoing bleeding, certain CNS malignancies, and failure of therapeutic anticoagulation. Additionally, filters may be indicated in patients with poor cardiopulmonary reserve who have substantial clot burden in the ilio-pelvic venous system. The only randomized prospective study of IVC filters showed that, although they are effective in preventing pulmonary embolism, they are associated with a doubling of the rate of deep venous thrombosis over the ensuing 2 years (35).

VIII. CONCLUSIONS

Massive pulmonary embolism requires rapid identification for optimal management. Submassive pulmonary embolism may be even more difficult to recognize, though elevated troponin levels and echocardiographic evidence of moderate or severe right ventricular dysfunction can be especially useful. Once such patients are identified, it is inadvisable to take a ''watch and wait'' approach based solely upon systemic arterial pressure, heart rate, and the need for pressors to maintain cardiac output. If they are followed with anticoagulation alone, their right ventricular function should be monitored frequently to ensure that right ventricular hypokinesis and dilatation are abating. However, these patients often do poorly with anticoagulation alone and should be considered for more aggressive intervention with thrombolysis or embolectomy.

REFERENCES

1. Levy SE, Simmons DH. Mechanisms of arterial hypoxemia following pulmonary thromboembolism in dogs. J Appl Physiol 1975; 39:41–46.
2. Levy SE, Simmons DH. Redistribution of alveolar ventilation following pulmonary thromboembolism in the dog. J Appl Physiol 1974; 36:60–68.
3. Alonzo GE, Bower JS, DeHart P, et al. The mechanisms of abnormal gas exchange in acute massive pulmonary embolism. Am Rev Dis 1983; 128:170–172.
4. Elliott CG. Pulmonary physiology during pulmonary embolism. Chest 1992; 101: 163S–171S.
5. Goldhaber SZ, Visani L, De Rosa M. Acute pulmonary embolism: clinical outcomes in the international cooperative pulmonary embolism registry (ICOPER). Lancet 1999; 353:1386–1389.

6. Kasper W, Konstantinides S, Geibel A, et al. Management strategies and determinants of outcome in acute major pulmonary embolism: results of a multicenter registry. J Am Coll Cardiol 1997; 30:1165–1171.

7. Horn H, Dack S, Friedberg CK. Cardiac sequelae of embolism of the pulmonary artery. Arch Intern Med 1939; 64:296–321.

8. Vlahakes GH, Turley K, Hoffman JIE. The pathophysiology of failure in acute right ventricular hypertension: hemodynamic and biochemical correlations. Circulation 1981; 63:87–95.

9. Giannitsis E, Muller-Bardorff M, Kurowski V, et al. Independent prognostic value of cardiac troponin T in patients with confirmed pulmonary embolism. Circulation 2000; 102:211–217.

10. Kasper W, Meinertz T, Henkel B, et al. Echocardiographic findings in patients with proved pulmonary embolism. Am Heart J 1986; 112:1284–1290.

11. Bounameauz H, de Moerloose P, Perrier A, Reber G. Plasma measurement of D-Dimer as a diagnostic aid in suspected venous thromboembolism: an overview. Thromb Haemost 1994; 71:1–6.

12. Bounameaux H, de Moerloose P, Perrier A, Miron MJ. D-Dimer testing in suspected venous thromboembolism: an update. QJ Med 1997; 90:437–441.

13. Goldhaber SZ, Simons GR, Elliot CG. Quantitative plasma d-dimer levels among patients undergoing pulmonary angiography for suspected pulmonary embolism. JAMA 1993; 270:2819–2822.

14. Kasper W, Kostantinides S, Geibel A, et al. Prognostic significance of right ventricular afterload stress detected by echocardiography in patients with clinically suspected pulmonary embolism. Heart 1997; 77:346–349.

15. McConnell MV, Solomon SD, Rayan ME, et al. Regional RV dysfunction detected by echocardiography in acute pulmonary embolism. Am J Cardiol 1996; 78:469–473.

16. Remy-Jardin M, Remy J, Wattine L, Giraud F. Central pulmonary thromboembolism: diagnosis with spiral volumetric CT with single-breath hold technique—comparison with pulmonary angiography. Radiology 1992; 185:381–387.

17. May JR, Remy-Jardin M, Muller NL, et al. Pulmonary embolism: prospective comparison of spiral CT with ventilation-perfusion scintigraphy. Radiology 1997; 205: 447–452.

18. Blum AG. Spiral-computed tomography versus angiography in the diagnosis of acute massive pulmonary embolism. Am J Cardiol 1994; 74:96–98.

19. Mullins MD, Becker DB, Hagspiel KD, Philbrick JT. The role of spiral volumetric computed tomography in the diagnosis of pulmonary embolism. Arch Intern Med 2000; 160:293–298.

20. Rathbun SW, Raskob GE, Whitsett TL. Sensitivity and specificity of helical computed tomography in the diagnosis of pulmonary embolism: A systematic review. Ann Intern Med 2000; 132:227–232.

21. Garg K, Sieler H, Welsh CH, Russ PD. Clinical validity of helical ct being interpreted as negative for pulmonary embolism: Implications for patient treatment. AJR 1999; 172:1627–1631.

22. Goodman LR, Lipchik RJ, Kuzo RS, Liu Y, McAuliffe TL, O'brien DJ. Subsequent pulmonary embolism: Risk after a negative helical CT pulmonary angiogram-prospective comparison with scintigraphy. Radiology 2000; 215:535–542.

23. Gupta A, Frazer CK, Ferguson JM, et al. Evaluation of pulmonary MR angiography in the diagnosis of acute pulmonary embolism. Radiology 1999; 210:353–359.

24. Meaney JFM, Weg JG, Chenevert TL, Stafford-Jonhnson D, Hamilton GH, Prinice MR. Diagnosis of pulmonary embolism with magnetic resonance angiography. N Engl J Med 1997; 336:1422–1427.

25. Yucel EK. Pulmonary MR angiography: Is it ready now? Radiology 1999; 210:301–303.

26. Zuckerman DA, Sterling KM, Oser RF. Safety of pulmonary angiography in the 1990s. JVIR 1996; 7:199–205.

27. Mercat A, Deihl J, Meyer G, Teboul J. Hemodynamic effects of fluid loading in acute massive pulmonary embolism. Crit Care Med 1999; 27:540–544.

28. Layish DT, Tapson VF. Pharmacologic hemodynamic support in massive pulmonary embolism. Chest 1997; 111:218–224.

29. Urokinase Pulmonary Embolism Trial: phase 1 results—a cooperative study. JAMA 1970; 214:2163–2172.

30. Arcasoy SM, Kreit JW. Thrombolytic therapy of pulmonary embolism. Chest 1999; 115:1695–1707.

31. Jerjes-Sanchez C, Ramirez-Rivera A, Garcia M de L, et al. Streptokinase and heparin versus heparin alone in massive pulmonary embolism: a randomized controlled trial. J Thromb Thrombolysis 1995; 2:227–229.

32. Goldhaber SZ, Haire WD, Feldstein ML, et al. Alteplase versus heparin in acute pulmonary embolism: randomize trial assessing right-ventricular function and pulmonary perfusion. Lancet 1993; 341:507–511.

33. Kasper W, Konstantitnides S, et al. Management strategy and prognosis of pulmonary embolism registry: results of a multi-center registry. J Am Coll Cardiol 1997; 30:1165–1173.

34. Verstralte M, Miller GAH, Bounameaux H, et al. Intravenous and intrapulmonary recombinant tissue-type plasminogen activator in the treatment of acute massive pulmonary embolism. Circulation 1988; 77:353–360.

35. Decousus H, et al. A clinical trial of vena caval filters in the prevention of pulmonary embolism in patients with proximal deep vein thrombosis. N Engl J Med 1998; 338: 409–415.

15

Thrombolysis in Pulmonary Embolism

Samuel Z. Goldhaber
*Brigham and Women's Hospital and Harvard Medical School,
Boston, Massachusetts*

Pulmonary embolism (PE) thrombolysis has remained controversial for the past 30 years. The major issues surrounding this controversy are listed in Table 1 and center around whether this strategy is effective, safe, and cost saving. Most studies of PE thrombolysis have been case series, undertaken without a prospective comparison group. The gold standard, however, remains the randomized clinical trial in which thrombolysis is compared with anticoagulation alone in a population of patients not tainted by selection bias.

I. EPIDEMIOLOGY

A. Mortality

PE can cause right ventricular failure, chronic pulmonary hypertension, and death. Acute right heart failure from PE can cause dyspnea, peripheral edema, and cardiogenic shock. Death may ensue due to right ventricular dilatation, compression of the left ventricle by the interventricular septum, and decreased forward cardiac output.

The mortality rate in the current era remains surprisingly high, approximately 15% according to a large international prospective registry of 2454 consecutive PE patients (1). In this registry, the International Cooperative PE Registry (ICOPER), most deaths occurred during the first 2 weeks after diagnosis. Other risk factors for PE mortality in ICOPER aside from right ventricular dysfunction included age >70 years, cancer, congestive heart failure, chronic obstructive pulmonary disease, and systemic arterial hypotension (1). Importantly, most patients who died had succumbed to PE, not to other comorbidities such as cancer. Nonfatal recurrent PE occurred in 4% of patients.

Table 1 Thrombolysis: Purported Pros and Cons

Pros	Cons
Reduce mortality by reversing right heart failure	Increase mortality with fatal bleeding complications
Prevent recurrent PE with medical embolectomy in situ of existing deep venous thrombosis	Cause recurrent PE by facilitating embolization of deep vein thrombi to the pulmonary arteries
Improve quality of life by reducing the frequency of chronic pulmonary hypertension	Impair quality of life by increasing the number of patients suffering from disabling strokes
Reducing costs by allowing more rapid and complete recovery	Increasing costs by using expensive thrombolytic agents

For patients with massive PE and cardiogenic shock, thrombolysis can be lifesaving (2). In a small clinical trial, patients with hypotension and heart failure due to PE were randomized to thrombolysis (streptokinase 1,500,000 U/1 h) plus anticoagulation versus anticoagulation alone. The trial was stopped after the first 8 of a planned 40 patients were enrolled, because all 4 patients allocated to the anticoagulation alone group died; in contrast, the 4 patients who received thrombolysis all survived. Of the 4 patients who died, 3 underwent postmortem examination and had right ventricular myocardial infarction (without significant coronary arterial obstruction) in addition to massive PE. Thus, these results support the argument that thrombolysis can help avert death from progressive right heart failure among PE patients in cardiogenic shock. This small trial, consisting of only 8 patients, is the sole investigation demonstrating that thrombolysis reduces mortality from PE.

B. Right Ventricular Dysfunction

A particularly problematic group of PE patients has impending hemodynamic instability—right ventricular dysfunction on echocardiogram but preserved systemic arterial pressure (3). In ICOPER, fewer than 5% presented in cardiogenic shock (1). Among the half who underwent baseline echocardiography, right ventricular hypokinesis was detected in 40%. Multivariate analysis in ICOPER indicated that right ventricular hypokinesis was independently associated with a doubling of the 3-month mortality rate. Similar observations were made in German (4) and Swedish (5) registries.

Moderate right ventricular hypertension can displace the interventricular septum toward the left ventricle, resulting in decreased left ventricular diastolic filling and end-diastolic volume, as well as right ventricular ischemia, infarction, and circulatory collapse (6). With underfilling of the left ventricle, systemic cardiac output and pressure both decrease, potentially compromising coronary perfusion and producing myocardial ischemia. By relieving obstruction to pulmonary artery blood flow, thrombolysis can theoretically lower abnormally elevated pulmonary artery pressure, thereby reversing cardiogenic shock and reducing the mortality rate from PE.

II. RISK STRATIFICATION

A. Clinical Evaluation

The benefit of PE thrombolysis is greatest among those patients at highest risk. Those rare patients who present to the hospital in cardiogenic shock, with poor tissue and organ perfusion, systemic arterial hypotension, and respiratory failure are at highest risk of death if treated solely with conventional anticoagulation. Those who are identified as having PE *in extremis* often die at home, en route to the hospital, or in the emergency department. In exceptional circumstances where the diagnosis of acute PE with cardiogenic shock is apparent, no additional testing is necessary prior to administration of a thrombolytic agent. However, in most situations, assessment of right ventricular function and troponin levels is warranted to provide a more sophisticated evaluation of the patient's risk.

Right ventricular dysfunction can be detected occasionally by physical examination. Clues include a left parasternal heave, distended jugular veins, and a systolic murmur of tricuspid regurgitation that increases with inspiration and that is best heard at the left lower sternal border. These findings, taken together with the observation of a new right bundle branch block or other evidence of evolution of right ventricular strain on the electrocardiogram, confirm the diagnosis of right ventricular dysfunction.

B. Echocardiography

Transthoracic echocardiography can help prognosticate and stratify clinical risk in patients who have been diagnosed with acute PE. In a cohort of 209 consecutive PE patients, there were no deaths among the subgroup with normal right ventricular function. Conversely, echocardiographic evidence of right ventricular dysfunction was present in 40% of all initially normotensive patients with PE in this case series. Right ventricular dysfunction was defined as the presence of right ventricular dilatation, paradoxical septal wall motion, or pulmonary hypertension. Among this latter group, 10% developed PE-related shock and 5% died (7).

In addition to right ventricular dysfunction, the presence of a patent foramen ovale, defined by contrast transthoracic echocardiography, is an important predictor of adverse outcome in patients with PE. After adjustment for baseline clinical characteristics, logistic regression analysis demonstrated that a patent foramen ovale was associated with a ninefold increase in mortality among patients with objectively confirmed PE (8).

Free-floating thrombi in the right heart are another echocardiographic predictor of a poor clinical outcome (9). The thrombus is typically wormlike and the echocardiogram usually demonstrates signs of cor pulmonale with right ventricular overload, paradoxical septal motion, and pulmonary hypertension. Almost half of the 38 patients in this series died during the index hospitalization.

For those patients who survive PE initially, the pulmonary artery systolic pressure appears to decrease exponentially until about 5 weeks after the acute episode. At that point, persistent pulmonary hypertension and right ventricular dysfunction tend to develop. An initial pulmonary artery systolic pressure that exceeds 50 mmHg is associated with disabling chronic pulmonary hypertension (10). Such patients may be suitable for PE thrombolysis when they initially present.

C. Troponin Levels

Recently, detection of cardiac troponin has been recognized as an adverse prognostic factor in patients with acute PE. Circulating troponin indicates irreversible myocardial cell damage and is much more sensitive than CK or CK-MB. Along with the electrocardiogram, this blood test is used routinely in patients who present to the Emergency Department with suspected acute myocardial infarction or acute coronary syndrome. Among PE patients, elevation of the troponin correlates with the presence of right ventricular dysfunction (11). This suggests that release of troponin from the myocardium during PE may result from acute right ventricular pressure overload, impaired coronary artery blood flow, or hypoxemia caused by the PE.

In a separate study of 56 patients, right ventricular dysfunction was more often found in patients with elevated troponin (12). These patients also had more frequent right bundle branch block and more frequent T-wave inversion in leads V1 through V4, indicators of right ventricular strain. The mortality rate from PE was 44% in troponin-positive patients, compared with 3% in troponin-negative patients. Interestingly, coronary angiography revealed obstructive coronary artery disease in an equal distribution of troponin-positive and troponin-negative patients. Furthermore, CK activity was not independently predictive of mortality (12). With respect to morbidity, troponin-positive patients more often required resuscitation, inotropic support, and mechanical ventilation.

Table 2 Adverse Outcomes During Hospitalization: MAPPET Registry

Event	Initial lysis ($n = 169$) n (%)	Heparin ($n = 550$) n (%)	p-value
All deaths	8 (4.7%)	61 (11.1%)	0.016
Death from PE	7 (4.1%)	58 (10.5%)	
Recurrent PE	13 (7.7%)	103 (18.7%)	<0.001
Major bleeding	37 (21.9%)	43 (7.8%)	<0.001
Intracranial bleeding	2 (1.2%)	2 (0.4%)	

Source: Modified from Ref. 15.

III. PROGNOSIS WITH HEPARIN ALONE

A. Registry Data

Among patients treated with heparin alone, the rate of death or recurrent PE within 2 weeks of diagnosis was 10% in the cohort of 399 patients followed by the Prospective Investigation of Pulmonary Embolism Diagnosis (PIOPED) group (13). Only 6% of the 399 PE patients received thrombolytic therapy. When 1-year mortality rates from all causes were assessed, patients who had received anticoagulation alone had a 19% mortality rate. In contrast, the lowest all-cause mortality rate (9%) was among those treated with thrombolytic therapy.

In the much larger Management Strategy And Prognosis of Pulmonary Embolism Registry (MAPPET), 1001 high-risk patients with right ventricular dysfunction were enrolled (14). Initial use of thrombolytic therapy among a subset of the 719 who presented with a normal systemic arterial pressure was associated with reduced in-hospital mortality and recurrent PE (Table 2) (15). After multivariate analysis, a marked benefit persisted for the thrombolysis-treated patients. Despite its limitations, MAPPET provides additional support for the hypothesis that thrombolysis will benefit PE patients who present with the combination of normal systemic arterial pressure and right ventricular dysfunction.

IV. INITIAL RANDOMIZED CONTROLLED CLINICAL TRIALS

The initial randomized controlled clinical trials of thrombolysis plus heparin versus heparin alone were cumbersome, complicated, and unwittingly predisposed PE patients to major bleeding. In the late 1960s and early 1970s, it was not appreciated that a high concentration of thrombolytic agent administered over a short duration was the best approach to maximizing efficacy and minimizing bleeding.

Urokinase (UK) was compared with heparin alone in 160 patients with angiographically documented PE who participated in Phase I of the Urokinase Pulmonary Embolism Trial (UPET) (16). The urokinase-dosing regimen was 4400 U/kg as a loading dose followed by 4400 U/kg/h for 24 h. Urokinase dissolved pulmonary arterial clot more rapidly than heparin alone and, in certain instances, reversed clinical shock. However, there was no difference in the rate of death or recurrent PE between the two groups.

More than 30 years after its inception, UPET remains the largest randomized controlled clinical trial that has ever been undertaken of PE thrombolysis versus anticoagulation alone. The lack of demonstration of a clinical benefit in the thrombolysis group in UPET is the most compelling argument that those who oppose PE thrombolysis can put forward.

Major hemorrhagic complications in UPET were frequent and occurred far more often among those patients randomized to urokinase than among those who received heparin alone. Thus, among skeptics, thrombolysis for PE was considered an unwieldy and expensive undertaking that consumed hospital resources and caused major bleeding complications in a large number of patients, without demonstrating a reduction in mortality or recurrent PE.

In the urokinase-streptokinase PE Trial (USPET) (17), 167 patients with angiographically documented PE were randomized to 1 of 3 different thrombolytic treatments: 12 h of urokinase, 24 h of urokinase, or 24 h of streptokinase. An important criticism of USPET is that it lacked a heparin-alone comparison group, so that the utility of thrombolysis versus heparin alone could not be evaluated. When the three thrombolytic regimens in USPET were compared, morbidity and mortality were similar as was the frequency of major bleeding complications. In a small ancillary study, acute thrombolysis followed by heparin improved pulmonary capillary blood volume at 2 weeks and at 1 year more than heparin alone (18). When followed for an average of 7 years, those assigned initially to thrombolysis appeared to have a more complete resolution of PE, as assessed by preservation of the normal pulmonary vascular response to exercise (19).

V. CONTEMPORARY CLINICAL TRIALS: EFFICACY AND SAFETY

PAIMS-2 investigators (20) randomized 36 patients with angiographically proven PE to 100 mg of rt-PA over 2 h or to heparin. Clot lysis at follow-up angiography occurred in the rt-PA group but not among heparin-alone patients. Mean pulmonary artery pressure decreased from 30 to 21 mmHg in the rt-PA group, but increased in patients who received heparin alone. Two rt-PA patients died (one from renal failure following cardiac tamponade and one from intracranial bleeding), and one patient who received heparin alone died from recurrent PE.

Goldhaber and colleagues tested the hypothesis that rt-PA followed by anticoagulation accelerates the improvement of right ventricular function and pulmonary perfusion more rapidly than anticoagulation alone (21). In this multicenter controlled trial, 101 patients were randomized: 46 to rt-PA 100 mg/2 h followed by heparin and 55 to heparin alone.

Based upon the number of patients enrolled, this PE trial is the second largest PE thrombolysis vs. heparin-alone randomized controlled trial that has ever been undertaken (with UPET being the largest). The trial tested the efficacy of thrombolytic therapy among a population of normotensive and "hemodynamically stable" patients. Most were enrolled on the basis of high-probability lung scans. Only 20% of the patients underwent diagnostic pulmonary angiograms, thus minimizing bleeding complications from groin hematomas (at the femoral vein puncture site used for angiography) among patients randomized to thrombolysis.

No clinical episodes of recurrent PE occurred among rt-PA patients, but there were 5 (2 fatal and 3 nonfatal) clinically suspected recurrent PEs within 14 days in patients randomized to heparin alone ($p = 0.06$). All five presented initially with right ventricular hypokinesis on echocardiogram, despite normal systemic arterial pressure at baseline. Thus, echocardiography helps identify a subgroup of PE patients with impending right ventricular failure who appear to be at high risk of adverse clinical outcomes if treated with heparin alone. Such patients, in particular, may be excellent candidates for thrombolytic therapy in the absence of contraindications.

Despite the risks of bleeding, the results from this clinical trial have modified our approach to PE thrombolysis. Based upon the available evidence, we believe that PE thrombolysis should be considered for patients with "impending hemodynamic instability," defined as normal systemic arterial pressure plus moderate or marked right ventricular dysfunction on echocardiogram.

Recently, our group showed quantitatively that most patients who receive thrombolytic therapy for PE achieve recovery of regional as well as global right ventricular function (22). At baseline, right ventricular areas were significantly larger than normal at end-diastole and at end-systole. Diastolic and systolic right ventricular areas decreased after thrombolysis. The area of the right ventricle most severely affected (and most improved after therapy) was the mid-right ventricular free wall.

A. Predictors of Efficacy

The appearance of the initial lung scan can help predict whether thrombolysis will be successful (23). Improvement in pulmonary perfusion after thrombolysis has been correlated with large initial perfusion defects that have a segmental appearance. These characteristics typically occur in patients who have anatomically extensive PE as well as a relatively short duration of symptoms.

There seems to be an inverse association between duration of symptoms and improvement on lung scan reperfusion after thrombolysis (24). After controlling for age and initial lung scan defect size, there was 0.7% less reperfusion per additional day of symptoms (95% CI; 0.2–1.2%; $p = 0.007$). Less clot lysis on angiography immediately following thrombolysis was observed in the quintile of patients with the longest duration of symptoms (>6 days; $p = 0.03$). Thus, delay will attenuate efficacy. Nevertheless, thrombolysis is still useful in patients who have had symptoms for up to 14 days.

VI. BLEEDING COMPLICATIONS

A. Clinical Trials Versus Registries

Catastrophic bleeding can occur with thrombolytic therapy, regardless of specific drug or specific indication. Therefore, *all* patients being considered for *any* thrombolytic regimen should be subjected to a meticulous evaluation for possible contraindications such as intracranial disease, recent surgery, or trauma. Randomized controlled trials tend to underestimate bleeding complication rates, because these trials usually have multiple safeguards to ensure appropriate exclusion of poor candidates for thrombolysis. However, registries that record ''real world'' results, including bleeding complications, may be much more realistic with respect to limitations and problems with thrombolysis.

B. Clinical Trials

Based on our series of 312 patients receiving thrombolysis for PE in five clinical trials, there is a 1.9% risk (95% CI, 0.7 to 4.1%) of intracranial bleeding (25). Two of the six patients received thrombolysis in violation of the trial protocol, because they had preexisting known intracranial disease. Two of the six intracranial hemorrhages probably were due to administration of heparin and not thrombolysis because they occurred late, 62 and 157 h after thrombolysis. Diastolic blood pressure on admission was significantly elevated in patients who developed intracranial hemorrhage compared with those who did not (90.3 vs. 77.6 mmHg; $p = 0.04$). No patient under age 55 was affected. These data reinforce the message that meticulous patient screening before administering thrombolysis is imperative.

C. Registries

In carefully conducted observational studies, thrombolysis for PE emerges as a strategy with a higher risk of major hemorrhagic complications than is reported in controlled clinical trials. At the Laennec Hospital in Paris, the group of Hervé Sors reviewed the bleeding complications in 132 consecutive patients who received rt-PA for massive PE (26). Two patients (1.5%) suffered intracranial bleeding, and one of the two died. Pericardial tamponade was equally problematic and occurred in two other patients (1.5%), one of whom died. Other major bleeding complications included 2 gastrointestinal hemorrhages, 3 cases of hemoptysis, and 11 hematomas at the puncture site for pulmonary angiography.

In ICOPER, the prospective registry of 2454 patients with PE conducted in 52 hospitals among 7 countries, 304 patients received thrombolytic therapy (1). An amazingly high 3.0% of patients who received thrombolysis suffered intracranial bleeding. Overall, 22% of those receiving thrombolysis had major bleeding and 12% required transfusions.

D. Predictors of Bleeding

In an overview of the five PE thrombolysis trials that we conducted (21,27–30), the mean age of patients with major bleeding was 63 years, while that of patients with no hemorrhagic complication was 56 years ($p = 0.005$). There was a 4% increased risk of bleeding for each additional year of age. Increasing body mass index and pulmonary angiography were also significant predictors of hemorrhage (31).

VII. PRACTICAL POINTS

The only FDA-approved contemporary dosing regimen for PE thrombolysis is rt-PA, given in a fixed dose of 100 mg as a continuous infusion over 2 h. There is no need to obtain laboratory tests during the thrombolytic infusion because no dosage adjustments are made. rt-PA administered locally within the pulmonary artery has never been shown to confer any advantage over peripheral administration of the drug (32).

A. PE Thrombolysis in Women

Data from 312 patients (144 women and 168 men) included in our group's PE trials (21,27–30) were analyzed to determine whether there were gender differences in the efficacy or safety of thrombolytic therapy (33). Our results indicated that women and men have a similar benefit and bleeding risk from PE thrombolysis. These findings suggest that thrombolytic therapy should be considered in the management of PE without regard to gender.

B. PE Thrombolysis in Cancer Patients

Although the initial angiographic response to thrombolysis is similar in cancer and noncancer patients, the magnitude of improvement among cancer patients becomes attenuated on perfusion scanning at 24 h. This observation suggests that cancer patients should receive maximally intensive anticoagulation immediately following thrombolysis in order to preserve their initial improvement from therapy. Fortunately, PE thrombolysis does not appear to be more hazardous in appropriately selected cancer patients than in patients without cancer (34).

VIII. CONTEMPORARY PE THROMBOLYSIS

Contemporary PE thrombolysis is safer, more streamlined, and more economical than classic PE thrombolysis (Table 3). Contemporary PE thrombolysis is characterized by a 2-week "time window," a brief infusion administered through a peripheral vein, and no special laboratory tests.

No ideal thrombolytic agent has yet been developed because of the continuing bleeding hazard posed by all lytic drugs. However, alternatives to rt-PA have been tested and appear in small series to be effective. All utilize high concentra-

Table 3 New Concepts in Pulmonary Embolism Thrombolysis

Variable	Old	New
Diagnosis	Mandatory pulmonary angiogram	High-probability lung scan, positive chest CT scan, echocardiogram showing isolated, severe right ventricular failure or pulmonary angiogram
Indications	Systemic arterial hypotension; hemodynamic instability	Hypotension *or* normotension with accompanying moderate or severe right ventricular hypokinesis
Time window	5 days or less	14 days or less
Route	Via pulmonary artery catheter	Via peripheral vein
Coagulation tests	"DIC screens" every 4–6 h during infusion	aPTT at conclusion of thrombolysis

tions of drug administered over a brief duration. They include urokinase 3,000,000 units over 2 h, with the first 1,000,000 units delivered as a 10-min bolus (29); streptokinase 1,500,000 units over 2 h (35), as well as the myocardial infarction dosing regimen of "double bolus" reteplase (36).

REFERENCES

1. Goldhaber SZ, Visani L, De Rosa M, for ICOPER. Acute pulmonary embolism: Clinical outcomes in the International Cooperative Pulmonary Embolism Registry (ICOPER). Lancet 1999; 353:1386–1389.
2. Jerjes-Sanchez C, Ramirez-Rivera A, Garcia M de L, Arriaga-Nava R, Valencia S, Rosado-Buzzo A, Pierzo JA, Rosas E. Streptokinase and heparin versus heparin alone in massive pulmonary embolism: A randomized controlled trial. J Thrombosis Thrombolysis 1995; 2:227–229.
3. Cannon CP, Goldhaber SZ. Cardiovascular risk stratification of pulmonary embolism in patients. Am J Cardiol 1996; 78:1149–1151.
4. Kasper W, Konstantinides S, Geibel A, Tiode N, Krause T, Just H. Prognostic significance of right ventricular afterload stress detected by echocardiography in patients with clinically suspected pulmonary embolism. Heart 1997; 77:346–349.
5. Ribeiro A, Lindmarker P, Juhlin-Dannfelt A, Johnsson H, Jorfeldt L. Echocardiography Doppler in pulmonary embolism: Right ventricular dysfunction as predictor of mortality. Am Heart J 1997; 134:479–487.
6. Goldhaber SZ. A contemporary approach to thrombolytic therapy for pulmonary embolism. Vasc Med 2000; 5:115–123.
7. Grifoni S, Olivotto I, Cecchini P, Pieralli F, Camaiti A, Santoro G et al. Short-term clinical outcome of patients with acute pulmonary embolism, normal blood pressure, and echocardiographic right ventricular dysfunction. Circulation 2000; 101:2817–2822.
8. Konstantinides S, Geibel A, Kasper W, Olschewski M, Blumel L, Just H. Patent foramen ovale is an important predictor of adverse outcome in patients with major pulmonary embolism. Circulation 1998; 97:1946–1951.
9. Chartier L, Bera J, Delomez M, Asseman P, Beregi JP, Bauchart JJ et al. Free-floating thrombi in the right heart: diagnosis, management, and prognostic indexes in 38 consecutive patients. Circulation 1999; 99:2779–2783.
10. Ribeiro A, Lindmarker P, Johnsson H, Juhlin-Dannfelt A, Jorfeldt L. Pulmonary embolism: one-year follow-up with echocardiography Doppler and five-year survival analysis. Circulation 1999; 99:1325–1330.
11. Meyer T, Binder L, Hruska N, Luthe H, Buchwald AB. Cardiac troponin I elevation in acute pulmonary embolism is associated with right ventricular dysfunction. J Am Coll Cardiol 2000; 36:1632–1636.
12. Giannitsis E, Muller-Bardorff M, Kurowski V, Weidtmann B, Wiegand U, Kampmann M et al. Independent prognostic value of cardiac troponin T in patients with confirmed pulmonary embolism. Circulation 2000; 102:211–217.

13. Carson JL, Kelley MA, Duff A, Weg JG, Fulkerson WJ, Palevsky HI, Schwartz JS, Thompson BT, Popovich J, Jr, Hobbins TE, Spera MA Alavi A, Terrin ML. The clinical course of pulmonary embolism. N Engl J Med 1992; 326:1240–1245.
14. Kasper W, Konstantinides S, Geibel A, Olschewski M, Heinrich F, Grosser KD, Rauber K, Iversen S, Redecker M, Kienast J. Management strategies and determinants of outcome in acute major pulmonary embolism: Results of a multicenter registry. J Am Coll Cardiol 1997; 30:1165–1171.
15. Konstantinides S, Geibel A, Olschewski M, Heinrich F, Grosser K, Rauber K, Iversen S, Redecker M, Kienast J, Just H, Kasper W. Impact of thrombolytic treatment on the prognosis of hemodynamically stable patients with major pulmonary embolism: Results of a Multicenter Registry. Circulation 1997; 96:882–888.
16. The Urokinase Pulmonary Embolism Trial. A national cooperative study. Circulation 1973; 47:1–108.
17. Urokinase-Streptokinase Embolism Trial. Phase 2 results. A cooperative study. JAMA 1974; 229:1606–1613.
18. Sharma GVRK, Burleson VA, Sasahara AA. Effect of thrombolytic therapy on pulmonary-capillary blood volume in patients with pulmonary embolism. N Engl J Med 1980; 303:842–845.
19. Sharma GVRK, Folland ED, McIntyre KM, Sasahara AA. Long-term benefit of thrombolytic therapy in patients with pulmonary embolism. Vasc Med 2000; 5:91–95.
20. Dalla-Volta S, Palla A, Santolicandro A, et al. PAIMS 2: Alteplase combined with heparin versus heparin in the treatment of acute pulmonary embolism. Plasminogen Activator Italian Multicenter Study 2. J Am Coll Cardiol 1992; 20:520–526.
21. Goldhaber SZ, Haire WD, Feldstein ML, Miller M, Toltzis R, Smith JL, Taveira da Silva AM, Come PC, Lee RT, Parker JA, Mogtader A, McDonough TJ, Braunwald E. Alteplase versus heparin in acute pulmonary embolism: randomised trial assessing right ventricular function and pulmonary perfusion. Lancet 1993; 341:507–511.
22. Nass N, McConnell MV, Goldhaber SZ, Chyu S, Solomon SD. Recovery of regional right ventricular function after thrombolysis for pulmonary embolism. Am J Cardiol 1999; 83:804–806.
23. Parker JA, Drum DE, Feldstein ML, Goldhaber SZ. Lung scan evaluation of thrombolytic therapy for pulmonary embolism. J Nucl Med 1995; 36:364–368.
24. Daniels LB, Parker JA, Patel SR, Grodstein F, Goldhaber SZ. Relation of duration of symptoms with response to thrombolytic therapy in pulmonary embolism. Am J Cardiol 1997; 80:184–188.
25. Kanter DS, Mikkola KM, Patel SR, Parker JA, Goldhaber SZ. Thrombolytic therapy for pulmonary embolism. Frequency of intracranial hemorrhage and associated risk factors. Chest 1997; 111:1241–1245.
26. Meyer G, Gisselbrecht M, Diehl JL, Journois D, Sors H. Incidence and predictors of major hemorrhagic complications from thrombolytic therapy in patients with massive pulmonary embolism. Am J Med 1998; 105:472–477.
27. Goldhaber SZ, Vaughan DE, Markis JE, Selwyn AP, Meyerovitz MF, Loscalzo J, Kim DS, Kessler CM, Dawley DL, Sharma GVRK, Sasahara A, Grossbard EB,

Braunwald E. Acute pulmonary embolism treated with tissue plasminogen activator. Lancet 1986; 2:886–889.

28. Goldhaber SZ, Kessler CM, Heit J, Markis J, Sharma GVRK, Dawley D, Nagel JS, Meyerovitz M, Kim D, Vaughan DE, Parker JA, Tumeh SS, Drum D, Loscalzo J, Reagan K, Selwyn AP, Anderson J, Braunwald E. A randomized controlled trial of recombinant tissue plasminogen activator versus urokinase in the treatment of acute pulmonary embolism. Lancet 1988; 2:293–298.

29. Goldhaber SZ, Kessler CM, Heit JA, et al. Recombinant tissue-type plasminogen activator versus a novel dosing regimen of urokinase in acute pulmonary embolism: A randomized controlled multicenter trial. J Am Coll Cardiol 1992; 20:24–30.

30. Goldhaber SZ, Agnelli G, Levine MN, on behalf of the Bolus Alteplase Pulmonary Embolism Group. Reduced dose bolus alteplase versus conventional alteplase infusion for pulmonary embolism thrombolysis. An international multicenter randomized trial. Chest 1994; 106:718–724.

31. Mikkola KM, Patel SR, Parker JA, Grodstein F, Goldhaber SZ. Increasing age is a major risk factor for hemorrhagic complications following pulmonary embolism thrombolysis. Am Heart J 1997; 134:69–72.

32. Verstraete M, Miller GAH, Bounameaux H, Charbonnier B, Colle JP, Lecorf G, Marbet GA, Mombaerts P, Olsson CG. Intravenous and intrapulmonary recombinant tissue-type plasminogen activator in the treatment of acute massive pulmonary embolism. Circulation 1988; 77:353–360.

33. Patel SR, Parker JA, Grodstein F, Goldhaber SZ. Similarity in presentation and response to thrombolysis among women and men with pulmonary embolism. J Thrombosis Thrombolysis 1998; 5:95–100.

34. Mikkola KM, Patel SR, Parker JA, Grodstein F, Goldhaber SZ. Attentuation over 24 hours of the efficacy of pulmonary embolism thrombolysis among cancer patients. Am Heart J 1997; 134:603–607.

35. Meneveau N, Schiele F, Metz D, Valette B, Attali P, Vuillemenot A, et al. Comparative efficacy of a two-hour regimen of streptokinase versus alteplase in acute massive pulmonary embolism: immediate clinical and hemodynamic outcome and one-year follow-up. J Am Coll Cardiol 1998; 31:1057–1063.

36. Tebbe U, Graf A, Kamke W, et al. Hemodynamic effects of double bolus reteplase versus alteplase infusion in a massive pulmonary embolism. Am Heart J 1999; 138: 39–44.

16

Optimal Duration of Anticoagulation Following Venous Thromboembolism Among Patients With and Without Inherited Thrombophilia

Gavin J. Blake and Paul M. Ridker
Brigham and Women's Hospital and Harvard Medical School,
Boston, Massachusetts

The optimal duration of oral anticoagulation following a venous thromboembolic event is controversial. The goal of therapy is to prevent recurrent events without exposing the patient to unnecessary hemorrhagic risk. Studies of the long-term clinical course of venous thromboembolism (VTE) suggest a high recurrence rate (1,2) particularly when the index event is idiopathic. However, the risk of bleeding while on oral anticoagulation is directly related to the length of exposure. Thus, at some point, the risk of treatment may outweigh the potential benefit.

Accumulating evidence indicates that VTE is a chronic, multicausal disease with genetic and acquired risk factors interacting in a dynamic manner to determine an individual's risk for VTE (3). Appropriate recommendations on the duration of anticoagulation following VTE should take these risk factors into account. Current recommendations of the American College of Chest Physicians suggest 3 to 6 months of oral anticoagulant therapy with warfarin, adjusted to a target International Normalized Ratio (INR) of 2–3, for the treatment of a first thromboembolic event in patients with reversible or time-limited risk factors (4). At least 6 months of therapy is recommended for patients with a first idiopathic event (4).

I. RANDOMIZED TRIALS OF ANTICOAGULATION FOLLOWING FIRST VTE

There are surprisingly few randomized trials assessing the optimal duration of anticoagulation following VTE. The Research Committee of the British Thoracic Society conducted a multicenter comparison of 4 weeks versus 3 months antico-agulation in 712 patients admitted with acute deep venous thrombosis (DVT), pulmonary embolism (PE), or both (5). After 12 months of follow-up, the recurrence rate was 7.8% in the group randomized to 4 weeks of anticoagulation compared to 4% in the 3-month group ($p = 0.04$). Regardless of duration of anticoagulation, there was only one recurrence (0.86%) among 116 patients who developed VTE postoperatively. By contrast, among nonsurgical patients, the recurrence rates were higher in the group treated for 4 weeks compared to the group treated for 3 months (9.1 vs. 4.7%; $p < 0.0002$).

This initial study has been criticized because objective methods were not used to confirm the diagnosis of recurrent VTE in the majority of patients (6). Nonetheless, these findings suggested that a short duration of anticoagulation may be adequate for patients with postoperative venous thrombosis, while a longer course of treatment is necessary for patients without a reversible risk factor such as recent surgery.

This concept is supported by the work of Levine et al., who conducted a randomized trial of placebo versus warfarin for 8 further weeks in patients who had completed 4 weeks of anticoagulation for VTE and who had a normal imped-ance plethysmogram at 4 weeks. One-hundred-five patients were randomized to placebo and 109 to warfarin with a target INR of 2–3, and these patients were followed for 11 months (7). Patients with two or more VTE, protein C deficiency, protein S deficiency, and antithrombin III deficiency were excluded.

During the first 8 weeks after randomization, 9 (8.6%) patients in the pla-cebo group developed VTE compared to 1 (0.9%) patient in the warfarin-treated group ($p = 0.009$). During the 9 months of follow-up beyond 8 weeks, 3 placebo-treated patients and 6 warfarin-treated patients developed VTE, so that over the total 11 months of follow-up, 12 (11.5%) in the placebo group and 7 (6.8%) in the warfarin group developed VTE ($p = 0.3$). All seven events in the warfarin group occurred in patients with continuing risk factors for VTE. These results suggested that more than 3 months of anticoagulation may be required for patients with continuing risk factors for VTE.

The Duration of Anticoagulation Trial Study Group (DURAC) conducted a comparison of 6 weeks versus 6 months of oral anticoagulant therapy after a first episode of VTE (8). Eight-hundred-ninety-seven patients were followed for 2 years, with a target INR of 2–2.85. The recurrence rate was 18.1% in the group treated for 6 weeks and 9.5% in the group treated for 6 months, giving an odds ratio for recurrence in the 6-week group of 2.1. There was a sharp increase in the recurrence rate in the group treated for 6 weeks after anticoagulation was stopped. The rate of recurrence remained nearly parallel for the 18 months thereafter, with a linear increase in cumulative risk for both groups, corresponding to 5 to 6% annually (Fig. 1).

In the DURAC trial, the overall rate of recurrence after 2 years was much lower among patients with temporary risk factors than among those with permanent risk factors (6.6 vs. 18%). Five episodes of major bleeding occurred in the 6-month group and one in the 6-week group, but this difference was not statistically different. Three of these patients were receiving excessive anticoagulation at the time of admission (INR 4–5.6).

Most recently, Kearon and colleagues randomly assigned 162 Canadian patients, who had completed 3 months of anticoagulant therapy for a first episode of idiopathic VTE, to receive either warfarin or placebo for a further 24 months (9). The target INR was 2–3. The trial was terminated early after an average follow-up of 10 months. The rate of recurrence was 1.3% per patient-year in the warfarin group and 27.4% per patient-year in the placebo group. Warfarin resulted in a 95% reduction in the risk of recurrent VTE (Fig. 2). There were three episodes of major bleeding in the warfarin group and one in the control group. None of the bleeds was fatal.

The authors conclude that patients with a first episode of idiopathic VTE should be treated with anticoagulation for longer than 3 months. The optimal duration of anticoagulation, however, remains unclear. Extended anticoagulant therapy is associated with a risk of major bleeding of about 3% per year (10). Although the risk of recurrence is high among patients without reversible risk factors, fatal pulmonary embolism, the most feared complication, is rare in these

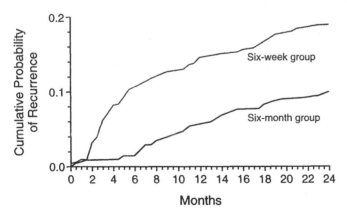

Figure 1 Cumulative probability of recurrent venous thromboembolism after a first episode, according to duration of anticoagulation. (Adapted from Ref. 8.)

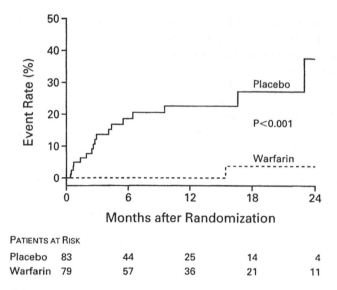

PATIENTS AT RISK

Placebo	83	44	25	14	4
Warfarin	79	57	36	21	11

Figure 2 Cumulative probability of recurrent venous thromboembolism in patients with a first episode of idiopathic thrombosis who were assigned to warfarin or placebo after an initial 3 months of anticoagulation. (Adapted from Ref. 9.)

patients providing they are not confined to bed. Schulman et al. reported only one fatal PE among 450 patients with idiopathic VTE, and Levine et al. reported none among 301 patients (7,8). Thus, there are insufficient data at this time to recommend lifelong anticoagulation to all patients with first idiopathic venous thrombosis.

II. RANDOMIZED TRIALS OF ANTICOAGULATION FOLLOWING RECURRENT VTE

The DURAC group have also conducted a trial comparing 6 months of oral anti-coagulation with indefinite anticoagulation in 227 patients with a second episode of VTE (11). The target INR was again 2–2.85 and the patients were followed for 4 years. The rate of recurrent VTE in the group treated for 6 months was 20.7% compared to 2.6% in the group treated indefinitely (Fig. 3). The relative risk for recurrence in the 6-month group was 8.0.

None of the recurrent episodes in the group assigned to indefinite anticoag-ulation actually occurred during anticoagulation; all three patients had discon-

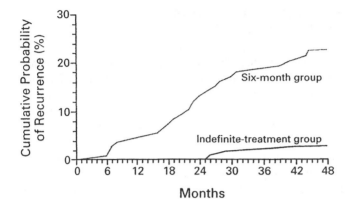

Figure 3 Cumulative probability of recurrent venous thrombosis in patients with a second episode, according to the duration of assigned anticoagulation therapy. (Adapted from Ref. 11.)

tinued their anticoagulation therapy prematurely; 8.6% of the group assigned to indefinite anticoagulation suffered a major hemorrhage compared to 2.7% of the 6 month group. This difference was not statistically significant ($p = 0.08$). The monthly incidence of major hemorrhage while on anticoagulation therapy was 0.20%, which compared favorably with older studies reporting major bleeding rates of 0.6 to 0.7% on oral anticoagulation.

This study showed that a target INR of 2–2.85 is effective in preventing recurrent VTE in individuals with a prior history of at least two events. The authors calculated that for every 100 patients with recurrent VTE receiving warfarin indefinitely compared to 6 months, 0.43 episodes of recurrent VTE would be averted per month at a cost of 0.2 major bleeds per month. Thus it would be of value to determine whether a lower intensity of anticoagulation could eliminate the risk of bleeding while still offering the same protective effect. This issue is being evaluated in the ongoing Prevention of Recurrent Venous Thromboembolism (PREVENT) trial, which will be discussed later in this chapter (12).

In view of the above data, it seems clinically appropriate to consider stratifying patients into those with low, intermediate, or high risk for recurrent VTE (13). The low-risk group, with temporary reversible risk factors for VTE such as trauma or surgery, can probably be treated for 4 to 6 weeks after the risk factor is removed. The intermediate-risk group, with a history of a first idiopathic event, should receive maintenance therapy with warfarin for at least 6 months. Indefinite anticoagulation should be reserved for the high-risk group, including those who already have recurrent VTE.

III. MULTICAUSAL MODEL FOR VENOUS THROMBOEMBOLIC RISK

Accumulating evidence suggests that VTE is a multicausal disease with gene–gene and gene–environment interactions playing a dynamic role. Rosendaal has recently proposed that a more precise model of VTE risk can be attained by considering the lifelong risk due to inherited defects along with a dynamically increasing risk with age (3). Superadded events such as pregnancy, trauma, or surgery may cause an individual to transiently exceed his or her thrombosis threshold and precipitate an acute event. In contrast, stopping oral contraception, increasing exercise, or folate supplementation may tip the balance away from thrombosis, and keep thrombosis-prone individuals below their thrombosis threshold.

However, several questions remain. As more genetic and acquired risk factors for VTE are discovered, which patients will be deemed intermediate or high risk? Should we screen for genetic risk factors in all patients with a first VTE? Could low-dose warfarin achieve the same beneficial effects in reduction of VTE risk without the accompanying risk of hemorrhage? The rest of this chapter will focus on these issues.

IV. INHERITED RISK FACTORS FOR VENOUS THROMBOEMBOLISM

Acquired reversible risk factors for VTE include surgery, trauma, immobilization, pregnancy, and the oral contraceptive pill (Table 1). Until recently, deficiencies

Table 1 Acquired and Genetic Risk Factors for Venous Thromboembolism

Acquired	Genetic
Surgery	Factor V Leiden
Trauma	Prothrombin G20210A mutation
Immobilization	Antithrombin deficiency
Obesity	Protein C deficiency
Pregnancy	Protein S deficiency
Oral contraception	Dysfibrinogenemia
Hormone replacement therapy	Dysfunctional thrombomodulin
Cancer	Hyperhomocysteinemia
Nephrotic syndrome	
Antiphospholipid antibody syndromes	
Hyperhomocysteinemia	

Table 2   Estimated Prevalence of Inherited Risk Factors for Venous Thrombosis in the General Population, Among Those with a History of Thrombosis, and Among Those with Familial Thrombophilia

Factor	General population	Patients with thrombosis	Familial thrombophilia
Protein C deficiency	<0.5	3	5
Protein S deficiency	<0.5	2	5
Antithrombin deficiency	<0.5	1	3
Factor V Leiden	5	20	50
Prothrombin G20210A	3	6	20
Hyperhomocysteinemia	5	10	15

of antithrombin, protein C and protein S, and the antiphospholipid syndrome were the only established thrombophilic syndromes. These deficiencies together, however, account for only 5 to 10% of familial VTE (3). Two recently discovered genetic defects, the factor V Leiden mutation and the prothrombin gene mutation, appear to account for a far greater proportion of thrombophilic syndromes (Table 2).

A.   Factor V Leiden

In 1993, Dahlbach first described resistance to breakdown by activated protein C which appeared to be characteristic of selected patients with VTE (14). This abnormality is caused by a single adenine for guanine point mutation in the gene coding for factor V, which leads to the substitution of glutamine for arginine at position 506, one of three cleavage sites on factor V for activated protein C (15). Thus, this mutation, known as factor V Leiden, makes factor V relatively resistant to degradation by protein C.

The significance of factor V Leiden as a risk factor for VTE was shown in the Leiden Thrombophilia study, a population-based study of 301 patients less than 70 years of age who had a first episode of VTE not related to malignancy (16). Resistance to protein C was detected in 21% of cases compared to 5% of age- and sex-matched controls (odds ratio 6.6). Subsequent analysis showed that 80% of the patients resistant to protein C were either heterozygous or homozygous for factor V Leiden. Factor V Leiden has since been shown to be the most common genetic mutation associated with VTE (17).

The association between factor V Leiden and risk of VTE was confirmed in a large prospective study of healthy U.S. males enrolled in the Physicians' Health Study (PHS) (18). The prevalence of the mutation was significantly higher among men who developed VTE than among controls (11.6 vs. 6%; $p = 0.02$). In adjusted analysis, the relative risk (RR) for VTE among men with the mutation was 2.7 ($p = 0.008$). The increased risk was seen in 63 patients with primary VTE (RR 3.5) but not in 58 patients with secondary VTE (RR1.7; $p = 0.3$). In men older than 70 years of age, the risk of primary VTE increased seven-fold.

The association between age, factor V Leiden, and the risk of VTE was analyzed in a further study from the PHS. For men <50 years old, those with the mutation had no increased risk of VTE compared to controls, but with increasing age the risk conferred by the mutation also increased (19). Incidence rate differences between affected and unaffected men were 1.23 for those aged 50 to 59; 1.61 for those aged 60 to 69; and 5.97 for those aged 70 or older. This trend was most pronounced for primary VTE (Fig. 4). No significant relationship was found for secondary events.

These findings strongly suggest that the pathogenesis of VTE is multifactorial and requires interactions between both inherited and acquired risk factors. One such interaction appears to be between factor V Leiden and homocysteine. In a further analysis from the PHS, it was shown that high homocysteine levels (>95th percentile) alone were not associated with a significantly increased risk of VTE but that, when present along with factor V Leiden, hyperhomocysteinemia conferred a 20-fold increased risk of idiopathic VTE (Fig. 5) (20).

Factor V Leiden also enhances the risk of VTE in patients with other thrombophilic states. In a study of patients with symptomatic protein C deficiency, the prevalence of factor V Leiden was 14% (21). In a study of seven families affected by both protein S deficiency and Factor V Leiden, 72% of individuals with both abnormalities had a thrombotic event compared to 19% of those with protein S deficiency alone and 19% of those with factor V Leiden alone (22).

In some reports, factor V Leiden has been associated with an increased risk of recurrent VTE (23). This would be an important finding as it would potentially identify patients who might benefit from prolonged anticoagulation. In the PHS, for example, 77 patients with idiopathic VTE were followed prospectively for an average of 68 months. Eleven patients (14.3%) developed recurrent VTE; seven cases (11.1%) among 63 patients who were not carriers of the mutation and four cases (28.6%) among 14 who were carriers of factor V Leiden. The incidence rate was 7.46 per 100 person-years among carriers and 1.82 per 100 person-years among those without the mutation. The crude RR was 4.1 ($p = 0.04$) and the age- and smoking-adjusted RR was 4.7 ($p = 0.047$). Among heterozygous men, 76% of recurrent events were attributable to the mutation.

This initial finding that factor V Leiden carries an increased risk for recurrent VTE is supported by a larger European study that followed 251 patients with VTE for up to 8 years (24). The recurrence rates were 39.5% in the group

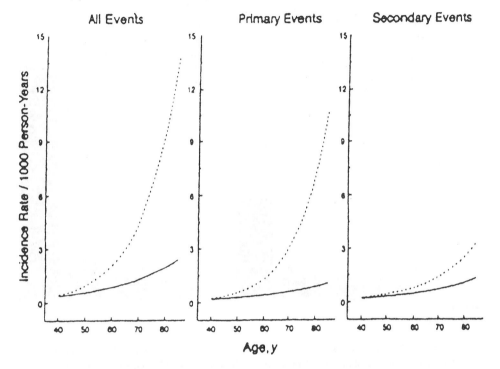

Figure 4   Estimated age-specific incidence rates for venous thromboembolism among men with (dashed lines) and without (solid lines) factor V Leiden mutation. Left: Any venous thromboembolism. Middle: Idiopathic venous thromboembolism. Right: Venous thromboembolism associated with cancer or surgery. (Adapted from Ref. 19.)

heterozygous for factor V Leiden, and 18.3% in those who were not carriers of the mutation, giving a relative risk of 2.4 for carriers of the mutation. Of note, factor V Leiden predicted risk of recurrence of both idiopathic and secondary VTE in this study.

Not all studies agree, however, that being a carrier for factor V Leiden confers an increased risk of recurrent VTE. Rintelen and colleagues conducted a retrospective study of Austrian patients with VTE and found that the risk of recurrence was increased only in those homozygous for factor V Leiden (9.5% per patient per year) (25). Those heterozygous for factor V leiden had a similar recurrence rate to controls (4.8% per patient per year and 5% per patient per year, respectively).

Workers in Milan have recently reported data regarding the frequency of

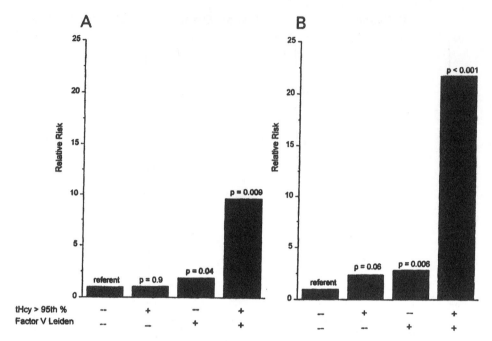

Figure 5   Interrelations of factor V Leiden mutation and hyperhomocysteinemia on risk of venous thromboembolism (+, present; −, absent). (Adapted from Ref. 20.)

recurrent VTE in 112 carriers of the factor V Leiden mutation alone, 17 patients heterozygous for both factor V Leiden and the prothrombin mutation, and 283 patients who had neither mutation (2). The cumulative incidence of recurrent VTE was 30% among carriers of factor V Leiden alone and 30% among patients with neither mutation. The cumulative incidence was 65% among the carriers of both factor V Leiden and the G20210A prothrombin mutation (RR 2.6). When only spontaneous recurrences were considered, the relative risk for carriers of both mutations was 3.7. No difference in recurrence rates was observed between patients heterozygous for factor V Leiden alone and those without either mutation. The authors conclude that a finding of heterozygosity for both factor V Leiden and the prothrombin mutation should prompt lifelong treatment with anticoagulants.

Thus, there remains disagreement whether factor V Leiden is associated with an increased risk of recurrent VTE. This issue merits further study as it has a potentially large impact on clinical practice.

B. Prothrombin Gene Mutation

Poort and colleagues have described a single point mutation in the prothrombin gene (G-to-A transition at position 20210) that appears to be associated with increased prothrombin levels (26). The G20210A allele is observed in 3–7% of cases and 1–3.9% of healthy subjects (27–30).

The association between the heterozygous state and VTE is controversial. A Swedish study from the DURAC group reported an odds ratio of 4.6 for first VTE in 28 carriers of the mutation, and other small studies have suggested a similar risk of VTE in heterozygous carriers of the mutation (27,28,31).

In contrast, a large American study of over 2000 men found only a weak association between the G20210A mutation and overall risk of VTE (30). The relative risk was 1.7 ($p = 0.08$). The relative risk for idiopathic VTE was 1.9 ($p = 0.1$). These effects were smaller in magnitude than those associated with factor V Leiden (RR 3 for overall VTE, RR 4.5 for primary VTE) (Fig. 6).

Other recent studies have sought to address the key question of whether patients who carry the G20210A transition are at increased risk of recurrent VTE. If this is the case, then carriers of the mutation who present with a first episode of VTE should be considered for more long-term anticoagulation.

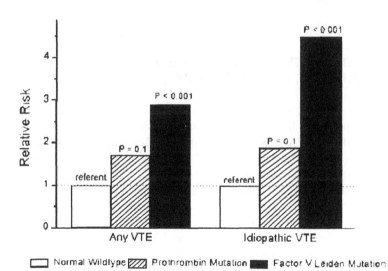

Figure 6 Relative risks of developing future venous thromboembolism (VTE) among participants in the Physicians' Health Study according to presence or absence of prothrombin or factor V Leiden mutations. Data are shown for any VTE and for events not associated with cancer, surgery, or trauma (idiopathic VTE). (Adapted from Ref. 30.)

A report from Austria found no association between the G20210A mutation and risk of recurrent VTE (27). Of 492 patients with documented VTE, 8.5% were carriers of the mutation. The recurrence rate was 7% in carriers versus 12% in those without the mutation. Similarly, a report from the DURAC group found no increased risk of recurrence in carriers of the prothrombin mutation (odds ratio 0.9) (31). In this study, the heterozygote state for factor V Leiden was not associated with an increased risk of recurrent VTE (17.8% in carriers vs. 17.6% in noncarriers). Those homozygous for the factor V Leiden, however, had a markedly increased risk of recurrence (odds ratio 4.8). By contrast, in the PHS, the prothrombin mutation was associated with an increased risk of recurrent events, particularly when coinherited with factor V Leiden.

How is this apparent discrepancy between risk for first and subsequent VTE explained? The average risk of a second episode of VTE is approximately 3 to 5% annually for all VTE patients, which is severalfold higher than the risk for carriers of the G20210A mutation for first VTE. Thus coexisting or unrecognized risk factors for recurrent VTE may overshadow the risk generated by this mutation alone. Recent data suggest that, when combined with other genetic mutations, the prothrombin gene mutation may greatly increase the risk of recurrent VTE. The Milan group reported a fourfold increased risk of recurrent idiopathic VTE in carriers of both factor V Leiden and the prothrombin gene mutation (2).

V. INTERACTION BETWEEN GENETIC MUTATIONS, ORAL CONTRACEPTION, AND PREGNANCY

Patients who carry factor V Leiden may be at increased risk of VTE when taking the oral contraceptive pill. In a case control study of women aged 15 to 49 from the Netherlands, the risk of VTE associated with the oral contraceptive pill (OCP) was 3.8, and with factor V Leiden was 7.9 (32). The risk of thrombosis for those with both risk factors increased by more than 30-fold.

Further evidence of gene–gene and gene–environment interactions comes from a recent study of VTE in pregnant women (33). Factor V Leiden was found in 43.7% of cases, compared to 7.7% of controls (RR 9.3), and the prothrombin gene mutation was found in 16.9% of cases and 1.3% of controls (RR 15.2). Remarkably, both abnormalities were detected in 9.3% of cases compared to none of the controls (estimated odds ratio 107).

There appears to be a relationship between the prothrombin gene mutation and pregnancy-related changes in fibrinolysis and coagulation, as the risk conferred by this mutation in pregnant women is greater than that observed in nonpregnant populations. Assuming an incidence of one thromboembolic event in 1500 pregnancies, the calculated probability of thrombosis among carriers of factor V Leiden was 0.25%, among those with the prothrombin mutation was 0.5%, and among those with both abnormalities was 4.6%. This finding has led to the controversial recommendation that all pregnant women with a personal or family history of VTE should be screened for these genetic abnormalities (34).

VI. HYPERHOMOCYSTEINEMIA

Patients with congenital forms of homozygous homocystinuria can have dramatically elevated plasma levels of homocysteine and are at markedly increased risk for both venous and arterial thrombosis. However, such severe forms of congenital hyperhomocysteinemia are rarely encountered in clinical practice. By contrast, modest elevations of plasma homocysteine (>17 μmol/L) are common, occurring in approximately 5% of the general population. Plasma homocysteine levels reflect both dietary intake of folic acid as well as inherited defects in the homocysteine metabolic enzymes cystathionine β-synthase and methylene-tetrahydrofolate reductase (MTHFR). Specifically, a common thermolabile (tl)-MTHFR variant caused by a C to T mutation at nucleotide 677 has been associated with elevated plasma homocysteine levels.

A recent metanalysis of nine clinical studies found that individuals with homocysteine levels in excess of the 95th percentile had an overall threefold increase in risk of VTE (Fig. 7) (35). As discussed above, risks associated with hyperhomocysteinemia are further increased in the presence of other inherited defects such as factor V Leiden.

VII. FACTOR XI

Factor XI is a component of the intrinsic pathway that contributes to thrombin generation. A recent study from the Leiden Thrombophilia group showed high plasma levels of factor XI are associated with an increased risk of VTE (36). Patients with factor XI levels above the 90th percentile were associated with an adjusted odds ratio of 2.2 for VTE when compared to those with levels below the 90th percentile. This risk was maintained when patients with known genetic risk factors for thrombosis were excluded. There was a linear relationship between increasing factor XI levels and risk of VTE.

The relative risk associated with factor XI did not vary according to age. The risk of VTE, however, is strongly associated with age, with an annual incidence of approximately 1 per 10,000 in the young increasing to nearly 1 in 100 in the elderly. Thus, in absolute terms, the effect of high factor XI levels is likely to be most important in the elderly.

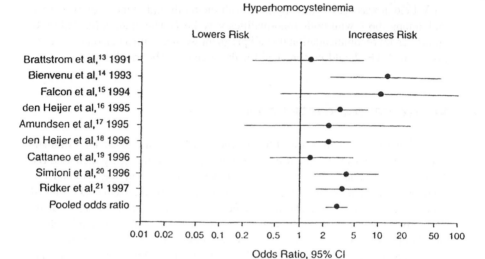

Figure 7   Overview of fasting hyperhomocysteinemia as a risk factor for venous thromboembolism. (Adapted from Ref. 35.)

VIII.   FACTOR VIII

Increased levels of factor VIII are also associated with an increased risk of first VTE (37). A recent study from the Vienna group examined the association between factor VIII levels and the risk of recurrent VTE (38). Three hundred sixty patients who had completed anticoagulation for a first thromboembolic event were followed for 30 months. Patients with previous recurrent or secondary VTE, lupus anticoagulant, known deficiency of antithrombin, protein C or protein S, cancer, or a long-term requirement for anticoagulation were excluded.

The overall recurrence rate was 10.6%. Patients with factor VIII levels >90th percentile had a recurrence rate of 37% at 2 years compared to a recurrence rate of 5% for those with levels <25th percentile. After adjustment for age, sex, duration of anticoagulation, and the presence or absence of factor V Leiden and G20210A, the relative risk for the group with factor VIII levels >90th percentile was 6.7 compared to those with levels <25th percentile. The relationship was nonlinear with a marked increase in risk for those over the 90th percentile. Other work has shown that the effect of factor VIII is independent of the acute phase response (39).

The overall recurrence rate in the Austrian study is approximately 5% per year. This is similar to that observed in the Swedish study by Schulman, but lower than that seen in the Canadian study of Kearon et al. which found a recurrence rate in of 20% in the first year (8,9). In contrast to the Canadian study, the Austrian study excluded patients at high risk for VTE, and consequently the lower recurrence rates reflect this.

IX. LABORATORY WORKUP FOR THROMBOPHILIA

A detailed personal and family history is a critical initial step in the evaluation of both acquired and inherited thrombotic risks in patients with early-onset, recurrent, idiopathic, or familial VTE. Specific laboratory tests may help guide the duration and intensity of anticoagulation. A typical thrombophilia workup should include tests to evaluate both acquired and inherited defects (Table 3). These tests will identify defects in approximately 40% of unselected patients with VTE and in the majority of patients with familial thrombophilia.

Screening programs to detect factor V Leiden carriers are controversial as the prevalence of the defect is high in the general population and most individuals never experience a thrombotic event. However, screening is likely to be indicated among patients with a first event. Those found to be carriers should consider nonpharmacological prophylactic measures on a long-term basis. Carriers of factor V Leiden should be prescribed alternative forms of birth control other than the oral contraceptive pill.

In many clinical settings, plasma-based testing for activated protein C (APC) resistance is used as an initial screening tool. This involves a modified assessment of activated partial thromboplastin time with and without APC. Although early assays for APC resistance were ineffective in the setting of anticoag-

Table 3 Laboratory Workup for Thrombophilic State

Thrombophilic condition	Laboratory test
APC resistance	APC resistance ratio
Factor V Leiden	Factor V Leiden DNA mutation test
Prothrombin mutation	Prothrombin G20210A DNA mutation test
Myeloproliferative disease	CBC and differential
Antiphospholipid antibody syndrome	aPTT, anticardiolipin antibodies
Hyperhomocysteinemia	Homocysteine
tl-MTHFR	tl-MTHFR DNA mutation test
Protein C deficiency	Protein C activity
Protein S deficiency	Protein S activity
Antithrombin III deficiency	Antithrombin III activity
Dysfibrinogenemia	Thrombin time, fibrinogen level

ulation, second-generation assays employing factor V–deficient plasma have largely overcome this problem. APC resistance ratios <2.0 are highly correlated with heterozygous carriers of factor V Leiden, while ratios <1.5 suggest homozygous defects. Genetic testing is recommended to confirm the suspected presence of factor V Leiden.

Formal screening for homocysteine levels in patients with VTE remains controversial. Homocysteine levels are easily reduced in most patients by the addition of folic acid to the diet; thus many clinicians favor the less expensive approach of giving patients with VTE a folate-containing multivitamin. There is also no currently available evidence that homocysteine reduction itself will reduce the risk of recurrent VTE.

Further work is required to define the value of measuring plasma levels of factor XI and VIII in patients with VTE. Testing for plasma factor XI and VIII levels may form part of the future thrombophilic workup in selected patients.

X. OPTIMAL DURATION OF ANTICOAGULATION: RISK OF BLEEDING VERSUS BENEFIT OF THERAPY

How long should a patient be treated with oral anticoagulants after VTE? The answer likely depends on a balance between the patient's risk of recurrence and risk of bleeding due to anticoagulation. The risk of hemorrhagic complications during warfarin therapy is related to several patient and treatment characteristics. A large prospective study from Italy recently reported the risk of hemorrhage among 2745 patients treated with warfarin (40). The overall risk of fatal, major, and minor bleeding was 0.25, 1.1, and 6.2 per 100 patient-years, respectively. These rates were lower that those previously reported in a large review of hemorrhagic complications in 1993 (41).

Patient characteristics that predicted increased risk of bleeding in the Italian study included age and the presence of cerebrovascular or peripheral vascular disease. The risk of hemorrhage was increased in the first 90 days after commencement of therapy and when the INR was >4.5.

Other studies have also found an increased risk early in the course of anticoagulation (42), and that the risk of bleeding increases with the intensity and duration of anticoagulation (9,43). A review by Levine et al. found that the frequency of major bleeding in patients randomly assigned to warfarin with a target INR of 2–3 was less than half that observed in those assigned to a target INR >3 (43). Other workers have reached similar conclusions (41).

Low-intensity warfarin (INR < 2) has been found to be safe. In a large-scale trial of several thousand men followed for over 10 years, no difference in bleeding rates has been documented between low-dose warfarin and low-dose aspirin (44). In the Coumadin Aspirin Reinfarction Study, mean hematocrit levels were similar between patients on low-dose warfarin and placebo (45). In two randomized trials of patients with malignancy, 1 mg of warfarin daily, and 1 mg of warfarin for 6 weeks followed by adjustment for an INR of 1.3 to 1.9 did not increase the risk of bleeding (46,47).

The duration of anticoagulation has been clearly associated with an increased risk of bleeding complications. In the study of Schulman et al., major bleeding occurred more commonly in those treated with warfarin indefinitely compared to those treated for 6 months (2.4 vs. 0.7% per year) after a recurrent thrombotic event (11). Kearon et al. have reported similar results in patients treated for a further 2 years after 3 months of anticoagulation for a first thrombotic event compared to those treated with placebo after 3 months of warfarin therapy (4.3 vs. 0% per year) (9). In these two studies combined, the case fatality rate with major bleeding was 15% (2 of 13 patients).

Most studies agree that patients with vascular disease, renal insufficiency, and a history of gastrointestinal bleeding carry an increased risk of bleeding on warfarin (43,48). Most studies have also found an increased risk of hemorrhage on warfarin with increasing age (40,48,49), although some have suggested that age is not an important determinant of risk of overall bleeding complications, but that patients >80 years old are at increased risk of fatal or life-threatening hemorrhagic complications (50).

Given these uncertainties about bleeding, several ongoing clinical trials are addressing the optimal duration of anticoagulation following VTE (Table 4). For example, PREVENT is a randomized double-blind, placebo-controlled trial of long-term low-dose warfarin among patients with a prior history of idiopathic venous thrombosis who have completed a standard course of 3 to 6 months of outpatient anticoagulation (12). Both men and women over 30 years old are included in the trial. Trial endpoints include recurrent VTE, major bleeding episodes, and all-cause mortality in the total patient population and separately in those who carry factor V Leiden.

The PREVENT trial has been designed to investigate directly two issues. First, with regard to concerns about the risk-benefit ratio of long-term anticoagulation therapy, PREVENT will evaluate a low intensity of warfarin (target INR 1.5–2), which, after initial titration, will require infrequent outpatient monitoring and has a proven safety profile (44,45). Second, to improve the future determination of patient-risk profile, PREVENT has been designed to address specifically the risk-to-benefit ratio of low-intensity warfarin among patients who carry factor V Leiden.

The limited clinical data regarding the use of low-dose warfarin for the prevention of VTE are encouraging. Very low doses of warfarin (1 mg) have been shown to prevent thrombosis of chronic indwelling central venous catheters

Table 4 Trials of Long-Term Anticoagulation to Prevent Recurrent VTE Following 3–6 Months of Full-Dose Warfarin

Trial (PI)	Study group	Randomized drug comparison		
PREVENT Ridker	Idiopathic VTE	INR 1.5–2.0	vs	Placebo
WODIT DVT Agnelli	Idiopathic DVT	INR 1.5–2.0	vs	No warfarin
WODIT PE Agnelli	Any PE	INR 2.0–3.0	vs	No warfarin
ELATE Kearon	Idiopathic VTE	INR 1.5–1.9	vs	INR 2.0–3.0
DURAC III Schulman	Any VTE + ACLA	INR 1.5–2.0	vs	INR 2.0–3.0
THRIVE III Schulman	Any VTE	Thrombin inhibitor	vs	Placebo

(47). Other studies have demonstrated that fixed minidose warfarin (1 mg) is effective in preventing VTE at the time of pelvic surgery, without any increase in surgical bleeding as compared to placebo (51).

Laboratory data are also available which suggest that low-dose warfarin has important inhibitory effects on hemostasis. Prothrombin F_{1+2} levels are a marker of prothrombin activation. Anticoagulation with warfarin to an INR of 1.3–1.6 results in a suppression of baseline F_{1+2} levels by approximately 50% (52). Low-dose warfarin (1 mg) has also been shown to reduce factor VII levels in normal volunteers (53).

Other trials are also investigating the optimal intensity and duration of anticoagulation following VTE. The WODIT DVT trial in Italy, similar to the PREVENT trial, is comparing low-dose warfarin with placebo after routine anticoagulation for deep venous thrombosis, while other studies in Canada and Europe are comparing long-term low-dose warfarin versus standard-dose anticoagulation, and long-term standard-dose warfarin versus placebo, all after an initial 3- to 6-month course of full-dose anticoagulation (Table 4).

XI. CONCLUSION

The optimal duration of anticoagulation following VTE remains controversial. Some patients, with transient risk factors for VTE, probably require only a short course of anticoagulation for 4 to 6 weeks. The risk of recurrence for individuals with an idiopathic thromboembolic event is determined by a dynamic interaction between genetic and acquired risk factors. Further studies are required to determine which subgroups of patients will benefit from lifelong anticoagulation, and whether long-term, low-dose warfarin will prove to be a safe and effective therapy for the prevention of recurrent venous thromboembolic disease.

REFERENCES

1. Prandoni P, Lensing AW, Cogo A, Cuppini S, Villalta S, Carta M, et al. The long-term clinical course of acute deep venous thrombosis. Ann Intern Med 1996; 125(1): 1–7.
2. De Stefano V, Martinelli I, Mannucci PM, Paciaroni K, Chiusolo P, Casorelli I, et al. The risk of recurrent deep venous thrombosis among heterozygous carriers of both factor V Leiden and the G20210A prothrombin mutation. N Engl J Med 1999; 341(11):801–806.
3. Rosendaal FR. Venous thrombosis: a multicausal disease. Lancet 1999; 353(9159): 1167–73.
4. Hyers TM, Agnelli G, Hull RD, Weg JG, Morris TA, Samama M, et al. Antithrombotic therapy for venous thromboembolic disease. Chest 1998; 114(5 suppl):561S–578S.
5. Optimum duration of anticoagulation for deep-vein thrombosis and pulmonary embolism. Research Committee of the British Thoracic Society. Lancet 1992; 340(8824):873–876.
6. Hirsh J. The optimal duration of anticoagulant therapy for venous thrombosis. N Engl J Med 1995; 332(25):1710–1711.
7. Levine MN, Hirsh J, Gent M, Turpie AG, Weitz J, Ginsberg J, et al. Optimal duration of oral anticoagulant therapy: a randomized trial comparing four weeks with three months of warfarin in patients with proximal deep vein thrombosis. Thromb Haemost 1995; 74(2):606–611.
8. Schulman S, Rhedin AS, Lindmarker P, Carlsson A, Larfars G, Nicol P, et al. A comparison of six weeks with six months of oral anticoagulant therapy after a first episode of venous thromboembolism. Duration of Anticoagulation Trial Study Group. N Engl J Med 1995; 332(25):1661–1665.
9. Kearon C, Gent M, Hirsh J, Weitz J, Kovacs MJ, Anderson DR, et al. A comparison of three months of anticoagulation with extended anticoagulation for a first episode of idiopathic venous thromboembolism. N Engl J Med 1999; 340(12):901–907.
10. Schafer AI. Venous thrombosis as a chronic disease. N Engl J Med 1999; 340(12): 955–956.
11. Schulman S, Granqvist S, Holmstrom M, Carlsson A, Lindmarker P, Nicol P, et al. The duration of oral anticoagulant therapy after a second episode of venous thromboembolism. The Duration of Anticoagulation Trial Study Group. N Engl J Med 1997; 336(6):393–398.

12. Ridker PM. Long-term, low-dose warfarin among venous thrombosis patients with and without factor V Leiden mutation: rationale and design for the Prevention of Recurrent Venous Thromboembolism (PREVENT) trial. Vasc Med 1998; 3(1):67–73.

13. Diuguid DL. Oral anticoagulant therapy for venous thromboembolism. N Engl J Med 1997; 336(6):433–434.

14. Dahlback B, Carlsson M, Svensson PJ. Familial thrombophilia due to a previously unrecognized mechanism characterized by poor anticoagulant response to activated protein C: prediction of a cofactor to activated protein C. Proc Natl Acad Sci USA 1993; 90(3):1004–1008.

15. Bertina RM, Koeleman BP, Koster T, Rosendaal FR, Dirven RJ, de Ronde H, et al. Mutation in blood coagulation factor V associated with resistance to activated protein C. Nature 1994; 369(6475):64–67.

16. Koster T, Rosendaal FR, de Ronde H, Briet E, Vandenbroucke JP, Bertina RM. Venous thrombosis due to poor anticoagulant response to activated protein C: Leiden Thrombophilia Study. Lancet 1993; 342(8886–8887):1503–1506.

17. Price DT, Ridker PM. Factor V Leiden mutation and the risks for thromboembolic disease: a clinical perspective. Ann Intern Med 1997; 127(10):895–903.

18. Ridker PM, Hennekens CH, Lindpaintner K, Stampfer MJ, Eisenberg PR, Miletich JP. Mutation in the gene coding for coagulation factor V and the risk of myocardial infarction, stroke, and venous thrombosis in apparently healthy men. N Engl J Med 1995; 332(14):912–917.

19. Ridker PM, Glynn RJ, Miletich JP, Goldhaber SZ, Stampfer MJ, Hennekens CH. Age-specific incidence rates of venous thromboembolism among heterozygous carriers of factor V Leiden mutation. Ann Intern Med 1997; 126(7):528–531.

20. Ridker PM, Hennekens CH, Selhub J, Miletich JP, Malinow MR, Stampfer MJ. Interrelation of hyperhomocyst(e)inemia, factor V Leiden, and risk of future venous thromboembolism. Circulation 1997; 95(7):1777–1782.

21. Gandrille S, Greengard JS, Alhenc-Gelas M, Juhan-Vague I, Abgrall JF, Jude B, et al. Incidence of activated protein C resistance caused by the ARG 506 GLN mutation in factor V in 113 unrelated symptomatic protein C-deficient patients. The French Network on behalf of INSERM. Blood 1995; 86(1):219–224.

22. Zoller B, Berntsdotter A, Garcia de Frutos P, Dahlback B. Resistance to activated protein C as an additional genetic risk factor in hereditary deficiency of protein S. Blood 1995; 85(12):3518–3523.

23. Ridker PM, Miletich JP, Stampfer MJ, Goldhaber SZ, Lindpaintner K, Hennekens CH. Factor V Leiden and risks of recurrent idiopathic venous thromboembolism. Circulation 1995; 92(10):2800–2802.

24. Simioni P, Prandoni P, Lensing AW, Scudeller A, Sardella C, Prins MH, et al. The risk of recurrent venous thromboembolism in patients with an Arg506-to-Gln mutation in the gene for factor V (factor V Leiden). N Engl J Med 1997; 336(6):399–403.

25. Rintelen C, Pabinger I, Knobl P, Lechner K, Mannhalter C. Probability of recurrence of thrombosis in patients with and without factor V Leiden. Thromb Haemost 1996; 75(2):229–232.

26. Poort SR, Rosendaal FR, Reitsma PH, Bertina RM. A common genetic variation in the 3'-untranslated region of the prothrombin gene is associated with elevated plasma prothrombin levels and an increase in venous thrombosis. Blood 1996; 88(10):3698–3703.

27. Eichinger S, Minar E, Hirschl M, Bialonczyk C, Stain M, Mannhalter C, et al. The risk of early recurrent venous thromboembolism after oral anticoagulant therapy in patients with the G20210A transition in the prothrombin gene. Thromb Haemost 1999; 81(1):14–17.

28. Hillarp A, Zoller B, Svensson PJ, Dahlback B. The 20210 A allele of the prothrombin gene is a common risk factor among Swedish outpatients with verified deep venous thrombosis. Thromb Haemost 1997; 78(3):990–992.

29. Cumming AM, Keeney S, Salden A, Bhavnani M, Shwe KH, Hay CR. The prothrombin gene G20210A variant: prevalence in a U.K. anticoagulant clinic population. Br J Haematol 1997; 98(2):353–355.

30. Ridker PM, Hennekens CH, Miletich JP. G20210A mutation in prothrombin gene and risk of myocardial infarction, stroke, and venous thrombosis in a large cohort of US men. Circulation 1999; 99(8):999–1004.

31. Lindmarker P, Schulman S, Sten-Linder M, Wiman B, Egberg N, Johnsson H. The risk of recurrent venous thromboembolism in carriers and non-carriers of the G1691A allele in the coagulation factor V gene and the G20210A allele in the prothrombin gene. DURAC Trial Study Group. Duration of Anticoagulation. Thromb Haemost 1999; 81(5):684–689.

32. Vandenbroucke JP, Koster T, Briet E, Reitsma PH, Bertina RM, Rosendaal FR. Increased risk of venous thrombosis in oral-contraceptive users who are carriers of factor V Leiden mutation. Lancet 1994; 344(8935):1453–1457.

33. Gerhardt A, Scharf RE, Beckmann MW, Struve S, Bender HG, Pillny M, et al. Prothrombin and factor V mutations in women with a history of thrombosis during pregnancy and the puerperium. N Engl J Med 2000; 342(6):374–380.

34. Greer IA. The challenge of thrombophilia in maternal-fetal medicine. N Engl J Med 2000; 342(6):424–425.

35. Ray JG. Meta-analysis of hyperhomocysteinemia as a risk factor for venous thromboembolic disease. Arch Intern Med 1998; 158(19):2101–2106.

36. Meijers JC, Tekelenburg WL, Bouma BN, Bertina RM, Rosendaal FR. High levels of coagulation factor XI as a risk factor for venous thrombosis. N Engl J Med 2000; 342(10):696–701.

37. Koster T, Blann AD, Briet E, Vandenbroucke JP, Rosendaal FR. Role of clotting factor VIII in effect of von Willebrand factor on occurrence of deep-vein thrombosis. Lancet 1995; 345(8943):152–155.

38. Kyrle PA, Minar E, Hirschl M, Bialonczyk C, Stain M, Schneider B, et al. High plasma levels of factor VIII and the risk of recurrent venous thromboembolism. N Engl J Med 2000; 343(7):457–462.

39. O'Donnell J, Mumford AD, Manning RA, Laffan M. Elevation of FVIII: C in venous thromboembolism is persistent and independent of the acute phase response. Thromb Haemost 2000; 83(1):10–13.

40. Palareti G, Leali, N, Coccheri S, Poggi M, Manotti C, D'Angelo A, et al. Bleeding

complications of oral anticoagulant treatment: an inception-cohort, prospective collaborative study (ISCOAT). Italian Study on Complications of Oral Anticoagulant Therapy. Lancet 1996; 348(9025):423–428.

41. Landefeld CS, Beyth RJ. Anticoagulant-related bleeding: clinical epidemiology, prediction, and prevention. Am J Med 1993; 95(3):315–328.

42. Landefeld CS, Anderson PA. Guideline-based consultation to prevent anticoagulant-related bleeding. A randomized, controlled trial in a teaching hospital. Ann Intern Med 1992; 116(10):829–837.

43. Levine MN, Raskob G, Landefeld S, Kearon C. Hemorrhagic complications of anticoagulant treatment. Chest 1998; 114(5 suppl):511S–523S.

44. Meade TW, Roderick PJ, Brennan PJ, Wilkes HC, Kelleher CC. Extra-cranial bleeding and other symptoms due to low dose aspirin and low intensity oral anticoagulation. Thromb Haemost 1992; 68(1):1–6.

45. Goodman SG, Langer A, Durica SS, Raskob GE, Comp PC, Gray RJ, et al. Safety and anticoagulation effect of a low-dose combination of warfarin and aspirin in clinically stable coronary artery disease. Coumadin Aspirin Reinfarction (CARS) Pilot Study Group. Am J Cardiol 1994; 74(7):657–661.

46. Levine M, Hirsh J, Gent M, Arnold A, Warr D, Falanga A, et al. Double-blind randomised trial of a very-low-dose warfarin for prevention of thromboembolism in stage IV breast cancer. Lancet 1994; 343(8902):886–889.

47. Bern MM, Lokich JJ, Wallach SR, Bothe A, Jr., Benotti PN, Arkin CF, et al. Very low doses of warfarin can prevent thrombosis in central venous catheters. A randomized prospective trial. Ann Intern Med 1990; 112(6):423–428.

48. Beyth RJ, Quinn LM, Landefeld CS. Prospective evaluation of an index for predicting the risk of major bleeding in outpatients treated with warfarin. Am J Med 1998; 105(2):91–99.

49. van der Meer FJ, Rosendaal FR, Vandenbroucke JP, Briet E. Assessment of a bleeding risk index in two cohorts of patients treated with oral anticoagulants. Thromb Haemost 1996; 76(1):12–16.

50. Fihn SD, Callahan CM, Martin DC, McDonell MB, Henikoff JG, White RH. The risk for and severity of bleeding complications in elderly patients treated with warfarin. The National Consortium of Anticoagulation Clinics. Ann Intern Med 1996; 124(11):970–979.

51. Poller L, McKernan A, Thomson JM, Elstein M, Hirsch PJ, Jones JB. Fixed minidose warfarin: a new approach to prophylaxis against venous thrombosis after major surgery. Br Med J (Clin Res Ed) 1987; 295(6609):1309–1312.

52. Millenson MM, Bauer KA, Kistler JP, Barzegar S, Tulin L, Rosenberg RD. Monitoring mini-intensity anticoagulation with warfarin: comparison of the prothrombin time using a sensitive thromboplastin with prothrombin fragment F_{1+2} levels. Blood 1992; 79(8):2034–2038.

53. Poller L, MacCallum PK, Thomson JM, Kerns W. Reduction of factor VII coagulant activity (VIIC), a risk factor for ischaemic heart disease, by fixed dose warfarin: a double blind crossover study. Br Heart J 1990; 63(4):231–233.

17

The Expanded Role of an Interdisciplinary Anticoagulation Service

Kanella V. Tsilimingras
Brigham and Women's Hospital, Boston, Massachusetts

Kristen Hallisey
Connecticut Surgical Group, Hartford, Connecticut

I. INTRODUCTION

Most anticoagulation services function in the setting of outpatient programs. At the Brigham and Women's Hospital Cardiac Center, the role of the anticoagulation service has been expanded to cover both inpatients as well as outpatients. Daily clinical anticoagulation rounds provide reinforcement of appropriate dosing guidelines for warfarin, low-molecular-weight heparins (LMWH), and other anticoagulants. The Anticoagulation Service serves as an educational resource as well as facilitating anticoagulation monitoring. A centralized anticoagulation service undertakes various levels of anticoagulation management, resulting in decreased hospital length of stay and improved patient outcomes. This model of care promotes a seamless transition for patients from the hospital to home.

The use of warfarin as an oral anticoagulant did not become commonplace until the 1950s following President Eisenhower's heart attack (1). Oral anticoagulation poses many challenges because warfarin is extremely difficult to regulate and has a narrow therapeutic index. Excessive anticoagulation predisposes to major hemorrhage. Subtherapeutic levels are associated with thrombosis and thromboembolism.

Our anticoagulation service functions as an interdisciplinary health-care team. Centralized anticoagulation management reduces the frequency of adverse clinical events compared with conventionally managed anticoagulation (Table 1). An anticoagulation service can also reduce use of the emergency department (2).

Table 1 Clinical Outcomes with an Anticoagulation
Service (ACS)

	UMC ($n = 145$)	ACS ($n = 183$)
Major/fatal bleeding	3.9%	1.6%
Thromboembolism	1.8%	3.3%
Warfarin/hospitalization	19%	5%
ED visits	22%	6%

Source: From Ref. 2.
UMC = usual medical care; ACS = anticoagulation service;
ED = emergency department.

There are 11 essential components in establishing and implementing a multidisciplinary anticoagulation service.

1. Mission statement, policies, and procedures
2. Qualified staff
3. Patient referrals
4. Initial patient assessment/dosing considerations
5. INR monitoring/laboratory results
6. Patient education
7. Proactive identification of potential warfarin–drug interactions
8. Computerized documentation of anticoagulation management
9. Decreasing hospital length of stay
10. Quality assurance and risk management
11. Exquisitely thorough and compulsive communication

II. MISSION STATEMENT, POLICIES, AND PROCEDURES

The mission statement characterizes the purpose of the anticoagulation service, staff structure, scope of services, and target patient population. The anticoagulation service policies and procedures provide the framework of daily activities, clinical guidelines, and quality assurance measurements. They clearly define the roles and responsibilities of the anticoagulation care providers and referring physicians.

III. QUALIFIED STAFF

The anticoagulation provider should hold a license in a patient-oriented health-related field (e.g., medicine, pharmacy, nursing) and meet minimum competencies and/or related work experience (3).

Currently, the University of Illinois at Chicago College of Pharmacy and the American Society of Health System Pharmacists Research and Education Foundation provide anticoagulation management traineeship programs for pharmacists. The National Certification Board for Anticoagulation offers on a quarterly basis, the Anticoagulation Care Provider (ACCP) Certification examination available to physicians, physician assistants, pharmacists, and nurses. For information contact *www.acforum.org*.

IV. PATIENT REFERRALS

The anticoagulation service obtains referrals from inpatients and outpatients. Mechanisms for efficient referrals must be established to avoid patients "falling through the cracks." An intake referral form is completed for each new patient. The form includes the patient's address, telephone number, referring physician, indication for anticoagulation, target INR, and duration of therapy. Pertinent current medication, recent lab data, and relevant past medical history are also listed (Fig. 1).

V. ANTICOAGULATION INITIAL PATIENT ASSESSMENT

The anticoagulation service should perform an initial patient assessment to ensure appropriate and effective warfarin therapy. The initial patient assessment should include but not be limited to the following:

Indication for anticoagulation
Intensity of anticoagulation
Duration of therapy
Age
History of bleeding events
Comorbid conditions
Drug–drug interactions
Nutritional status

ANTICOAGULATION SERVICE

INTAKE/REFERRAL FORM

NAME_____DOB_____MR#_____

ADDRESS_____

CITY_____STATE_____ZIP CODE_____

TELE#_____ALTERNATIVE#_____

CARDIOLOGIST/CARD.SURGEON_____TELE#_____

PCP_____TELE#_____

ADDRESS_____

DIAGNOSIS_____

START DATE_____TARGET INR_____DURATION_____

LAB AGENCY_____TELE#_____

VNA/HOME CARE_____TELE#_____

PAST MEDICAL HISTORY   CURRENT MEDS

_____   _____

_____   _____

_____   _____

INITAIL NOTE_____

DOSE/INR BEFORE D/C_____

FOR OFFICE USE ONLY   DATE ACTIVATED_____

ADMIT TO   DISCH FROM

BICS _____   _____ MET PT IN HOSP/OR AMB_____

COUMA_____   _____ SPOKE ON THE PHONE_____

ACCESS_____   _____ GIVEN/SENT ED. MAT._____

Figure 1   Anticoagulation service referral form.

VI. INDICATION FOR ANTICOAGULATION

Each anticoagulation service should have guidelines that include: (1) indication for anticoagulation; (2) the International Normalized Ratio (INR) target range; and (3) duration of therapy. These guidelines (4) should encompass: atrial fibrillation; prosthetic heart valves; deep vein thrombosis; pulmonary embolism; valvular heart disease; and cardiomyopathies.

Table 2 Initiating Warfarin at 5 mg versus 10 mg

INR	Day #5 INR Warfarin 5 mg ($n = 31$)	Warfarin 10 mg ($n = 21$)
<2.0	8%	15%
2.0–3.0	88%	69%
>3.0	4%	15%

Source: From Ref. 5.

VII. DOSING CONSIDERATIONS

In most instances, the initial dose of warfarin should be 5 mg followed by subsequent INR monitoring for appropriate dose adjustments. A clinical trial indicates that initiating 5 mg of warfarin daily is more likely to achieve a target INR of 2.0–3.0 in 5 days than initiating warfarin at a dose of 10 mg daily (Table 2) (5). However, lower starting doses of less than 5 mg may be appropriate in the elderly and patients at high risk of bleeding (6).

A genetic mutation in the cytochrome P450 system in the liver results in slow metabolism of the warfarin in 1 to 3 % of the population (7). Warfarin is a racemic mixture of an S- and R-enantiomer metabolized by this cytochrome. The S-enantiomer exhibits 2 to 5 times more anticoagulation activity than the R-enantiomer. The cytochrome P450 CYP2C9 is responsible for the metabolism of the S-warfarin. Patients with a CYP2C9 genetic mutation require a maintenance dose of 1.5 mg or less of warfarin, with no other apparent cause for low-dose requirement (Fig. 2).

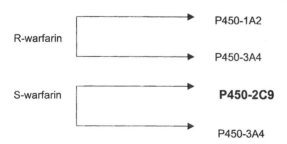

Figure 2 Oxidative metabolism of warfarin enantiomers.

VIII.   PATIENT EDUCATION

The anticoagulation service educates the patient regarding anticoagulants, including low-molecular-weight heparin and subcutaneous self-injections. Patients and/or family members are required to perform injections prior to discharge to ensure proper administration and adherence after discharge.

In general, the rate of nonadherence to medication regimens ranges from 30 to 70%, directly related to the number of prescribed medications (8). Most elderly patients on warfarin take more than four prescribed medications a day, which fosters the possibilities of nonadherence and medication errors. Therefore, patient education is the rate-limiting factor in the success of anticoagulation management (9). The initial educational meeting with the patient and family is ex-

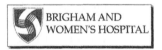 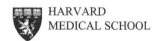

BRIGHAM AND WOMEN'S HOSPITAL

HARVARD MEDICAL SCHOOL

Anticoagulation Service
75 Francis Street
Boston, Massachusetts 02115
Tel: 617-732-8887
FAX: 617-975-0989

IMPORTANT

ANTICOAGULATION DISCHARGE SHEET

1. Visiting Nurse's
    Association:_____
2. Laboratory where blood will be processed:_____
3. Progression of blood work:
    __ Daily x 3
    __ Twice a week
    __ Once a week
    __ Once every two weeks
    __ Once a month
4. INR range: ____ - ____
5. Duration of treatment:_____
6. We will call you within 24 hours of your blood test.

Pharmacist: Kim Tsilimingras B.S.Pharm
Nurse: Kris Hallisey RN, BSN, CVN
Admin. Assistant: Kate Connell
Medical Director: Samuel Z. Goldhaber M.D.

Under the auspices of the Cardiac Center

Figure 3   Brigham and Women's Hospital Cardiac Center anticoagulation discharge sheet.

tremely important and helps foster compliance and trust. Our educational policy mandates that we

1. Personally meet with the patient and/or family.
2. Discuss and provide the patient with the written discharge plan of his/her anticoagulation therapy and follow-up.
3. Provide reading material and videotapes.

The details of our management plan are summarized on a discharge sheet (Fig. 3). One copy of the discharge sheet is given to the patient, and the other copy is placed in the patient's medical record. The discharge sheets assist the hospital staff, such as nurses and discharge care coordinators, in appropriate discharge planning.

IX. INR MONITORING AND LABORATORY RESULTS

Effective control of INR monitoring requires a rapid process of obtaining laboratory results for appropriate interpretation and subsequent patient management. Initially, an INR is obtained at least twice weekly. The anticoagulation service should coordinate INR testing, reporting, and ordering dosing changes (Fig. 4). Locations for INR testing include local laboratories, physicians' offices, hospital laboratories, or point-of-care self-testing. Octogenarians or homebound patients may require home phlebotomy performed by a laboratory technologist or by a visiting nurse.

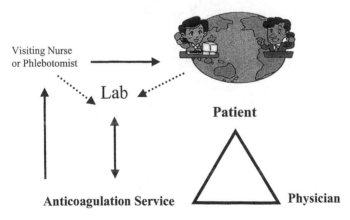

Figure 4 Communication scheme for the anticoagulation service.

The INR results are either called or faxed to the anticoagulation service for interpretation and dosing recommendations. On a daily basis, the anticoagulation service also calls those laboratories that fail to report expected results. Brigham and Women's Hospital's Cardiac Center's anticoagulation service accommodates anticoagulation monitoring for patients living or traveling out of state or internationally.

A. Patient Self-Monitoring of Anticoagulation

The Coagu-Chek (Roche Diagnostics) is a point-of-care testing device to monitor INRs (Fig. 5). In the treatment of diabetes mellitus, self-monitoring and self-adjustment of medication combined with a structured patient treatment program have resulted in major improvements in patient adherence, outcomes, and quality of life (10). Insurance companies are beginning to cover the use of self point-of-care testing devices, but at this time widespread coverage is not available (11).

Though studies have shown that self-management can be as effective and safe as conventional management, a specific teaching program is necessary to certify that patients can use the self point-of-care testing device. Cromheecke and colleagues (12) performed a crossover randomized study that revealed that self-management of oral anticoagulation results in control of anticoagulation that

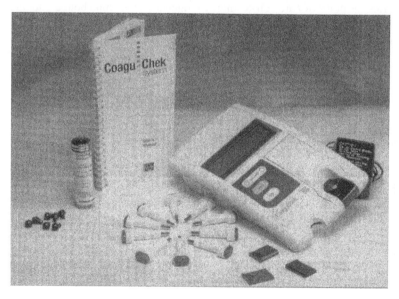

Figure 5   Roche diagnostic Coagu-Chek machine and supplies.

is at least as good and potentially superior to control by an anticoagulation service. Quality of life was improved in the self-care group. However, the percentage of patients within the target INR range was similar in both groups. Despite the ability of patients to self-manage oral anticoagulation, adequate education and structure remain necessary.

X. PROACTIVE IDENTIFICATION OF WARFARIN–DRUG INTERACTIONS

Initial assessment of the patient should include a medication history to identify potential drug–drug interactions with warfarin. Warfarin can be inhibited or potentiated by other drugs, resulting in an enhanced or decreased anticoagulant effect (Table 3). The anticoagulation care provider should be able to identify potential drug interactions and suggest dose adjustments with respect to the magnitude of response, time of onset, and the duration of the effect. The provider should also warn all patients about potential hazards, and instruct against taking any drug, including nonprescription products, without the advice of a physician or anticoagulation service.

Patients should be instructed to notify the Anticoagulation Service of changes or addition of other medication. Drugs can influence the pharmacokinetics of warfarin either by decreasing the absorption from the intestine or altering its metabolic clearance. Amiodarone and warfarin are one of the most commonly

Table 3 Most Common Warfarin–Drug Interactions

Drugs that increase the anticoagulant effect of warfarin	Drugs that decrease the anticoagulant effect of warfarin
Amiodarone	Rifampin
Fluconazole	Dicloxacillin
Quinolones	Nafcillin
(Levofloxacin, ciprofloxacin)	Sucralfate
Bactrim	Cholestyramine
Metronidazole	Carbamazepine
Cimetidine	
Acetaminophen	
Omeprazole	
Propafenone	
Rofecoxib (Vioxx)	
Celecoxib (Celebrex)	
NSAIDs	

seen drug interactions that require warfarin dose reduction upon initiation of amiodarone. Amiodarone appears to inhibit the hepatic metabolism of warfarin, resulting in 50 to 100% increase in the INR in patients previously stabilized on warfarin therapy. Careful monitoring and appropriate dosage reduction permits combination therapy.

XI. COMPUTERIZED DOCUMENTATION

Documentation of coordinated patient services is required by JCAHO (Joint Commission on Accreditation of Healthcare Organization). The Brigham and Women's Hospital's Cardiac Center's anticoagulation service uses a virtually paperless computerized system. Documentation of patient anticoagulation management is entered in the CoumaCare program and the centralized hospital computer system. CoumaCare is one of many computerized programs currently available that is specifically designed for anticoagulation management. This facilitates access to INR results, previous dosing regimens, and future scheduled laboratory test dates.

XII. DECREASING HOSPITAL LENGTH OF STAY

The anticoagulation service at the Brigham and Women's Hospital has decreased the hospital length of stay with respect to anticoagulation management (Fig. 6). A prospective quality assurance analysis of approximately 400 cardiac patients managed by the ACS from April 1999 to August 2000 reflects a decreased hospital length of stay in approximately one-fourth of patients.

XIII. QUALITY ASSURANCE

Brigham and Women's Hospital utilizes a daily prospective computerized tracking system to document patients outside the target INR range, as well as the clinical complications of bleeding and thrombosis. Whenever an adverse event occurs, we analyze it as part of our continuous quality improvement.

XIV. COMMUNICATION

Communication is the key to a successful anticoagulation service. We orient the patient and family to the process in which INRs will be obtained and how we will communicate dosing changes.

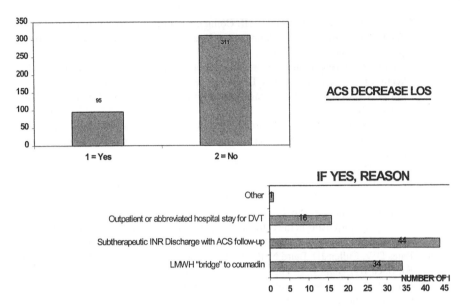

Figure 6 Anticoagulation service decreases hospital length of stay.

XV. CONCLUSION

At the Brigham and Women's Hospital's Cardiac Center's anticoagulation service, education and communication are the keys to our success. The Brigham and Women's Cardiac Center helps to provide a seamless transition in anticoagulation monitoring from hospital to home. The expanded role allows us to function as a hospital-wide educational resource for patients as well as hospital staff. The educational areas include medication use, drug interactions, dosing requirements, and use of self point-of-care testing devices. In addition to the educational activities, we round daily on the cardiac surgery units to assist with appropriate postoperative warfarin dosing. A multidiscipline centralized anticoagulation service enhances the efficacy and safety of both the inpatient and outpatient anticoagulation management.

REFERENCES

1. Ansell J. Historical developments in oral anticoagulation: managing oral anticoagulation therapy clinical and operational guidelines. Hist Devel Oral Anticoagulation 2000; 1A-1:1S.

2. Chiquette E, Amato MG, Bussey HI. Comparison of an anticoagulation clinic with usual medical care: Anticoagulation control, patient outcomes, and health care costs. Arch Intern Med 1998; 158:1641–1647.

3. Oertel L. Anticoagulation services. Quality improvement direction—pursuing a certification process. J Thrombosis Thrombolysis 1999; 7:153S–156S.

4. Fifth ACCP Consensus Conference on Antithrombotic Therapy. Chest 1998; 114: 439S–748S.

5. Crowther MA, Ginsberg JB, Kearon C, Harrison L, Johnson J, Masicotte MP, Hirsh J. A randomized trial comparing 5 mg and 10 mg warfarin loading doses. Arch Intern Med 1999; 159:46–48.

6. Hirsh J, Dalen JE, Anderson DR, Poller L, Bussey H, Ansell J, Deykin D, Brandt JT. Oral anticoagulants mechanism of action, clinical effectiveness, and optimal therapeutic range. Chest 1998; 114:443S–454S.

7. Aithal P, Guruprasad, Day P, Christopher, Kesteven JL, Patrick, Daly AK. Association of polymorphisms in the cytochrome P450 CYP2C9 with warfarin dose requirement and risk of bleeding complications. Lancet 1999; 353:717–719.

8. Bates DW, Cullen JD, Laird N, Petersen LA, Small SD, Servi D, Laffel G, Sweitzer BJ, Shea BF, Halliey R, Vliet MV, Nemeskal R, Leape LL. Incidence of adverse drug events and potential adverse drug events. JAMA 1995; 274:29–34.

9. Gibbar-Clements T, Shirrell D, Dooley R, Smiley B. The challenge of warfarin therapy. Am J Nursing 2000; 3:38–40.

10. Zimmerman C. The pole of point-of-care anticoagulation monitoring in arterial and venous thromboembolic disorders. J Thrombosis Thrombolysis 2000; 5:87S–198S.

11. Sawicki PT. A structured teaching and self-management program for patients receiving oral anticoagulation. A randomized controlled trial. JAMA 1999; 281:145–150.

12. Cromheecke EM, Levi M, Colly L, deMol B, Prins M, Hutten B, Mak R, Keyzers K, Buller H. Oral anticoagulation self-management and management by a specialist anticoagulation clinic: a randomised cross-over comparison. Lancet 2000; 356:97–102.

18

Interventional Venous Angiography

Gordon Haugland
SUNY–Downstate Medical Center, Brooklyn, New York

Stephen Bravo
St. Francis Hospital, Roslyn, New York

Michael F. Meyerovitz
St. Vincent's Hospital, Worcester Medical Center, Worcester, Massachusetts

The role of the interventional angiographer in the care of patients with venous thrombosis, stenosis, and occlusion continues to expand. Over the past several years, the application of endovascular techniques to the treatment of venous abnormalities has resulted in advances paralleling those achieved in the arterial system.

I. INFERIOR VENA CAVAL FILTERS

Deep venous thrombosis (DVT) and pulmonary embolism (PE) represent a continuum of the same disease process. DVT and PE account for hundreds of thousands of hospitalizations and tens of thousands of deaths annually in the United States (1,2). Most PEs arise from the deep venous system of the lower extremities, with the remainder arising within the inferior or superior vena cava, upper extremities, ovarian veins, and right atrium (3).

Mechanical interruption of the inferior vena cava (IVC) by filter devices has become a well-established technique. When the source of emboli is identified as the upper extremities and certain other indications are met, filter devices may be placed in the superior vena cava.

The indications for IVC interruption after the confirmation of the diagnosis of deep venous thrombosis or pulmonary embolism include: a contraindication to or a complication from anticoagulation (recent hemorrhagic stroke, active gastrointestinal bleeding, etc.); failure of anticoagulation (progression of deep venous thrombosis or recurrent pulmonary embolism despite anticoagulation); free-floating thrombus within the IVC; preoperative placement during surgical pulmonary embolectomy or severe pulmonary disease, or prior history of pulmonary embolism and subsequent limited pulmonary reserve in whom a new PE might be fatal (4–6). Prophylactic IVC filter placement in patients at high risk of DVT and PE (primarily in the setting of multiple trauma–pelvic fracture, head/spinal injury) has been the subject of much debate. Several authors advocate the early prophylactic caval filter placement to minimize post-trauma morbidity and mortality from pulmonary embolism (7,8).

The development of IVC filters that can be deployed through relatively small venous sheaths (6–14 Fr.) has led to the routine percutaneous placement of these devices via a common femoral, internal jugular, or, in the case of one device (Simon-Nitinol), an antecubital venous approach. Prior to filter placement, an inferior vena cavagram is routinely performed to assess caval patency, to define any anomalies, and to determine the level of the renal vein inflow as well as the caudal termination of the IVC. Optimal placement of the filter is below the level of the renal veins. This allows for the preservation of renal venous outflow in the event of caval thrombosis, a complication of filter placement. Furthermore, this minimizes the volume of cava above the filter that may be filled with thrombus in the setting of caval thrombosis and act as a source for continued PE. However, when infrarenal placement is not possible, usually because of caval thrombus, filter placement in the suprarenal IVC is acceptable.

There are currently seven filter devices approved for clinical use in the U.S. These are the Greenfield filter (Boston Scientific, Natick, MA) in both stainless steel and titanium, the Gianturco-Roehm Bird's Nest filter (Cook, Inc., Bloomington, IN), the Simon-Nitinol filter (C.R. Bard Inc., Covington, GA), the LGM-Vena Tech filter (B. Braun Medical Inc., Evanston, IL), the TrapEase filter (Cordis, Miami, FL), and the Gunther Tulip filter (Cook, Inc., Bloomington, IN). The long-term clinical and radiographic outcome of patients undergoing insertion of these filters has been excellent with superior clinical efficacy in the prevention of recurrent PE. A summary of available data demonstrates recurrent pulmonary embolism rates ranging from 3 to 4% and inferior vena caval patency rates ranging from 90 to 97% (6,9–14). It is difficult to ascertain in the individual patient whether caval thrombosis is due to efficient trapping of emboli by the filter or to in situ thrombosis. It is believed that the former is more common. The most common complication of filter insertion is venous thrombosis at the insertion site or in the ipsilateral lower extremity (approximately 22%) (15–17). Less common complications include bleeding, arteriovenous fistula, air embolus, malposition, and filter migration. Caval penetration, filter fracture, and caval thrombosis have also rarely been reported (9–14).

Temporary filters might be useful in patients when the risk of thromboembolism is high (e.g., perioperatively) or in whom short-term suspension of anticoagulation is necessary. Temporary filters are designed for short-term use (less than 2 weeks) and generally have an external component at the access site that allows for easy removal of the device. Retrievable filters, on the other hand, can be permanent devices but have designs that permit removal at a later date. The accumulation of thrombi and the intimal incorporation of the filter can make retrieval challenging beyond 14 to 16 days.

The Amplatz and Gunther Tulip (William Cook Europe, Bjaerverskov, Denmark) are two retrievable-type filters. Early experience with the Amplatz filter in Europe has demonstrated a recurrent pulmonary embolism rate of approximately 7% in a small series of patients (18). In another small series, there was a relatively high rate of occlusion of the IVC (17.5%) (19). The implantation period for these filters is on the order of 14 to 16 days (20–22). Percutaneous removal of the Amplatz filter appears to be relatively traumatic (20). A spontaneous migration rate of 43% and a disruption and fragmentation rate of 77% plagued the Gunther Tulip filter in early experience, although revision of the prototype has shown promise (21).

Temporary filters include the Gunther temporary filter, Protect Infusion catheter (a similar device in Europe is known as the Prolyser), Another filter, and the Tempofilter. A multicenter registry in Europe has revealed that the main indication for temporary filter use was protection during pelvic/lower extremity thrombolysis (53.1%) (23). The average time of implantation was 5.4 days. The Antheor filter was utilized in 56.4% of cases. The major complications reported were thrombosis (16%) and dislocation (4.8%). Four of 188 patients died from pulmonary embolism during filter protection. The Tempofilter has been retrieved up to 55 days after implantation (24).

II. VENOUS THROMBOLYSIS: PHARMACOLOGICAL AND MECHANICAL

The use of pharmacological thrombolytic therapy in patients with acute myocardial infarction has lead to the application of lytic therapy for DVT and massive acute PE (25). Thrombolytic therapy and mechanical embolectomy are often used as complementary techniques in acute massive PE, peripheral and central venous thromboses, and thrombosed dialysis shunts. Pharmacological thrombolysis utilizes lytic agents such as streptokinase, urokinase (no longer available in the U.S.), alteplase (rt-PA, Activase; Genentech, Inc., South San Francisco, CA) or a newer agent, reteplase (Retavase, Centocor, Inc., Malvern, PA). Mechanical thrombectomy and embolectomy physically disrupts the thrombus with devices such as a ''propellor'' (Amplatz ''Clot-buster''), rotating wires (Trerotola device) to macerate the clot, or a high-speed jet of saline to create a Venturi effect that disrupts and aspirates thrombus (Angiojet, Oasis, and Hydrolyser devices).

Thrombolytic therapy has been especially advocated in the management of patients presenting with documented massive acute PE and hypotension or evidence of right ventricular dysfunction (26). Though earlier trials evaluating the percutaneous treatment of pulmonary embolism with urokinase were performed in the early 1970s, it has been the introduction of rt-PA which has renewed interest in thrombolytic therapy for massive PE (27).

Whether local catheter-directed thrombolytic therapy demonstrates any benefit over the systemic administration of thrombolytic agents for PE is uncertain. Although a randomized trial comparing the intravenous administration of rt-PA for pulmonary embolism to intrapulmonary administration demonstrated similar efficacy, it should be noted that the intrapulmonary administration of lytic agent was into the main pulmonary artery and not directly into the clot (i.e., not catheter-directed thrombolytic therapy) (28). It is generally accepted that for efficient and effective clot dissolution, at least in systemic venous thrombosis, the lytic agent should be delivered directly into the thrombus. Percutaneous embolectomy procedures can be performed utilizing a combination of mechanical disruption of the thrombus by pigtail catheter, guidewire, or mechanical thrombectomy device such as the Angiojet, Hydrolyser, or Amplatz, followed by catheter-directed thrombolytic infusion, if necessary.

The authors have employed percutaneous pulmonary arterial thromboembolectomy on selected patients at our institution for the past 6 years, using either catheter aspiration thrombectomy with a 8-10 Fr. guiding catheter, or the Amplatz or Angiojet devices. This procedure has been used for patients with massive PE who present in extremis (severe right heart failure, pulmonary arterial hypertension, or systemic hypotension) and have a contraindication to systemic thrombolytic therapy. Our anecdotal experience has been that this procedure can be lifesaving, although the amount of thrombus removed is usually relatively small. Clearly, the ideal device for percutaneous pulmonary embolectomy is not yet available. The Amplatz "Clot Buster" and the Angiojet devices work best on very fresh thrombus. Surgical pulmonary embolectomy should be considered in the setting of failed pharmacological/mechanical thrombolysis or impending cardiac arrest.

Thrombolytic therapy is also used to treat thrombosed hemodialysis accesses and symptomatic peripheral and central venous occlusions (29–34).

Aggressive thrombolytic therapy with the goals of rapid dissolution of thrombus and reduced extremity swelling and pain may be superior to intravenous heparin therapy alone in treating extensive DVT (35). The long-term goal of aggressive therapy is to preserve valvular function. The peripheral intravenous administration of thrombolytic agents, however, is hampered by the inability of the lytic agent to reach the bulk of the thrombus, particularly in completely occluded veins (36). For this reason, catheter-directed therapy to deliver the thrombolytic agent directly into the thrombus has become more widely practiced. Technical success rates in the delivery of thrombolytic therapy via catheter-directed technique range from 80 to 85% (31–34). The acuity of thrombosis helps determine the immediate technical success of lytic therapy. The best results are seen with thrombus of 7 to 10 days duration. Patients with duration of symptoms of greater than 4 weeks prior to intervention have lower technical success, though some advocate intervention up to 6 weeks after onset of thrombus. Further evidence that thrombolytic therapy is superior to heparin anticoagulation in achieving early lysis of the deep veins has been demonstrated in a national multicenter registry. A total of 473 patients were enrolled with acute (<4 weeks) and chronic lower extremity DVT. Patients were treated with urokinase. Complete or partial lysis was achieved in 84% of patients. Overall complete/partial lysis was associated with a primary patency of 60% at 1 year, while those patients who experienced complete lysis demonstrated a 1-year primary patency rate of 79%. Primary patency is higher at 1 year in the iliofemoral venous system (79%) than in the femoro-popliteal venous system (64%) (32).

Absolute contraindications to thrombolytic therapy include active internal bleeding, recent (less than 2 months) cerebral vascular accident, other active intracranial processes such as tumor, recent ocular surgery, and severe allergic reaction to thrombolytic agent. Major relative contraindications include recent (less than 10 days) major surgery, recent GI bleeding, recent serious trauma, or severe arterial hypertension (greater than or equal to 200 mmHg systolic or greater than or equal to 100 mmHg diastolic), bacterial endocarditis, and pregnancy. Risk–benefit analysis needs to be performed on an individual basis in these underlying circumstances (37).

The most serious major complication associated with thrombolytic therapy is intracranial bleeding, which occurs in approximately 1% of patients. Other complications include bleeding at sites remote from the primary access, allergic or idiosyncratic drug reactions, and pericatheter thrombosis (37). Pericatheter thrombosis, a frequent problem in the early experience with thrombolytic therapy, has been virtually eliminated with concomitant systemic heparin therapy (37).

Thrombolytic therapy has played an increasing role in the salvage of hemodialysis access grafts. These access grafts typically demonstrate 1 year patency rates ranging from 60 to 70% (38). Several studies have demonstrated the efficacy of thrombolytic therapy in preserving long-term patency and viability of the access grafts (38–40). Long-term results for dialysis grafts demonstrate primary and secondary patency rates at one year of 26% and 51%, respectively (40). These results are comparable to the 60–70% patency rate reported for surgical revision at one year (41). Thrombolytic therapy facilitates clot dissolution and subsequent detection and treatment of the most common cause of graft failure, venous outflow stenosis.

The current management of Paget-Schroetter syndrome (effort vein thrombosis, primary axillosubclavian vein thrombosis) now incorporates thrombolytic therapy, either mechanical and/or pharmacological, as first-line therapy (30,42,43). The timely initiation of thrombolytic therapy can reestablish patency of the subclavian vein and confirm the underlying etiology. Balloon angioplasty is not advocated by most authors in the acute setting because of inflammation at the site of stenosis but is instead reserved for restenosis after surgery (44). Postlysis management is controversial, but most treatment algorithms involve long-term anticoagulation (6 weeks to 3 months) followed by definitive surgical correction of the underlying structural abnormality (44). Thrombolytic therapy with delayed surgical decompression has demonstrated long-term benefit in greater than 75% of these patients (45).

III. MECHANICAL THROMBECTOMY DEVICES

The simplest method of removing thrombus percutaneously involves aspiration through a non-tapered 6–10 Fr. guiding catheter with a 50- or 60-mL syringe. However, there is an increasing number of mechanical thrombectomy devices available for the percutaneous removal or fragmentation of thrombus. These devices have been approved by the FDA for use in clotted dialysis shunts. The Angiojet device has also been recently approved for peripheral arterial occlusions. The ''Clot Buster'' Amplatz Thrombectomy Device (Microvena Corp., White Bear Lake, MN) is an 8-Fr. catheter with an enclosed impeller at the end, driven at 150,000 rpm by an air turbine. This spinning impeller creates a recirculating vortex, macerating acute thrombus into very small particles. The Arrow-Trerotola Percutaneous Thrombolytic Device (Arrow International, Inc., Reading, PA) is an expandable basket introduced through a 5-Fr. sheath and attached to a disposable drive unit that rotates the wire basket at 3000 rpm. This results in fragmentation of acute thrombus into particles that are larger than the Amplatz device and should be aspirated through the introducer sheath. The Angiojet Rapid Thrombectomy System (Possis Medical, Inc., Minneapolis, MN) is a 5- or 6-Fr. catheter which creates a strong Venturi effect at its tip by virtue of a high-velocity saline jet directed back through the catheter shaft. It employs a dedicated and expensive drive unit to create the high-pressure saline jet to remove acute thrombus. The 6-Fr. version of this device has only recently become available and promises to be effective and can be used in larger vessels as well (Fig. 1). The Cordis Hydrolyser Thrombectomy Catheter (Cordis, Miami, FL) and the Oasis Thrombectomy Catheter (Boston Scientific, Watertown, MA) both employ a similar principle to the Angiojet but utilize a standard angiographic power injector rather than a dedicated drive unit to create a lower pressure jet.

IV. VENOUS ANGIOPLASTY

Percutaneous balloon angioplasty (PTA) has often been utilized in the venous system, predominately in the setting of venous stenoses secondary to arteriovenous dialysis shunt creation, central venous stenoses from both benign and malignant causes, and in venous bypass grafts.

The creation of an arteriovenous connection for dialysis access leads to arterialization of the venous limb. Stenoses commonly develop due to intimal hyperplasia in the outflow veins. Stenoses may also occur in the central veins, particularly the subclavian veins if these have been used for prior catheter insertions. The largest study of angioplasty in dialysis access grafts reported a 1-year primary patency rate of 41% and a secondary patency rate of 65% for venous limb and central venous stenoses treated solely with angioplasty (46). Serial venous angioplasty procedures may help prolong the life of the shunt. Increasingly, central venous stenoses are being treated with angioplasty in combination with stent placement.

When operative reconstruction is compared with percutaneous balloon dilatation for central venous obstruction, primary symptomatic relief at 1 year occurred in 88% of the surgical group versus 36% in the angioplasty group (47). However, with repeated angioplasty, secondary 1- and 2-year patency rates approach those of operative reconstruction at 86% and 66%, respectively. In the nonoperative candidate, serial angioplasty with stent placement for those lesions demonstrating elastic recoil appears to offer excellent 1- to 2-year patency rates.

Balloon angioplasty has been used to salvage saphenous venous arterial bypass grafts. The most recent long-term study of transluminal angioplasty of distal venous bypass grafts demonstrates assisted primary patency, cumulative patency, and limb salvage rates at 65%, 91%, and 100% at 1 year and 53%, 72%, and 96% at 2 years (48). There appears to be little difference in patency rates with regard to the location of the stenosis. The stenoses themselves have improved response if less than 5 cm in aggregate length. The results in PTFE grafts appear to be less impressive, although the primary and secondary patency rates at 1 year do mimic those of surgical repair.

V. VENOUS STENTING

Expandable metallic stents have been placed with increasing frequency in the venous system (49–59). Stents hold the potential for longer term relief in the setting of recoil or external compression. There is, however, the risk of restenosis or occlusion secondary to intimal hyperplasia within the stent as well as from extrinsic compression of the stent by an adjacent mass lesion, for example (49–51).

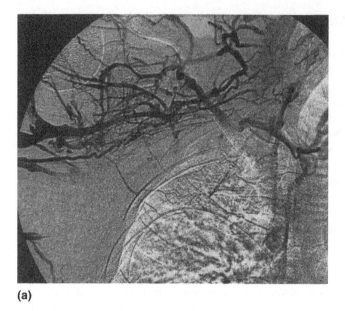

(a)

Figure 1 (a) A 51-year-old weightlifter with right upper extremity swelling for 8 days. Complete thrombosis of the right axillary and subclavian veins with collateral flow. (b) After mechanical thrombectomy with a 6-Fr. Angiojet device, the axillary and distal subclavian veins are patent with some residual thrombus, but there is a complete mid-subclavian vein occlusion. (c) Following transcatheter lysis with rt-PA, axillary, subclavian, and brachiocephalic veins are all patent with good flow into the SVC. There is a stenosis in the brachiocephalic vein due to extrinsic compression which was then surgically treated.

In the United States, there are currently a variety of FDA-approved stents that may be divided into two broad categories—self-expanding stents and balloon expandable stents. Self-expanding stents include the Wallstent (Schneider Inc., Minneapolis, MN), the SMART stent (Cordis Corp., Miami, FL), the Memotherm FLEX stent (C.R. Bard Inc., Covington, GA), the Z-stent (Cook Inc., Bloomington, IN), and the Symphony stent (Boston Scientific, Natick, MA). Balloon expandable stents include the Palmaz and the Corinthian stents (Cordis, Miami, FL), the Megalink and Herculink stents (Guidant Inc., Temecula, CA), the AVE stent (Medtronic AVE, Santa Rosa, CA), the IntraStent (Intra Therapeutics, St. Paul, MN) and the VistaFlex stent (Angiodynamics Inc., Queensbury, NY). These stents are mostly FDA approved for biliary use only (the large-diameter Z stents are approved for tracheobronchial use), but many are nevertheless commonly used in the arterial and venous systems.

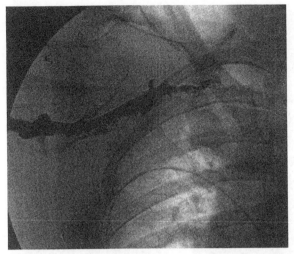

(b)

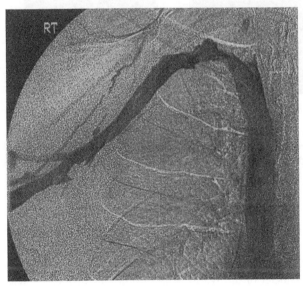

(c)

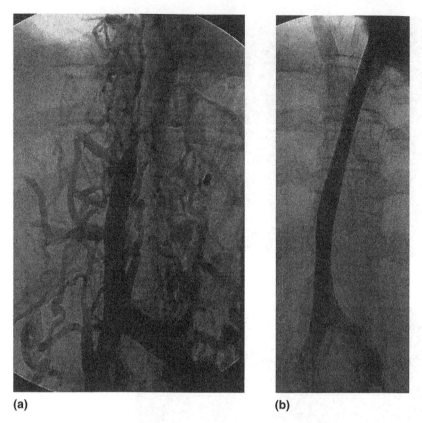

(a)   (b)

Figure 2   (a) A 30-year-old female with SLE and Budd-Chiari syndrome. Inferior vena cavogram demonstrates completely occluded intrahepatic IVC with numerous collateral veins. (b) After balloon dilatation and placement of a Wallstent in the IVC, the IVC is widely patent and there is no longer collateral flow evident.

None of these stents are FDA approved for intravenous use, although the Palmaz stent and Wallstent are FDA approved for intra-arterial use. The Wallstent is also approved for creation of percutaneous transjugular portosystemic shunts (TIPS). The maximal diameter of the Wallstent is 24 mm. The balloon-expandable Palmaz stent is available up to 12 mm, but this stent can be overdilated slightly. The advantages of the balloon-expandable stents for venous use include larger available diameters, flexibility, and resistance to permanent deformation from external compressive forces. The major disadvantages of the balloon-expandable stents in the venous system are their lack of availability in large diameters and their susceptibility to deformation by external compressive forces. As

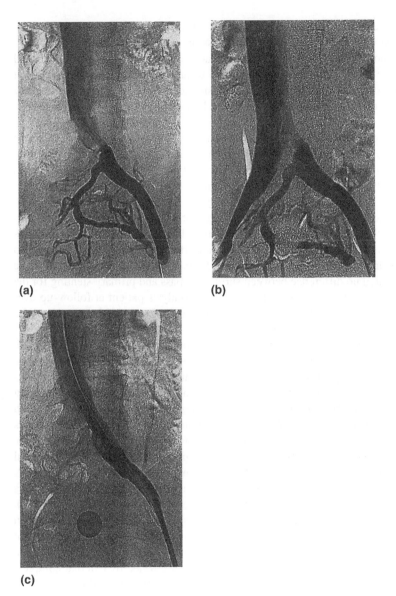

(a)

(b)

(c)

Figure 3   (a) A 31-year-old female previously treated with transcatheter thrombolytic therapy for left lower extremity DVT. Left iliac venogram demonstrates left common iliac vein stenosis with collateral flow to the opposite side. (b) Bilateral simultaneous iliac venography demonstrates the left common iliac vein stenosis at the site where the right common iliac artery crosses the vein (May-Thurner syndrome). (c) After balloon dilatation and placement of a 14 mm × 4 cm Wallstent, the left common iliac vein is widely patent.

such, placement of balloon-expandable stents in the subclavian or arm veins, where the vein may be subject to compression, is not recommended (51,55).

Venous stenoses amenable to stent placement can be divided into two broad categories: (1) related and (2) not related to arteriovenous hemodialysis shunt creation. Stenoses unrelated to hemodialysis include upper and lower extremity as well as central venous obstruction from benign or malignant etiologies (Figs. 2 and 3).

Procedural success rates of approximately 96% are achieved when stents are used to treat hemodialysis access-related venous stenoses and occlusions that are deemed untreatable with balloon angioplasty (49). These are mainly lesions that have been dilated by balloon but exhibit elastic recoil when the balloon is deflated. Cumulative primary patency rate has been demonstrated at 50% at 6 months and 20% at 12 months. However, repeat treatment increased the cumulative assisted patency rate to 76% at 6 months and 33% at 12 months. Other studies have demonstrated improved shunt function after stent placement, with up to 77% of shunts functioning at 2 years (52,53). In addition, Bhatia et al. have demonstrated no difference between surgical bypass and primary stenting for the treatment of central venous obstruction in the dialysis patient at follow-up over a 1-year period (51). It is clear that judicious use of stents helps to extend the life of the dialysis access shunt.

Stent placement in nonhemodialysis venous stenoses continues to expand. Central venous stenoses secondary to benign etiologies demonstrate improved short-term patency rates compared to malignant etiologies (54). Studies demonstrate up to 82% primary patency and 94% secondary patency at 2 years following stent placement (56–60). There are few studies assessing long-term patency in stenting of benign venous stenoses. Wohlgemuth et al. reported on 35 patients followed for an average of 4 years after stenting for pelvic venous stenoses. They were able to stratify patients on the basis of angioscopy into those with abnormal veins (usually after surgical thrombectomy) and normal veins (after lytic therapy). The primary patency rate for the group with abnormal veins was 43 versus 86% for those with normal veins after thrombectomy and stent placement (57).

Complications of venous stenting are unusual but include vessel perforation and disruption, venous thrombosis, and stent migration. The risk of migration can be minimized by using self-expanding stents that are appropriately oversized. Balloon-expandable stents may become kinked or crushed by external compression and should not be placed in the subclavian or arm veins (59).

REFERENCES

1. Ferris EJ. Deep venous thrombosis and pulmonary embolism: correlative evaluation and therapeutic implications. AJR 1992; 159:1149–1155.

2. Harmon B. Deep vein thrombosis: a perspective on anatomy and venographic analysis. J Thorac Imaging 1989; 4:15–19.

3. Morse KM. Pulmonary embolism. Am Rev Respir Dis 1977; 115:829–852.

4. Hirsh J. Treatment of pulmonary embolism. Ann Rev Med 1987; 38:91–105.

5. Carter BL, Jones ME, Waikman LA. Pathophysiology and treatment of deep venous thrombosis and pulmonary embolism. Clin Pharmacol 1985; 4:279–296.

6. Becker DM, Philbrick JT, Selby JB. Inferior vena cava filters. Indications, safety, effectiveness. Arch Intern Med 1992; 152(10):1985–94.

7. Patton JH, Fabian TC, Croce MA, et al. Prophylactic Greenfield filters: acute complications and long-term follow-up. J Trauma 1996; 41(2):231–237.

8. Rodriguez JL, Lopez JM, Proctor MC. Early placement of prophylactic vena caval filters in injured patients at high risk for pulmonary embolism. J Trauma 1996; 40(5): 797–802.

9. Starok MS, Common AA. Follow-up after insertion of bird's nest inferior vena cava filters. Can Assoc Radiol J 1996; 47(3):189–94.

10. Ferdani M, Rudondy P, Caburol G et al. In vitro testing of six vena cava filters: filtering efficiency and pressure measurements. J Cardiovasc Surg 1995; 36(2):127–133.

11. Schwarz RE, Marrero AM, Conlon KC, Burt M. Inferior vena cava filters in cancer patients: indications and outcome. J Clin Oncol 1996; 14(2):652–657.

12. Mohan CR, Hoballah JJ, Sharp WJ, et al. Comparative efficacy and complications of vena cava filters. J Vasc Surg 1995; 21(2):235–245.

13. Ferris EJ, McCowan TC, Carver DK, McFarland DR. Percutaneous inferior vena cava filters: follow-up of seven designs in 320 patients. Radiology 1993; 188(3):851–856.

14. Ascer E, Gennaro M, Lorensen E, Pollina RM. Superior vena cava Greenfield filters: indications, techniques, and results. J Vasc Surg 1996; 23(3):498–503.

15. Molgaard CP, Yucel EK, Geller SC, et al. Access site thrombosis after placement of inferior vena cava filters with 12-14F delivery sheaths. Radiology 1992; 185: 257–261.

16. Mewissen MW, Erickson SJ, Foley WD, et al. Thrombosis at venous insertion site after inferior vena caval filter placement. Radiology 1989; 173:155–157.

17. Blebea J, Wilson R, Waybill P et al. Deep venous thrombosis after percutaneous insertion of vena caval filters. J Vasc Surg 1999; 30(5):821–8.

18. McCowan TC, Ferris EJ, Carver DK, Baker ML. Amplatz vena cava filter: clinical experience in 30 patients. AJR 1990; 155:177–81.

19. Epstein DH, Darcy MD, Hunter DW, et al. Experience with the Amplatz retrievable vena cava filter. Radiology 1989; 172:105–110.

20. Hunter DW, Lund G, Rysany JA, et al. Retrieving the Amplatz retrievable vena cava filter. Cardiovasc Intervent Radiol 1987; 10:32–36.

21. Becker CD, Hoogewoud HM, Felder P et al. Long-term follow-up of the Gunther basket inferior vena cava filter: does mechanical instability cause complications. Cardiovasc Intervent Radiol 1994; 17:247–251.

22. Millward SF, Bhargava A, Aquino J Jr, et al. Gunther Tulip filter: preliminary experience with retrieval. J Vasc Intervent Radiol 2000; 11(1):75–82.

23. Lorch H et al. Current practice of temporary vena cava filter insertion: a multicenter registry. J Vasc Interven Radiol 2000; 11(1):83–88.

24. Bovyn G, Gory P, Reynaud P et al. The Tempofilter: a multicenter study of a new

temporary caval filter implantable for up to six weeks. Ann Vasc Surg 1997; 11: 520–528.

25. Levine MN. Thrombolytic therapy for venous thromboembolism: Complications and contradictions. Clin Chest Med 1995; 16:321–328.

26. Goldhaber SZ. Thrombolytic therapy in venous thromboembolism. Clinical trials and correct indications. Clin Chest Med 1995; 16:307–320.

27. Goldhaber SZ, Kessler CM, Heit J, et al. Randomized controlled trial of recombinant tissue plasminogen activator versus urokinase in the treatment of acute pulmonary embolism. Lancet 1988; 2:293–298.

28. Verstraete M, Miller AH, Bounameaux H et al. Intravenous and intrapulmonary recombinant tissue-type plasminogen activator in the treatment of acute massive pulmonary embolism. Circulation 1988; 77:353–60.

29. Markel A, Manzo RA, Strandness DE. The potential role of thrombolytic therapy in venous thrombosis. Arch Intern Med 1992; 152:1265–1267.

30. Landercasper J, Gall W, Fischer M, et al. Thrombolytic therapy of axillary-subclavian venous thrombosis. Arch Surg 1987; 122:1072–1075.

31. Semba CP, Dake MD. Catheter-directed thrombolysis for iliofemoral venous thrombosis. Semin Vasc Surg 1996; 9:26–33.

32. Comerota AJ, Aldridge SC. Thrombolytic therapy for deep venous thrombosis, a clinical review. Can J Surg 1992; 36:359–364.

33. Semba CP, Dake MD. Iliofemoral deep venous thrombosis: aggressive therapy with catheter-directed thrombolysis. Radiology 1994; 191:487–494.

34. Bjarnason H, Kruse JR, Asinger DA, et al. Iliofemoral deep venous thrombosis: safety and efficacy outcome during five years of catheter-directed thrombolytic therapy. J Vasc Intervent Radiol 1997; 8:405–418.

35. Francis CW, Marder VJ. Fibrinolytic therapy for venous thrombosis. Prog Cardiovasc Dis 1991; 34:193–204.

36. Meyerovitz MF, Polak JF, Goldhaber SZ. Short-term response to thrombolytic therapy in deep venous thrombosis: predictive value of venographic appearance. Radiology 1992; 184:345–348.

37. Valji K, Bookstein JJ. Thrombolysis: clinical applications. In: Baum S, Pentecost M, eds. Abrams' Angiography: Interventional Radiology. Boston: Little Brown, 1997:132–157.

38. Kumpe DA, Cohen MAH. Angioplasty/thrombolytic treatment of failing and failed hemodialysis access sites: comparison with surgical treatment. Prog Cardiovasc Dis 1992; 34:263–278.

39. Valji K, Bookstein JJ, Roberts AC, et al. Pulse-spray pharmacomechanical thrombolysis of thrombosed hemodialysis access grafts: long term experience and comparison of original and current techniques. AJR 1995; 1654:1495–1500.

40. Valji, K, Bookstein JJ, Roberts AC, et al. Pharmacomechanical thrombolysis and angioplasty in the management of clotted hemodialysis grafts: early and late clinical results. Radiology 1991; 178:243–247.

41. Palder SB, Kirkman RL, Whittemore AD, et al. Vascular access for hemodialysis: patency rates and results of revisions. Ann Surg 1985; 202:235–239.

42. Grassi CG, Bettman MA. Effort thrombosis: role of interventional therapy. Cardiovasc Intervent Radiology 1990; 13:317–322.

43. Frankuchen EI, Neff RA, Collins RA et al. Urokinase perfusions for axillary-subclavian vein thrombosis. Cardiovasc Intervent Radiol 1984; 7:90–93.

44. Machleder HI,. Evaluation of a new treatment strategy for Paget-Schroetter syndrome: spontaneous thrombosis of the axillary-subclavian vein. J Vasc Surg 1993; 17:305–315.

45. Malcynski J, O'Donnell TF, Mackey WC, et al. Long-term results of treatment for axillary-subclavian vein thrombosis. Can J Surg 1993; 36:365–371.

46. Kanterman RY, Vesely TM, Pilgram TK, et al. Dialysis access grafts: anatomic location of venous stenosis and results of angioplasty. Radiology 1995; 195:135–139.

47. Wisselink W, Money SR, Becker MO, et al. Comparison of operative reconstruction and percutaneous balloon dilatation for central venous obstruction. Am J Surg 1993; 166:200–205.

48. Favre JP, Malovki I, Sobhy M, et al. Angioplasty of distal venous bypasses: is it worth the cost? J Cardiovasc Surg 1996; 37(suppl 1):59–65.

49. Gray RJ, Horton KM, Dolmatch BL, et al. Use of Wallstents for hemodialysis access-related venous stenoses and occlusions untreatable with balloon angioplasty. Radiology 1995; 195:479–484.

50. Quinn SF, Schuman ES, Hall L, et al. Venous stenoses in patients who undergo hemodialysis: treatment with self-expandable endovascular stents. Radiology 1992; 183:499–504.

51. Nazarian GK, Austin WR, et al. Venous recanalization by metallic stents after failure of balloon angioplasty or surgery: four year experience. Cardiovasc Intervent Radiol 1996; 19:227–233.

52. Vorwerk D, Guenther RW, Mann H, et al. Venous stenosis and occlusion in hemodialysis hunts: follow-up results of stent placement in 65 patients. Radiology 1995; 195:140–146.

53. Bhatia DS, Money SR, Ochsner JL,. Comparison of surgical bypass and percutaneous balloon dilatation with primary stent placement in the treatment of central venous obstruction in the dialysis patient: one year follow-up. Ann Vasc Surg 1996; 10: 452–455.

54. Nazarian GK, Bjarnason H, Dietz CA, et al. Iliofemoral venous stenosis: effectiveness of treatment with metallic endovascular stents. Radiology 1996; 200:193–199.

55. Elson JD, Becker GJ, Wholey MH, Ehrman KO. Vena caval and central venous stenoses: management with Palmaz balloon-expandable intraluminal stents. J Vasc Intervent Radiol 1991; 2:215–223.

56. Neglen P, Raju S. Balloon dilation and stenting of chronic iliac vein obstruction: technical aspects and early clinical outcome. J Endovasc Ther 2000; 7(2):79–91.

57. Wohlgemuth WA, Weber H, Loeprecht H et al. PTA and stenting of benign venous stenoses in the pelvis: long-term results. Cardiovasc Intervent Radiol 2000; 23(1): 9–16.

58. Lakin PC. Venous thrombolysis and stenting. In: Baum S, Pentecost M, eds. Abram's Angiography: Interventional Radiology. Boston: Little Brown, 1997:1046–1057.

59. Marache P, Asseman P, Jabinet JL, et al. Percutaneous transluminal venous angioplasty in occlusive iliac vein thrombosis resistant to thrombolysis. Am Heart J 1993; 125:362–366.

19

Catheter-Directed Thrombolysis for Lower Extremity Deep Vein Thrombosis

Mark W. Mewissen
Wisconsin Heart and Vascular Clinics and Medical College of Wisconsin, Milwaukee, Wisconsin

I. INTRODUCTION

Elimination of the embolic potential of existing thrombus, restoration of unobstructed flow, prevention of further thrombosis, and preservation of venous valve function are the ideal goals of therapy for acute deep vein thrombosis (DVT). Meeting these goals will not only prevent pulmonary embolism (PE) but will also minimize the long-term sequelae of venous hypertension and the development of the post-thrombotic syndrome (PTS). Treatment strategies aimed at eliminating or reducing the risk of PTS should focus on preserving valvular function and eliminating the risk of continued venous obstruction following acute DVT. Thrombolytic agents are an attractive form of early therapy because they have the ability to eliminate obstructive thrombus in the deep veins and should, therefore, help provide protection against the PTS. The perceived benefits of early and rapid recanalization in preserving valve function has been the basis for the use of lytic therapy to treat acute DVT. As with any therapy, the risks and incremental cost of thrombolysis must be considered when devising a patient's management strategy.

The therapeutic goals for treating the patient with acute DVT include preventing pulmonary embolus, restoration of unobstructed blood flow through the thrombosed segment, prevention of recurrent thrombosis, and preservation of venous valve function. Success in achieving these clinical goals will minimize the

morbidity and mortality of pulmonary embolism and will also diminish the sequelae of the postthrombotic syndrome. As shown by Johnson, it is the combination of reflux and obstruction that correlates with the severity of PTS, as opposed
to either alone (1). Up to two-thirds of the patients with iliofemoral DVT will
develop edema and pain, with 5% developing ulcers in spite of adequate anticoagulation (2).

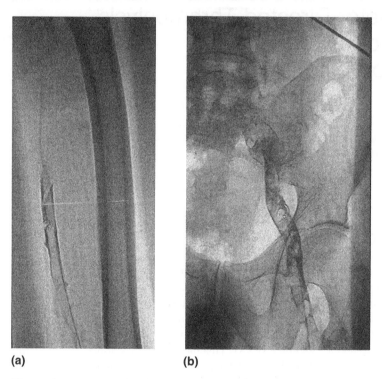

(a)   **(b)**

Figure 1   A 45-year-old man who presented with a 1-week history of worsening pain
and swelling of the left lower extremity. Duplex study revealed DVT extending from the
popliteal vein to the common iliac vein. Following catheterization of the left posterior
tibial vein at the ankle under ultrasound guidance, the noninvasive studies are confirmed
at venography: there is thrombosis of the superficial femoral, common femoral, external,
and common iliac veins (a, b). Following administration of 20 units of retavase over 20
h directly into the thrombus with a 5- Fr. coaxial infusing system, there is complete lysis
demonstrated in all previously thrombosed veins (c,d). Note uncovered stenosis in proximal common iliac vein (e, magnified view), successfully treated with a self-expanding
stent (f). At 6 months' follow-up, the deep veins remain patent and the patient is asymptomatic.

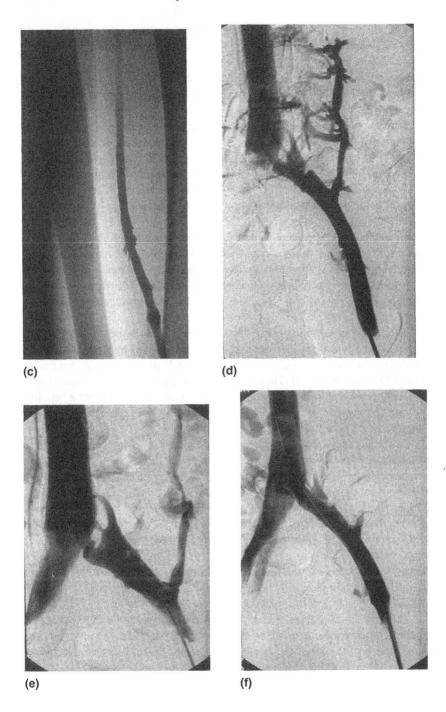

(c)   (d)

(e)   (f)

The standard of care at the moment includes systemic anticoagulation with heparin followed by warfarin therapy (3). Such a regimen, however, does not promote lysis to reduce the thrombus load nor does it contribute to restoration of venous valvular function. Anticoagulation alone, therefore, does not protect the limb from PTS, which can occur months to years following the acute thrombotic event (2).

Thrombolysis is a potentially attractive form of therapy since it provides the opportunity for promptly restoring venous patency and preserving venous valve function. This therapy provides the potential for preventing the long-term sequelae of DVT. There is published evidence that thrombolytic agents, even administered systemically, are superior to standard anticoagulation therapy in achieving early lysis of thrombus. In a pooled analysis of 13 randomized studies, Comerota and Aldridge found that only 4% of patients treated with heparin had significant or complete lysis compared with 45% of patients randomized to systemic streptokinase therapy (4). Similarly, in reviewing pooled data from six trials judged to have proper randomization, systemic thrombolysis was 3.7 times more effective in producing some degree of lysis than was heparin (5). However, the risk of major bleeding tripled in patients receiving thrombolysis.

With systemic administration, the drug does not reach the thrombus in sufficient concentration to provide optimal results. The report by Semba and Dake in 1994 provided the first insight on the potential role of catheter-directed thrombolytic (CDT) techniques (6). They reported complete lysis in 72% of the patients with concomitant resolution of symptoms. Only one patient suffered a bleeding complication of hemepositive stools. After the drug was discontinued, there were no significant adverse sequelae.

Delivering the thrombolytic agent directly into the thrombus offers significant advantages over systemic therapy, which may fail to reach and penetrate an occluded venous segment. Because thrombolytic agents activate plasminogen within the thrombus, delivery of the drug to that site enhances its effectiveness. By focusing the delivery of higher concentrations of drug, lysis rates can be improved, the duration of treatment can be reduced, and complications associated with the exposure of the patient to systemic thrombolytic therapy may be reduced. The progress of CDT can be monitored by direct imaging techniques, and lesions potentially contributing to the thrombosis can be identified. These defects, such as stenosis of the common iliac vein, can be treated by balloon angioplasty with or without the placement of endovascular stents (Fig. 1).

The removal of urokinase from the United States market in 1999 secondary to manufacturing concerns raised by the Food and Drug Administration has limited the choice of thrombolytic therapy for catheter-directed thrombolysis. Currently, available agents for noncoronary lytic therapy include alteplase (rt-PA) and reteplase (r-PA). Their optimal dose, use of concomitant heparin, and the technique of catheter-directed treatment are undergoing evaluation.

II. TECHNIQUE OF CATHETER-DIRECTED THROMBOLYSIS

With the patient prone on the angiographic table, we prefer the ipsilateral popliteal venous approach. It is often difficult to penetrate an occluded superficial femoral vein from the internal jugular vein or the contralateral common femoral vein, due to venous valves that may prevent safe catheter and guidewire manipulations. Should the popliteal vein be thrombosed, the ipsilateral posterior tibial vein is cannulated. The venous access site should be accessed under ultrasound guidance with a small-gauge echogenic needle. A 5-Fr. short sheath is then introduced, through which all subsequent catheters can be exchanged. Following baseline venography obtained via the venous sheath, the occluded venous segment is crossed with a straight-tip 5-Fr. catheter and a 0.035-in. curved-tip glidewire. Venography is then repeated to confirm intraluminal passage of the catheter, which is then exchanged for a 5-Fr. infusing coaxial system, consisting of a proximal multisidehole catheter and a distal infusing wire. It is critical to position the system directly into the thrombus, to maximize plasminogen activation at the site of obstruction. If urokinase is being used, this agent should be initiated at 150,000 to 200,000 units per hour, evenly split between the infusing ports. Currently, anecdotal experience with reteplase and alteplase would suggest that 1 unit per hour for the former and 0.5 mg per hour for the latter are a safe and effective strategy. Intravenous heparin is concomitantly administered via the popliteal (or tibial) sheath at a rate of 500 to 1000 units per hour following a 5000-unit bolus of heparin. Patients are monitored in the ICU or a step-down unit, similar to those receiving thombolytic treatment for acute PE or an arterial occlusion. Because the duration of therapy may be in excess of 24 h, it is not necessary to frequently assess the progress of lysis. The frequency of follow-up venograms should be every 12 h, primarily to reposition the infusion devices into the remaining thrombus. Gentle thrombus maceration with a 6-mm balloon angioplasty catheter may be helpful, particularly in the superficial femoral vein, where focal narrowings are at times encountered, probably representing sites of organized thrombus. Typically, unless a complication would dictate otherwise, lytic therapy should be continued until complete lysis is achieved, unless no discernible progress is venographically demonstrated from the previous venogram obtained 12 h prior. Since the grade of thrombolysis has been shown in the Thrombolysis Registry (7) to be a strong predictor of continued patency, it is critical that a complete lysis venogram be achieved. Lesions uncovered in the iliac venous segments should probably be treated with stents, although the long-term benefits of such devices are not known. However, if left untreated, there appears to be a significant risk of early rethrombosis.

III. RESULTS OF THE VENOUS REGISTRY

Clearly, the initial report by Semba and Dake suggested that CDT can be effective in achieving significant lysis of thrombus and may be associated with low complication rates. This experience stimulated the development of a multicenter registry with enrollment of almost 500 patients within over 50 North American centers (7). Complete data with follow-up of at least 6 months were available on nearly 300 patients, 70% of whom had iliofemoral DVT (IFVT). Treatment duration averaged more than 48 h with close to 7 million units of urokinase administered in those with direct intrathrombus delivery. One-third of the patients received adjunctive stenting for residual narrowing, but this was close to 40% in the IFVT group and close to half of those with left-sided involvement. The difference between the pre- and postlytic thrombus scores divided by the prelytic score resulted in a percentage of thrombolysis achieved, which was then classified into three groups for analysis: Grade I, <50% lysis; Grade II, >50% lysis; and Grade III, 100% or complete lysis (Table 1). Grades II and III lysis were achieved in over 80% of cases. Complete lysis was achieved in close to one-third.

The degree of lysis was found to be a significant predictor of early and continued patency (Fig. 2). Seventy-five percent of limbs with complete lysis remained patent at 1 year, compared to only 32% for limbs with insignificant lysis (<50%). In general, acute DVT (<10 days) predicted a better lysis grade

Table 1 Example of Pre- and Postlysis Thrombus Scores and Calculation of Lysis Grade in a Patient with Iliofemoral DVT

	IVC	CIV	EIV	CFV	pSFV	dSFV	PopV	Score
Prelysis	0	2	2	2	2	0	0	8
Postlysis	0	0	0	1	1	0	0	2

Thrombus score: 0 = patent; 1 = partially occluded; 2 = complete occlusion. Venous segments: IVC = inferior vena cava; CIV = common iliac vein; EIV = external iliac vein; CFV = common femoral vein; pSFV = proximal superficial femoral vein; dSFV = distal superficial femoral vein; PopV = popliteal vein.
Prelysis venographic evaluation of a patient with iliofemoral DVT, extending into the proximal superficial femoral vein. Following lysis, residual partially occluding thrombus remains in the common femoral and proximal superficial veins. The lysis grade is calculated as follows: (8-2)/8 = 0.75, resulting in Grade II lytic grade.

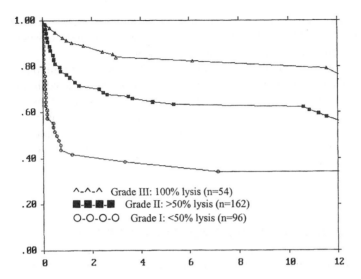

Figure 2 Long-term patency in relation to initial degree of thrombolysis achieved.

when compared to chronic DVT (>10 days), although significant lysis could be achieved in patients with chronic IFDVT. When isolated femoropopliteal DVT was present for more than 10 days, none achieved complete lysis. Reflux at 6 months follow-up was less than 30% in those with complete lysis, around 45% in those with >50% lysis, but over 60% in those with <50% initial lysis, again showing the greater protective effect of complete clot removal. Longer follow-up, including those who still had incomplete data at 6 months, should provide more definitive recommendations based on careful subgroup analysis and functional evaluation. There were only two deaths in the entire study (0.4%), one from intracranial hemorrhage and one from PE. Overall, in the Registry, six patients suffered a PE (1.2%).

Because the Registry was not designed to be a controlled trial, no restrictions were imposed on patient enrollment such as duration of symptoms, location of thrombus, prior history of DVT, or technique of thrombolysis. Therefore, patients with a variety of these features were prospectively enrolled. This may help explain a relatively low overall yield of complete lysis (31%). However, when analyzed by subgroups, several important observations can be made. For example, for a patient with acute IFDVT and no prior history of previous DVT, when CDT was performed via the popliteal vein (without a pedal infusion), complete lysis occurred 65% of the time and the 1-year patency was 96%. At the other extreme, complete lysis never occurred in any patients with chronic femoropopliteal DVT. Analysis of groups with particular combinations of features, while not always numerous for statistical comparison, provides a useful perspective of what can be expected from CDT in different settings and can serve as a guide to patient selection for this potentially effective form of treatment.

Based on health-related quality of life (HRQOL) evaluation, Comerota et al. recently reported on the benefits of catheter lysis in patients entered in the venous registry with iliofemoral DVT (8). After lytic treatment, patients reported better overall physical functioning, less stigma, less health distress, and fewer post-thrombotic symptoms, compared with similar patients treated with anticoagulation alone. Successful lysis was directly correlated with improved HRQOL, with patients who were classified as lytic failures having similar outcomes to patients treated with heparin alone.

IV. PATIENT SELECTION FOR LOWER EXTREMITY DVT

Patients with acute iliofemoral DVT and a life expectancy not hampered by fatal illness are likely to suffer from severe post-thrombotic sequelae and should benefit most from lytic therapy. Any patient who presents with phlegmasia cerulea dolens, regardless of age or underlying disease, should be considered for treatment unless a contraindication is obvious. Final analysis of the Venous Registry data will hopefully identify variables that will impact upon late outcome, and help better define patients who will most benefit from lytic therapy.

V. CONCLUSION

CDT can safely and effectively dissolve thrombus from the deep veins of identifiable groups of patients with symptomatic lower limb DVT. The best results can be anticipated in patients with acute symptoms without a prior history of DVT, who are treated with CDT without systemic infusion. In contrast, results of CDT are marginal among those patients with chronic femoropopliteal DVT. The long-term benefits of CDT are uncertain and cannot be conclusively derived from available data. A controlled trial comparing CDT to anticoagulation will be necessary to validate the long-term benefits of CDT and its application for the prevention of the post-thrombotic syndrome.

REFERENCES

1. Johnson BF, Manzo RA, Bergelin RO, Srandness DE Jr. Relationship between changes in the deep venous system and the development of the post-thrombotic syn-

drome after an acute episode of lower limb deep venous thrombosis: A one- to six-year follow-up. J Vasc Surg 1995; 21:307.

2. Strandness DE, Langlois Y, Cramer M, Randkett A, et al. Long-term sequelae of acute venous thrombosis. JAMA 1983; 250:1289–92.

3. Hull RD, Raskob GE, Rosenbloom D, Panju AA, Brill-Edwards P, Ginsberg JF, Hirsch J, Martin GJ, Green D. Heparin for 5 days as compared with 10 days in the initial treatment of proximal venous thrombosis. N Engl J Med 1990; 322(18):1260–1264.

4. Comerota A, Aldridge SC. Thrombolytic therapy for deep venous thrombosis: a clinical review. CJS 1993; 36:359–364.

5. Goldhaber SZ, Buring JE, Lipchick RJ, et al. Pooled analysis of randomized trials of streptokinase and heparin in phlebographically documented acute deep venous thrombosis. Am J Med 1984; 76:393–397.

6. Semba CP, Dake MD. Catheter directed thrombolysis for iliofemoral venous thrombosis. Radiology 1994; 191:487–494.

7. Mewissen MW, Seabrook GR, Meissner MH, Cynamon J, Labroupoulos N, Haughton SH. Catheter-directed thrombolysis for lower extremity deep venous thrombosis: report of a national multicenter registry. Radiology 1999; 211:39–49.

8. Camerota AJ, Throm RC, Mathias SD, Haughton SH, Mewissen MW. Catheter-directed thrombolysis for iliofemoral deep vein thrombosis improves health-related quality of life. Vasc Surg 2000; 32:130–137.

20

Surgical Embolectomy for Pulmonary Embolism

Lishan Aklog
*Brigham and Women's Hospital and Harvard Medical School,
Boston, Massachusetts*

Surgical pulmonary embolectomy has played a central role in the history of cardiac surgery. It was one of the first cardiac surgical procedures performed in humans and inspired the development of the heart–lung machine, the cornerstone of modern cardiac surgery. Despite its historical importance and the fact that its modern version was developed 40 years ago, its role in the management of patients with acute pulmonary embolism (PE) has been controversial. This controversy has persisted despite major advances in the safety and availability of cardiac surgery, our understanding of the biology of thomboembolic disease, and the emergence of alternative therapies such as thrombolysis and catheter-based embolectomy.

The challenge of determining the appropriate role for surgical embolectomy arises from the nature of the disease itself. Acute pulmonary embolism is fairly common, affecting at least 100,000 patients each year in the United States (1). It, however, spans a broad spectrum of patients from those who are relatively stable to those who present in full cardiac arrest. Although the overall 90-day mortality rate has been reported to be about 15%, with 75% of patients dying during the initial hospital admission (2), the actual risk in a given patient is directly related to the clinical presentation and the degree of underlying cardiopulmonary disease. In stable patients, without significant cardiopulmonary disease, this 90-day mortality can be well under 5% while patients who present in cardiac arrest have an in-hospital mortality of at least 50 to 60% even with surgical intervention (2,3).

Given this heterogeneous picture, it is not surprising that pulmonary embolectomy has been so controversial. Skeptics tend to emphasize the overall operative mortality of about 30% reported in the literature while dismissing the handful of reports with above-average results by saying that they ". . . merely reflected their better preoperative condition . . ." (4). Proponents, on the other hand, lament "negative literature . . . that has promoted a nihilistic attitude . . . currently many physicians never even consider the possibility of pulmonary embolectomy" (5) and emphasize that embolectomy has become a relatively simple and widely available procedure which, if performed before cardiovascular collapse, provides immediate, dramatic relief of the obstruction with good short- and long-term results.

Recent developments in early risk stratification (2) and rapid, noninvasive diagnosis with spiral CT scanning and echocardiography (6–8) may improve patient selection and decrease the interval between presentation and embolectomy to the point where more patients with large, central pulmonary emboli can be successfully treated surgically *before* cardiovascular collapse.

The goals of this chapter are to:

1. Review the history of the procedure and the principles that guided its pioneers.
2. Analyze the surgical results of the major surgical series over the past 30 years.
3. Review the preoperative evaluation of these patients, including indications for surgery.
4. Review the intra- and postoperative management of these patients in some detail.
5. Briefly present our most recent results at the Brigham and Women's Hospital in Boston.

I. HISTORY

A. The Trendelenburg Procedure

When Professor Friedrich Trendelenburg of Leipzig, Germany, presented his new operation for acute pulmonary embolism to the German Surgical Association in 1908 (9), the only successful cardiovascular operations to date had been suturing traumatic wounds of the heart. Diseases of the heart and great vessels were still considered off-limits to surgical treatment. He was motivated by the observation that, contrary to prevailing wisdom, most pulmonary emboli were not instantly fatal. He estimated that he would have on the order of 15 min from the time of diagnosis to relieve the obstruction (including the 8-min taxi ride from his home to the hospital!). His account of his bold effort is striking for the obvious necessity for speed in an era without circulatory support (10).

After perfecting his techniques in the laboratory on dogs, he made his first attempt on a 70-year-old woman who collapsed 6 days after fracturing her hip. The operation began with a small left anterior thoracotomy in the second intercostal space through which the aorta and main pulmonary artery were exposed and snared. He then extracted the embolus with forceps through a small arteriotomy that he sutured closed under a clamp. Although he completed this in less than 6 min, the patient died of hemorrhage from the back of the pulmonary artery. His two subsequent attempts were also unsuccessful. It was not until 1924 that his former trainee, Professor Martin Kirschner, performed the first successful Trendelenburg procedure in a 38-year-old woman who collapsed after hernia surgery (11).

Although Trendelenberg and Kirschner demonstrated that the hemodynamic insult of a massive pulmonary embolism could be reversed by direct surgical removal of the emboli, the operation did not enjoy widespread success. Alton Ochsner, in discussing a paper at the American Surgical Association in 1944, expressed his hope that ''. . . we will not have any more papers on the removal of pulmonary emboli before this organization'' (12). It was not until 1958 that R.W. Steenburg and Richard Warren of the Peter Bent Brigham Hospital (currently Brigham and Women's Hospital) in Boston reported the first successful Trendelenburg procedure in the United States (13). In their report they were only able to find 12 patients in the literature who had undergone successful pulmonary embolectomies.

B.   Inspiration for the Heart–Lung Machine

In 1930, Edward Churchill, Surgeon-in-Chief at the Massachusetts General Hospital, diagnosed a massive pulmonary embolism in a middle-aged woman following a cholecystectomy. John Gibbon was a research fellow studying pulmonary embolism in cats in Dr. Churchill's laboratory. He was assigned to monitor the patient's vital signs every 15 min for the next 17 h. She eventually deteriorated and Dr. Churchill performed an unsuccessful emergency Trendelenburg procedure (14). This vigil was the sentinel event that inspired Dr. Gibbon to spend the next 23 years of his professional life perfecting the heart–lung machine. He wrote the following in the patient's chart:

> During the long night's vigil, watching the patient struggle for life, the thought naturally occurred to me that the patient's life might be saved if some of the blue blood in her veins could be continuously withdrawn into an extracorporeal blood circuit, exposed to an atmosphere of oxygen, and then returned to the patient by way of a systemic artery in a central direction. Thus some of the patient's cardiorespiratory functions might be temporarily performed by the extracorporeal blood circuit while the massive embolism was surgically removed.

In 1953, he performed the first operation on cardiopulmonary bypass, an atrial septal defect repair, ushering in the modern era of cardiac surgery (15).

C. Venous Inflow Occlusion and the Modified Trendelenburg Procedure

Further laboratory work demonstrated that venous inflow occlusion was better tolerated than arterial outflow occlusion and that brief periods of circulatory arrest were well tolerated, especially if systemic hypothermia was added (16,17). In 1958, P.S. Allison from Oxford University performed a successful pulmonary embolectomy using venous inflow occlusion and systemic hypothermia (18). A few years later, Richard Sautter performed the same procedure under normothermic conditions using multiple, very short (less than 2-min) periods of circulatory arrest followed by periods of recovery (19).

Although the first reports of embolectomy with cardiopulmonary bypass would soon follow, the normothermic inflow occlusion technique continued to have its proponents, especially in the United Kingdom, with reports appearing as recently as 1994 (20–25). Other nonbypass techniques also appeared, including clot extraction without circulatory arrest through the right ventricular outflow tract or one of the branch pulmonary arteries (17,26–34). These techniques could, in theory, be performed rapidly by any surgeon at any hospital without the need to set up a heart–lung machine. Although they were a significant improvement over the classic Trendelenburg procedure, with its dismal 50-year record, they were unable to salvage more than 30 to 40% of patients or compete with the control and visualization that embolectomy on cardiopulmonary bypass offered the surgeon. They are now primarily of historical interest except in the most

Table 1   Historical Highlights in the Development of Pulmonary Embolectomy

Year	Surgeon	Event
1908	Trendelenburg	First attempted pulmonary embolectomy
1924	Kirschner	First successful Trendelenburg procedure
1930	Gibbon	Inspired to develop heart–lung machine after witnessing unsuccessful Trendelenburg procedure
1953	Gibbon	First cardiac operation on cardiopulmonary bypass
1958	Steenburg and Warren	First successful Trendelenburg procedure in the United States
1958	Allison	First embolectomy using hypothermic inflow occlusion
1962	Sautter	First embolectomy using intermittent normothermic inflow occlusion
1961	Cooley and Sharp	First embolectomies using cardiopulmonary bypass

desperate situations where a dying patient requires emergency embolectomy and cardiopulmonary bypass is not immediately available.

D. Embolectomy on Cardiopulmonary Bypass

In 1961, Denton Cooley, then at Baylor University in Houston, and Edward Sharp from Johns Hopkins University in Baltimore, independently performed the first pulmonary embolectomies using cardiopulmonary bypass within 6 weeks of each other (35,36). Both patients were in cardiogenic shock on vasopressors and underwent removal of the emboli from both pulmonary arteries using forceps and suction during a brief period of cardiopulmonary bypass. They were both easily weaned from bypass with excellent hemodynamics off vasopressors and underwent ligation of the inferior vena cavae to prevent recurrent embolization. Both were discharged from the hospital in good condition. The key elements of these procedures—cardiopulmonary bypass, pulmonary arteriotomy, complete evacuation of emboli under direct vision, and consideration of vena caval interruption— have been preserved over the past 40 years.

These two successes led to a flurry of activity with multiple centers reporting on embolectomy with bypass in the next few years (12,37–47). The poor results from the classic Trendelenburg procedure and the lack of alternatives in this highly lethal condition made the 40 to 60% mortality rates in these early series appear quite acceptable. In 1967, a survey of 40 North American surgeons at 28 centers found a total of 137 embolectomies, over 80% on cardiopulmonary bypass, with an operative mortality of 57%. The enthusiasm for this procedure was reflected in review articles and editorials pronouncing a ''new era'' of active therapy for pulmonary embolism (48–52). Efforts to improve these results concentrated on decreasing the delay between diagnosis and the institution of bypass by developing miniaturized heart–lung machines that could be attached to a gurney and brought to the patient (46,53). Partial femoral bypass would be instituted at the bedside and would support the patient while he or she was transported to the angiography suite for confirmation of the diagnosis or to the operating room.

E. Debates on Indications for Embolectomy

By the late 1960s and early 1970s the basic techniques of embolectomy on cardiopulmonary bypass were well established. The debate on the indications for embolectomy, however, continued during this period, flaring up regularly in the editorial pages and letters to the editor in response to a provocative article. In 1969, a large autopsy series found that two-thirds of patients with pulmonary embolism on autopsy either died within 1 h of the onset of symptoms or did not have symptoms suggestive of a pulmonary embolism. Most of the remaining patients who survived long enough to have potentially undergone angiography and embolectomy had terminal cancer, irreversible neurological injury, or were "too ill" for surgery. They concluded that only about 5% of patients would have benefited from embolectomy. This and other similar studies (54–56) led skeptics to claim that the patients who would benefit from surgery die before they could undergo the procedure and those who survive long enough do not need it.

In 1973, Berger reported improved results with aggressive use of preoperative circulatory support and encouraged more liberal use of the procedure (57). An accompanying editorial by Sasahara and Barsamian argued that patients who respond to medical resuscitation "do well" and should not be referred for embolectomy (58). Alpert concurred, presenting mortality data on patients with pulmonary embolism and concluding that although embolectomy is potentially life-saving ". . . it is rarely technically feasible *and* clinically appropriate" (59). Beall and Collins, however, objected vigorously, comparing this to "the approach 5000 years ago . . . whereby the physician only selects for treatment those patients who will probably live and leaves to a Greater Being responsibility for those who will probably die . . ." (60). Similar debates continued into the late 1980s without resolution (61–64).

II. MAJOR SURGICAL SERIES

A. Overview

We were able to identify 22 unique reports of at least 10 pulmonary embolectomies, incorporating a total of 837 patients, published since 1970 either in English or with a substantive English abstract (Table 2). Over half of these reports were published since 1990, accounting for two-thirds of the patients. Only four reports (none since 1981) are from centers in the United States. The remaining 18 (and all recent) reports are from European centers with Germany (six) and France (three) particularly well represented.

Nearly all of these series cover at least 10 years (mean 15.7, range 4–25), with the average center performing only 2.9 embolectomies per year (range 0.8–7.1) and only four centers averaging more than four per year. The largest series from Strasbourg, France, averaged 7.1 procedures per year over 19 years for a total of 139 patients (24). Three centers included a total of 100 patients undergoing embolectomy with the inflow occlusion technique (23–25). The remaining were performed on cardiopulmonary bypass.

B. Operative Mortality Rates

1. Overall

There were 261 operative deaths among 837 patients for an overall operative mortality of 31%, with nearly all centers reporting mortality rates of 20 to 40%.

Table 2 Surgical Series of Pulmonary Embolectomy

Lead author	Country	Publication date	Years covered	Number of years	Number of patients	Cases per year	Operative deaths	Operative mortality
Doerge (65,67)	Germany	1999	1979–1998	19	41	2.2	12	29%
Ullman (66)	Germany	1999	1989–1997	8	40	5.0	14	35%
Jakob (68)	Germany	1995	1988–1994	7	25	3.6	6	24%
Gulba (104)	Germany	1994	1988–1993	5	13	2.6	3	23%
Stulz (25)	Switzerland	1994	1968–1992	26	50	1.9	23	46%
Laas, Schmid (69,72)	Germany	1993	1975–1992	17	34	2.0	15	44%
Meyns (70)	Belgium	1992	1973–1991	18	30	1.7	6	20%
Bauer (71)	Switzerland	1991	1978–1990	12	44	3.7	9	20%
Kieny (24)	France	1991	1970–1989	19	134	7.1	21	16%
Meyer (73)	France	1991	1968–1988	20	96	4.8	36	38%
Morshuis (74)	Netherlands	1990	1975–1988	13	16	1.2	6	38%
Gray (75)	England	1988	1964–1986	22	71	3.2	21	30%
Clarke (23)	England	1986	1960–1985	25	55	2.2	24	44%
Jaumin (105)	Belgium	1986	1969–1984	15	23	1.5	7	30%
Stalpaert (106)	Belgium	1986	1970–1984	14	29	2.1	10	34%
Mattox (79)	United States	1982	1961–1981	20	35	1.8	17	49%
Soyer (84)	France	1982	1977–1980	14	17	1.2	4	24%
Glassford (76)	United States	1981	1969–1979	10	20	2.0	8	40%
Tschirkov (77)	Germany	1978	1972–1976	4	24	6.0	7	29%
De Weese (78)	United States	1976	1961–1975	14	11	0.8	7	64%
Berger (57)	United States	1973			17		4	24%
Heimbecker (47)	Canada	1973			12		1	8%
Overall.					837	2.9	261	31%

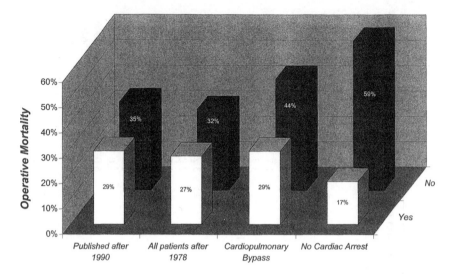

Figure 1   Average operative mortality after pulmonary embolectomy in major surgical series listed in Table 2 as a function of publication date, inclusion of patients from prior to 1978, use of cardiopulmonary bypass (CPB), and preoperative cardiac arrest (CPR).

Although there is a trend toward slightly improved results in recent years, the operative mortality rate remains high (Fig. 1). It was 29% among reports published since 1990, compared to 35% for the older reports. It was 27% in those studies which only included patients since 1978 compared to 32% for those including patients from the remote past.

2. Cardiopulmonary Bypass Versus Inflow Occlusion

Embolectomy under cardiopulmonary bypass appears to have a lower operative mortality (29%) than with normothermic inflow occlusion (44%) (Fig. 1), probably reflecting the fact that, at most centers, inflow occlusion is used only in desperate situations. In fact, 46% of patients undergoing inflow occlusion had suffered a preoperative cardiac arrest compared to 24% of the cardiopulmonary bypass group. Technical differences may also have contributed. Bypass provides more control, less time pressure, and better visualization than inflow occlusion and should permit a more complete embolectomy. Incomplete embolectomy can prevent normalization of pulmonary artery pressures and lead to right heart failure. Bypass may also be important in resuscitating the acutely failing right ventricle by unloading it and providing a good coronary perfusion pressure during the embolectomy. This may be most important in those patients with the most severe cardiac insults, those in severe shock or cardiac arrest.

C. Risk Factors for Operative Death

1. Preoperative Cardiac Arrest

Among the 15 reports with preoperative hemodynamic data, the operative mortality among the 26% of patients who suffered a preoperative cardiac arrest was a staggering 59% (23–25,65–78). The results in this high-risk group have not changed much over the years. It was 54% in the reports published since 1990 and 61% among those reports that only included patients since 1978. Although many of the remaining patients without preoperative arrest were in shock, their mortality was 17% overall and 10% if operated on cardiopulmonary bypass after 1978. Figure 2 demonstrates that operative mortality correlates fairly well with preoperative cardiac arrest. Hence, the centers that were able to operate prior to cardiac arrest, such as the Strasbourg group, generally had the best operative results (24).

Three of the more recent reports performed uni- or multivariate analyses to determine risk factors for operative mortality (25,66,73). Preoperative cardiac arrest was clearly the most important independent risk factor with odds ratios of 6.3 and 3.2 in the two multivariate analyses (66,73).

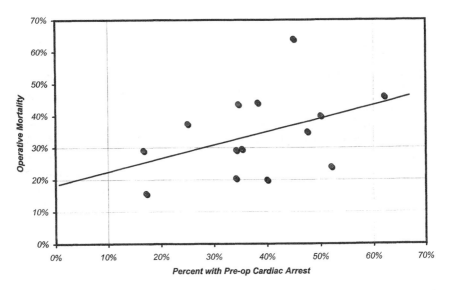

Figure 2 Relationship between operative mortality after pulmonary embolectomy and proportion of patients presenting with preoperative cardiac arrest requiring cardiopulmonary resuscitation. Each point represents a published report from Table 2 that documents the preoperative hemodynamic status of the patient.

2. Underlying Cardiopulmonary Disease

Both multivariate analyses also found underlying cardiopulmonary disease to be an independent risk factor for operative death with odds ratios of 3.7 and 4.7, respectively (66,73). Patients with limited cardiopulmonary reserve are more likely to present with hemodynamic instability, shock, or cardiac arrest even with relatively low embolic burdens. They may be more likely to have smaller, more distal emboli that are more difficult to completely extract. Increased pulmonary vascular resistance from incomplete embolectomy or underlying cardiopulmonary disease makes them more prone to postoperative right heart failure. Thus, these patients start off sicker and tend to have a less effective embolectomy. Patients with normal heart and lungs, on the other hand, need larger, central emboli to develop significant hemodynamic compromise. These patients are, therefore, ideal candidates for embolectomy and can expect complete normalization of pulmonary artery pressures and right heart function.

D. Causes of Operative Mortality

Ten reports document the cause of death after embolectomy (24,25,65,66,68–73,75,79) Although these are not always well defined and the categories differ among studies, certain trends are clearly apparent. Figure 3(a) summarizes the leading causes of operative death in these studies.

1. Heart Failure

Heart failure accounts for approximately 44% of all operative deaths with up to one-half of these resulting from failure to wean from cardiopulmonary bypass. The vast majority of both the intra- and postoperative cardiac deaths are from *right* heart failure from severe preoperative right heart injury combined with underlying cardiopulmonary disease or incomplete embolectomy. Left heart failure only occurs in those patients with underlying heart disease, prolonged preoperative hypotension, or long aortic cross-clamp times. The risk of heart failure may be minimized by intervening before the onset of irreversible myocardial injury, assuring complete evacuation of all emboli and avoiding aortic cross-clamping and myocardial ischemia that may exacerbate the underlying myocardial injury. Operating on the beating, unloaded heart may be the best means of resuscitating the injured right ventricle.

2. Severe Neurological Injury

Severe neurological injury accounted for 22% of all deaths. This is usually a diffuse, anoxic injury resulting from preoperative shock or cardiac arrest with hypoxemia as an exacerbating factor. An occasional patient survives the injury but ends up in a persistent vegetative state. The incidence of neurological injury

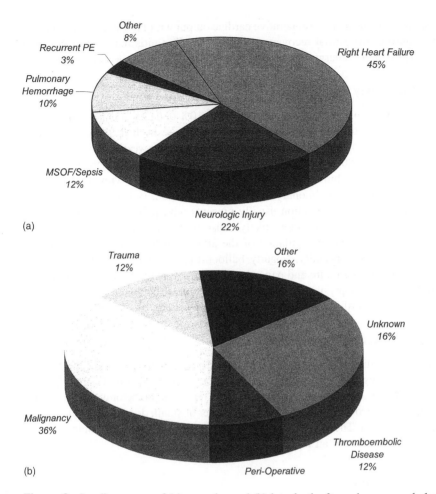

Figure 3 Leading causes of (a) operative and (b) late death after pulmonary embolectomy in those major surgical series listed in Table 2 which report cause of death. PE, pulmonary embolism; MSOF, multisystem organ failure.

may be minimized by intervening before cardiovascular collapse and aggressively treating with pressors to maintain adequate cerebral perfusion during the preoperative evaluation.

3. Multisystem Organ Failure and Sepsis

Multisystem organ failure and sepsis accounted for 12% of deaths. Many of these are probably secondary to prolonged pre- or postoperative low cardiac output.

Maintaining adequate postoperative cardiac output with inotropic agents and volume during myocardial recovery is critical. Mediastinitis may also occur in an arrested patient undergoing stereotomy under less than sterile conditions.

4. Pulmonary Hemorrhage

Massive pulmonary hemorrhage accounts for 10% of deaths and is the only major cause of death directly attributable to the procedure itself. It typically presents as massive hemorrhage from the endotracheal tube with weaning from cardiopulmonary bypass (80–82). Although some have attributed this to ischemia-reperfusion injury of the lung, this seems unlikely since patients with central emboli usually do not have pulmonary ischemia or infarction. Ischemia-reperfusion injury after lung transplantation usually presents with pulmonary edema and not massive hemoptysis. The more likely cause is direct pulmonary artery trauma from overaggressive manipulation of the arteries or blind passes with forceps, suction tips, or, especially, Fogarty balloon-tipped catheters. This can lead to pulmonary artery rupture and parenchymal hemorrhage or bronchial fistulization and massive hemoptysis. In my opinion, blind clot extraction of any type is never necessary or worth the risk of this lethal complication.

5. Recurrent Pulmonary Embolism

Recurrent pulmonary embolism is occasionally reported as a cause of death, typically occurring within hours or days of the original procedure. It is poorly tolerated in these already tenuous patients and repeat embolectomy is often futile because the second embolism may be a shower of small, distal emboli that are not easily extracted. The most common way to avoid this often lethal complication is routine placement of an inferior vena caval filter.

E. Late Follow-Up

Patients surviving embolectomy appear to have a good long-term outlook, which is primarily determined by their underlying condition (malignancy, heart and lung disease, etc.) and not by their history of pulmonary embolism and embolectomy. Although formal follow-up is limited, some studies do present causes of late death, actuarial survival, functional class, and follow-up diagnostic studies.

1. Survival Data

Ten centers report on 298 patients who underwent pulmonary embolectomy and were followed for 16 to 127 months (mean 71) (25,65,66,68–73,75,83–85) (Table 3). The 25 late deaths result in an overall late mortality rate of 8% and a linearized rate of 1.4% per year. Causes of death were documented in all 25 patients (Fig. 3b) and only 20% could be attributed to the history of pulmonary embolism—two following perioperative neurological injury, two from recurrent pulmonary embolism, and one from anticoagulation-related hemorrhage. Four deaths from unknown causes may have been related to pulmonary embolism. The majority of deaths, however, were from unrelated causes, mostly cancer (36%) and trauma (16%).

Four studies report actuarial survival data (65,66,71,85) These survival curves all show a steep initial decline reflecting the 20 to 40% operative mortality and a very flat portion thereafter reflecting the excellent mid- and long-term survival in operative survivors (Fig. 4). Medium-term (4–5 year) survival was 65 to 80% (65,66,71,85) and long-term (8–10 year) survival was 62 to 71% (65,66). Even patients who had suffered preoperative cardiac arrest and survived to discharge had excellent long-term survival (66).

2. Recurrent Pulmonary Embolism

Clinically significant recurrent pulmonary embolism appears to be rare. Two patients, noted above, died from recurrent embolism. There was only one additional report of a nonfatal embolism (71). Although these retrospective studies might underestimate the incidence, they are consistent with the relatively low rate of recurrent thromboembolism in patients treated medically after pulmonary embolism (86). In addition, most, but not all, centers routinely performed inferior vena

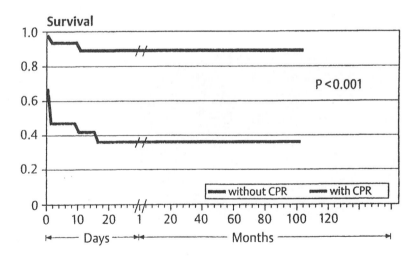

Figure 4 Actuarial survival after pulmonary embolectomy with and without cardiopulmonary resuscitation (CPR). (From Ref. 66.)

caval interruption to protect against recurrent embolism. The three patients who did suffer recurrent embolism had not undergone inferior vena caval interruption either as a matter of policy (75) or for technical reasons (71).

3. Functional Status

Six studies document New York Heart Association functional class in 176 hospital survivors at a mean follow-up of 71 months (65,66,71,73,83,85). Nearly all (98%) were in Class I or II (Fig. 5). One nonrandomized study from the mid-1980s compared late functional status among patients treated with heparin, streptokinase, or embolectomy (85). Although the surgical patients were more ill at presentation, their late functional status was better with 45% in Class I compared to 17% of medical patients. No surgical patient was in Class III or IV compared to 10% of medical patients.

A recent study sought to correlate late functional status with objective diagnostic studies in 19 of 21 survivors of embolectomy at a mean follow-up of 8.4 years (83). All patients underwent physical examination, ventilation-perfusion scintigraphy, echocardiography, and pulmonary function testing. Class III patients also underwent right heart catheterization and pulmonary arteriography. Using an explicit set of criteria, three-fourths of patients had at least one minor abnormality and one-fourth had a major abnormality. The presence of minor or major abnormalities correlated well with the patient's functional status, with major abnormalities occurring in only 12% of Class I or II patients but all Class III patients. Eighty percent of patients with no abnormalities were in Class I.

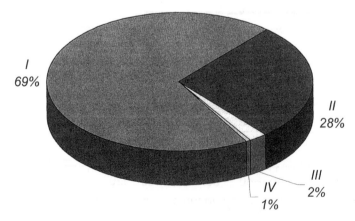

Figure 5   Late functional status after pulmonary embolectomy in those major surgical series listed in Table 2 that report New York Heart Association (NYHA) functional class.

Table 3 Late Mortality Among Survivors of
Pulmonary Embolectomy

Total Number of patients	298 patients
Follow-up period	
Mean	71 months
Range	16–127 months
Number of late deaths	25 deaths
Overall late mortality rate	8%
Linearized late mortality rate	1.4% per year
Actuarial survival	
Medium-term (4–5 years)	65–80%
Long-term (8–10 years)	62–71%

Interestingly, the three Class III patients were found to have abnormalities unrelated to their history of pulmonary embolism.

Another study found a similar incidence of minor abnormalities in 10 of 12 survivors of embolectomy (84) that the authors attributed to incomplete embolectomy, intraoperative trauma with thrombosis, or small recurrent emboli. Two patients, both with a preoperative history of prior embolism, had major residual perfusion defects and pulmonary hypertension. They conclude that patients with underlying, chronic pulmonary thromboembolic disease have significantly worse long-term outcome.

III. PREOPERATIVE EVALUATION

A. Surgical Indications and Timing

1. Overall Strategy

There is no consensus on the indications for surgery in acute pulmonary embolism (Table 4). The decision is fairly straightforward at either extreme. A stable patient with multiple peripheral perfusion defects is clearly not a surgical candidate. On the other hand, a patient in refractory cardiogenic shock with a documented saddle embolus, and a contraindication to thrombolysis, is certainly best served by emergency embolectomy. Most patients, however, fall between these two extremes and require careful individualized assessment to determine the optimal management. The indications for surgery should be part of a multidisciplinary strategy that seeks to minimize *overall* morbidity and mortality using all available modalities. Embolectomy should be considered one tool which, if applied before severe hemodynamic compromise, can provide excellent short- and long-term results. A strategy that positions it as a treatment of last resort, to be avoided

Table 4 Factors to Consider in the Decision to Proceed with Surgical Pulmonary Embolectomy

Possible indications for embolectomy	Contraindications to thrombolysis	
	Absolute	Relative
Embolus in the central pulmonary arteries	Active internal bleeding	Age over 75
Over 50% obstruction of pulmonary vasculature	Intracranial neoplasm, vascular malformation, or aneurysm	Recent (less than 10 days) major surgery, puncture of noncompressible puncture, or organ biopsy
Refractory cardiogenic shock	Neurosurgical procedure or stroke within 2 months	Pregnancy or early postpartum
Right atrial or ventricular thrombus	Severe uncontrolled hypertension	Recent trauma, including chest compressions
?Severe right heart dysfunction	Known bleeding diathesis	Recent GI bleeding or active ulcer disease (less than 10 days)
?Elevated cardiac troponin	Known allergy to thrombolytic agents	Known coagulation defects, including anticoagulant therapy and significant liver dysfunction
?Moderate hemodynamic compromise or right heart dysfunction with contraindication to thrombolysis		High likelihood of left heart thrombus (e.g., mitral stenosis with atrial fibrillation)

unless other options have failed or are unavailable, is doomed, in my opinion, to provide suboptimal results.

2. Location of Pulmonary Emboli

The classic anatomical criteria for embolectomy have been over 50% obstruction of the pulmonary vascular tree by pulmonary angiography. The location of the emboli, however, may be as important as the degree of obstruction. The ideal patient has large emboli in the central pulmonary arteries (at times accompanied by right atrial thrombus) that can be completely removed in a few pieces resulting in normalization of the pulmonary artery pressures and restoration of right heart function. A patient who has showered multiple emboli may also demonstrate vascular obstruction approaching 50% but is not as good a surgical candidate. Complete embolectomy may not be possible in these patients without traumatic maneuvers such as massaging the lungs, blind passage of instruments into the periphery, or retrograde perfusion of the lungs through the pulmonary veins.

3. Hemodynamic Status

As we have seen from the results of the major surgical series, a specific center's results will primarily depend on its hemodynamic threshold for intervening surgically. If surgery is limited to those patients *in extremis*, one can expect mortality rates over 50%. If surgery is applied more liberally with every effort to intervene *before* the onset of shock or cardiac arrest, one can expect mortality rates as low as 10%, comparable to patients undergoing thrombolysis (87). This dichotomy is understandable given that the leading causes of operative death—right heart failure, neurological injury, and multisystem organ failure—are a result of the patient's preoperative hemodynamic condition and not to the procedure itself. Pulmonary embolectomy, if applied with attention to minimizing pulmonary artery trauma, is a relatively simple procedure that should carry little inherent risk of death. Cardiopulmonary bypass times should be short; cardioplegic arrest should be unnecessary; and bleeding complications should be minimal.

That some patients will always present with sudden cardiovascular collapse may make it impossible to lower the overall mortality rate to less than 5 to 10% unless patients *in extremis* are simply not offered surgery. However, as Trendelenburg observed nearly a century ago, most patients have between 15 min and several hours before severe hemodynamic compromise ensues. Utilizing this time period effectively is the most critical challenge, with high stakes on both sides. Delaying surgery for a trial of medical therapy may avoid a major operation but may risk converting a stable patient with an operative mortality of 5 to 10% to one in severe cardiogenic shock or cardiac arrest with a mortality of 40 to 60%.

Sasahara's classic hemodynamic criteria for embolectomy include refractory cardiogenic shock (systolic pressure less than 90 mmHg) and oliguria (less than 20 mL/h) despite *maximal* medical therapy or when thrombolytic therapy is contraindicated (88). These stringent criteria, however, may withhold a potentially life-saving procedure until irreversible cardiac and end-organ injury has occurred. In my opinion, all patients with a hemodynamically significant central embolus should be considered for surgery. If the patient stabilizes with volume and low-dose inotropic support, then thrombolytic therapy may be appropriate, but the surgical team must be kept on alert and notified early if the patient deteriorates. Invasive monitoring of cardiac output may permit intervention before end-organ injury. The use of high-dose pressors during thrombolytic therapy to avoid surgery at all costs is inappropriate.

4. Right Ventricular Function

Goldhaber (2) and others (89) have clearly demonstrated that right ventricular hypokinesis without systemic hypotension is a strong, independent risk factor for early mortality and that this finding can be used to triage patients to more aggressive treatment. In a large registry report, the 14-day mortality among the 40% of patients with right ventricular hypokinesis was double that in those without this finding (2). This risk stratification has typically been applied in selecting patients for thrombolysis but may also be used in recommending embolectomy in those patients with contraindications to thrombolysis, even if they are hemodynamically stable. Evidence of severe right ventricular dysfunction might justify proceeding with embolectomy even if thrombolytic therapy is not contraindicated.

5. Right Atrial or Ventricular Thrombus

Mobile thrombus or "in-transit" emboli within the right atrium or right ventricle may occur in up to 10 to 15% of patients with pulmonary embolism (90,91). Even modest-sized thrombi can be fatal if they embolize in a patient with moderate degrees of vascular obstruction and right heart dysfunction. Because they are associated with a high (>40%) mortality rate, their presence is generally considered a strong indication for aggressive intervention. Although thrombolysis has been advocated for this condition (90,92,93), embolectomy may be the most appropriate treatment. These thrombi can embolize at any time (94) and thrombolysis may require several hours to achieve its maximal effect and might actually promote embolization. In my opinion, the presence of mobile thrombi in the right heart in a patient with documented central pulmonary emboli is a strong indication for emergency surgery.

6. Cardiac Enzymes

A recent report demonstrated that an elevated cardiac troponin T was present in 32% of patients with pulmonary embolism, correlated well with the severity of presentation, and was a strong predictor of in-hospital mortality—44% vs. 3% (95). On multivariate analysis, it was the only remaining independent predictor of death (adjusted odds ratio 15.2). Although these results need confirmation, cardiac troponins may supplement echocardiography in triaging patients to aggressive treatment.

7. Contraindications to Thrombolytic Therapy

Thrombolytic therapy has been shown to accelerate the resolution of emboli, the normalization of pulmonary artery pressures and right heart function, and lower mortality in selected patients (96–98). The risk of intracranial hemorrhage is 1 to 3% and the risk of other major hemorrhage is 10 to 20%. Some patients, however, have significantly higher risks of complications and thrombolytic therapy is contraindicated in them (Table 4). Patients with central pulmonary emboli who have contraindications to thrombolytic therapy should be considered for surgical embolectomy.

B. Diagnostic Studies

1. Overall Strategy

A streamlined diagnostic approach, focusing on documenting central emboli as rapidly as possible, is critical to achieving good results in patients being considered for embolectomy. Once this has been done, the patient should be transported to the operating room *immediately* even if relatively stable. Echocardiography, pulmonary angiography, and CT scanning all play important roles, but the specific tests performed depend on the patient's clinical presentation, location, and what is available. Although many patients will have undergone ventilation-perfusion scintigraphy at some point, this study is not particularly helpful in this setting. Large perfusion defects may suggest central emboli but their actual location cannot reliably be determined without a chest CT scan, pulmonary angiogram, or echocardiogram that shows thrombus in the main pulmonary arteries.

2. Chest CT Scanning

Contrast-enhanced spiral chest CT has become increasingly popular in evaluating pulmonary embolism (99,100). Its accuracy has been well documented in recent years and is comparable to other noninvasive tests. It may, in fact, be the ideal study in Emergency Department patients with suspected major pulmonary embolism. Although spiral CT is usually necessary to document peripheral emboli, large central emboli are usually well visualized with a standard chest CT scan. CT scanning is usually readily available, often in the Emergency Department itself, and can be performed in 10 to 15 min. If central emboli are visualized in the main or proximal branch pulmonary arteries, and if the patient is a candidate for surgical embolectomy by clinical criteria, no further confirmatory testing is necessary, and the patient can be immediately transported to the operating room.

3. Echocardiography

Echocardiography, transthoracic and transesophageal, is also playing an increasing role in the diagnosis and risk stratification of patients with pulmonary embolism (6,7,99,101,102). Although the pulmonary arteries themselves are often not well visualized, echocardiography provides important prognostic information to help determine whether aggressive treatment should be considered. Right heart function can be assessed, pulmonary artery pressures can be estimated, and mobile thromboemboli in the right atrium or ventricle can be visualized. Right ventricular hypokinesis is a strong predictor of poor outcome and may justify aggressive treatment—thrombolysis or surgery—even if the patient is hemodynamically stable.

Echocardiography may also be helpful as an initial study in a patient with some hemodynamic compromise in whom the diagnosis of pulmonary embolism is being considered. If the echocardiogram is suggestive but not definitive, a confirmatory CT scan or, more likely, pulmonary angiogram would be indicated. A tenuous patient, with clear-cut echocardiographic findings of a major pulmonary embolism, who is considered a candidate for surgical embolectomy, could be taken to the operating room without further testing. Intraoperative transesophageal or surface echocardiography could then confirm the presence of central emboli. Intraoperative TEE is also the only available test in the occasional patient who suffers a major pulmonary embolism on the operating room table during another operation. Evidence of a major embolism by TEE may justify immediate sternotomy and embolectomy.

4. Pulmonary Angiography

Although pulmonary angiography remains the gold standard for diagnosing pulmonary embolism, its role in evaluating patients for embolectomy should be limited. With spiral CT and echocardiography, most embolectomy patients will not need preoperative angiography. Clinically stable patients, with intermediate- to high-probability ventilation-perfusion scans, may undergo confirmatory angiography where unsuspected, massive central pulmonary embolism requiring surgery is discovered. Other patients, with echocardiographic findings suggestive of a large embolism, might need angiography to define the anatomical distribution of emboli and to determine whether surgical embolectomy is appropriate.

IV. INTRA- AND POSTOPERATIVE MANAGEMENT

A. Basic Principles

Patients selected for embolectomy should be immediately transported to the operating room even if they "appear" relatively stable. In our hospital, patients go directly from the radiology suite or ward to the operating room without stopping in the intensive care unit for "stabilization." Resuscitation can be performed *en route* and in the operating room. Patients from outside hospitals are transferred directly to the operating room by helicopter. In the operating room, teamwork is critical and only essential preoperative maneuvers are performed so the patient can be placed on cardiopulmonary bypass without delay.

B. Anesthesia

Patients with large central pulmonary emboli are very tenuous, even if awake and appearing relatively clinically stable. The failing right ventricle is dependent on elevated preload to maintain flow through the obstructed pulmonary vasculature. The underfilled left ventricle is dependent on increased peripheral vascular tone to maintain systemic blood pressure. Although compensatory mechanisms can maintain normal blood pressure and tissue perfusion, small hemodynamic perturbations, such as venous and arterial vasodilatation from general anesthesia, can reverse these mechanisms and lead to hemodynamic collapse. This has been well appreciated in the earliest days of surgical embolectomy when femoral cannulation for cardiopulmonary bypass under local anesthesia was quite popular. That is now rarely necessary with modern anesthetic techniques, including awake fiberoptic intubation and the use of new agents with minimal hemodynamic effects. Nonetheless, anesthesia should not begin until the perfusionist is present with the heart–lung machine primed and ready. Prepping and draping the patient before induction may also be prudent as this will allow the surgeon to open the chest and be on bypass within 60 to 90 s.

Although an arterial monitoring line and large-bore venous access are necessary prior to induction, central venous access can be deferred until after the patient is on bypass. A pulmonary artery catheter is critical for weaning from bypass and postoperative management but the dilated right heart can make advancing the catheter difficult and time-consuming. The introducer sheath can be inserted and the catheter advanced with the surgeon's guidance *after* embolectomy and prior to weaning from bypass.

C. Transesophageal Echocardiography

Intraoperative transesophageal echocardiography (TEE) is a useful tool during embolectomy. Although placement of the probe should not be a high priority in an unstable patient, imaging of the right atrium and ventricle prior to cannulation for bypass is helpful. Visualization of mobile thromboemboli in the right heart can help determine whether right heart exploration is necessary and guide venous cannulation. Assessment of right heart function can help anticipate difficulties with weaning from bypass. TEE can often visualize emboli in the central pulmonary arteries in a patient who has come to the operating room without good visualization of these structures. Surface scanning of the right heart and pulmonary arteries is very simple and can be used in the occasional patient who cannot undergo TEE or in whom adequate images cannot be obtained (103). Persistent right heart dysfunction can make postbypass hemodynamic management difficult. TEE can assess the degree of residual right heart dysfunction as well as ventricular volumes to help determine whether to treat the patient with volume, inotropic agents, pulmonary vasodilators, or systemic vasoconstrictors.

D. Surgical Technique

1. Incision and Cardiopulmonary Bypass

Embolectomy is performed through a full median sternotomy that provides good exposure of the pulmonary arteries, vena cavae, and right heart chambers. After pericardiotomy and full heparinization, the patient is cannulated for cardiopulmonary bypass. Arterial cannulation is usually performed in the distal ascending aorta. The most common technique for venous cannulation is to place separate cannulae in the superior and inferior vena cavae with tourniquets to prevent air from entering the venous line when the pulmonary artery or right heart is opened. The availability of intraoperative TEE has allowed us to simplify our venous cannulation technique. We explore the right atrium and ventricle only if the TEE (or surface echo) demonstrates mobile thromboemboli. In addition, we routinely employ vacuum-assisted venous drainage that is not affected by moderate amounts of air in the venous line. This allows us to rapidly cannulate the right atrium through the appendage using a standard two-stage venous cannula. This technique works even in situations where right heart exploration is necessary. With vacuum-assisted venous drainage, the right atrium can be explored without separately controlling the vena cavae.

Although some authors report using aortic cross-clamping and cardioplegic or fibrillatory arrest, this is, in my opinion, never necessary and always potentially detrimental. Pulmonary embolectomy and right heart exploration can easily be performed with the heart beating under normothermic conditions. Some degree of right heart stunning is almost always present and aortic cross-clamping and cardiac arrest add an additional ischemic insult that risks further stunning and right heart dysfunction. Performing the operation on the unloaded, well-perfused beating heart not only avoids any further ischemic insult but also provides time for the heart to recover and regenerate its depleted energy stores.

2. Exploration of the Right Atrium and Ventricle

If echocardiography demonstrates mobile thromboemboli in the right atrium or right ventricle, exploration of these chambers is mandatory and should be performed prior to embolectomy. Cannulating the right atrium and inferior vena cava in patients with right atrial thrombus must be performed with caution to prevent dislodging the thrombus or aspirating it into the venous line. In these situations we cannulate the right atrium while visualizing it and the thrombus by TEE. The cannula is advanced just far enough to achieve adequate venous drainage to initiate bypass. The right atrium is then opened and explored with the venous cannula on vacuum suction. The right ventricle is inspected through the tricuspid valve and later through the pulmonary valve. The venous cannula is repositioned after confirming that the right heart is completely free of clot by TEE.

3. Pulmonary Arteriotomy and Embolectomy

Once cardiopulmonary bypass has been established, the actual embolectomy begins with an incision over the main pulmonary artery. Some surgeons use a longitudinal incision starting just below the pulmonary valve, but we find that a very low transverse incision provides better visualization and can be extended onto the branch pulmonary arteries if necessary. The proximal portion of the clot is usually immediately apparent, especially if a saddle embolus is present. The clot is then gently extracted in a hand-over-hand fashion using simple gallbladder stone forceps. If this is done carefully, the clot can usually be removed en bloc, emerging as a cast of the femoral vein. Once the large central clots have been removed, the entire pulmonary vascular tree is inspected. With good head-mounted lighting and firm anterior retraction of the aorta, all segmental pulmonary artery branches, except, occasionally, the individual basal segments, can be cleared of emboli *under direct vision* using the stone forceps or a small suction-tipped catheter.

Many other techniques for clot extraction have been utilized and advocated in the literature. I believe that these techniques are not only unnecessary but excessively traumatic and potentially dangerous. The pulmonary arteries are very fragile and trauma to these vessels from overaggressive or blind instrumentation can lead to pulmonary hemorrhage, which is usually fatal. If patients for embolectomy are carefully selected to include only those with large central emboli, then simple extraction of all *visible* central and distal clots will result in nearly complete normalization of pulmonary artery pressures. Leaving small, peripheral emboli behind is preferable to performing dangerous blind maneuvers to achieve a perfectly complete embolectomy. The pulmonary vasculature is known to possess a great capacity for fibrinolysis and may clear these peripheral emboli over time.

Among these adjunctive techniques, blind Fogarty balloon catheter embolectomy is particularly worthy of criticism. Even if this technique did not risk pulmonary artery perforation and fatal pulmonary hemorrhage, it is unlikely to be particularly effective. The likelihood of advancing the catheter into each segmental branch, without visual guidance, is very low. Several Japanese centers have advocated using fiberoptic angioscopy to help visualize and extract small peripheral emboli. Although theoretically attractive, this technique can be time-consuming and requires additional equipment that might not be available during the off-hours. Again, the benefit of extracting a few more peripheral emboli is unlikely to be worth the effort. Massaging the lungs to dislodge peripheral emboli is also potentially traumatic and may promote postoperative pulmonary edema. Without active retrograde blood flow, it seems unlikely that a significant amount of dislodged clot would find its way back to the central pulmonary arteries. Retrograde perfusion of the lungs through the pulmonary veins, although theoretically attractive, requires aortic cross-clamping, cardioplegic arrest, opening of the left atrium, and deairing the left heart. The cumulative risk of these maneuvers does not justify the theoretical benefit of extracting a few more peripheral emboli.

4. Weaning from Cardiopulmonary Bypass

The primary issue in weaning patients from cardiopulmonary bypass after embolectomy is right ventricular function. Although most patients will demonstrate immediate, often dramatic, improvements, some residual dysfunction or stunning is common. Accurate right atrial and pulmonary artery pressures are critical and TEE is helpful. Volume loading to a right atrial pressure of 15 to 25 cm of water and inotropic agents may be necessary. If the pulmonary artery pressure has normalized, we prefer dopamine, dobutamine, or low-dose epinephrine. The chronotropic effects of these agents may be beneficial in the stroke-volume-limited, stunned right ventricle. Persistent elevation of pulmonary artery pressures must be investigated and treated expeditiously. Inadequate ventilation or oxygenation is sometimes the culprit and normal arterial blood gases should be documented before weaning begins. The heparin antagonist, protamine, is a known pulmonary vasoconstrictor and should be administered cautiously. The possibility of residual or recurrent emboli should be considered and, if echocardiography is suggestive, the pulmonary arteries should be reexplored. Phosphodiesterase inhibitors such as milrinone may be the ideal inotropic class of agents in this setting but systemic vasodilatory effects may need to be counteracted with other agents. Inhaled nitric oxide or intravenous prostacyclin can be life-saving in severe cases.

E. Inferior Vena Caval Filters

The role of inferior vena caval (IVC) filters in pulmonary embolectomy is controversial. About two-thirds of the reports advocate IVC interruption to avoid the uncommon, but often fatal, complication of early recurrent embolization. The alternative, early anticoagulation with heparin, does not completely eliminate the risk and may increase postoperative bleeding complications, particularly in patients with contraindications to thrombolytic therapy. The immediate postoperative period, before heparin can be safely initiated, may also be the period of greatest risk for reembolization. For these reasons, and from a personal experience with a fatal recurrent embolus, I believe most patients should undergo placement of an IVC filter. The low, but finite, incidence of filter complications (IVC thrombosis with recurrent embolization, migration, and chronic venous stasis) must, however, be considered, especially in younger patients in whom their cumulative incidence can be significant over a lifetime.

We usually place the filter in the operating room just prior to sternal closure. It is advanced through the right atrial appendage venous pursestring into the infrarenal vena cava, guided by a portable "C-arm" fluoroscope. Occasionally, a stable patient who is already in the angiography suite for a pulmonary angiogram will undergo preoperative filter placement if the procedure can be completed with minimal delay. Some centers transfer the fresh postoperative patient to the angiography suite on the way to the intensive care unit but this seems more complicated and potentially dangerous.

F. Postoperative Management

Right ventricular function may take several days to normalize, and aggressive support may be necessary during this period. Right atrial and pulmonary artery pressure, cardiac output, and mixed venous oxygen saturation should be carefully monitored. Strict attention to adequate ventilation and oxygenation is critical to avoid even transient pulmonary vasoconstriction. Inotropic agents should be weaned slowly. If a prolonged wean is anticipated, adding milrinone can permit catecholamines to be withdrawn. If an IVC filter has been placed, postoperative heparin can be delayed for 24 to 48 h and started gently, without a bolus, to maintain a partial thromboplastin time of 50 to 60 s. Warfarin can be initiated, with a target International Normalized Ratio (INR) or 2.0 to 2.5, once the patient is able to take oral medications. Long-term anticoagulation is usually continued for at least 6 months. A baseline echocardiogram and quantitative ventilation-perfusion scan are performed prior to discharge and repeated at 6 months to document resolution of any residual small perfusion defects and normalization of right heart function.

V. RECENT BRIGHAM AND WOMEN'S HOSPITAL EXPERIENCE

In the fall of 1999 we embarked on a multidisciplinary program at Brigham and Women's Hospital in Boston to improve our results with acute pulmonary embolectomy. The team consisted of a single cardiologist and surgeon in close collaboration with interventional cardiology and radiology. Our goal was to identify candidates for surgical embolectomy soon after presentation by emphasizing rapid diagnosis and triage. Our indications for embolectomy are similar to those described above and include all patients with large central pulmonary emboli who have contraindications to thrombolysis, are in severe cardiogenic shock, or have mobile right heart thromboemboli. Once the patient has been selected for embolectomy, the team is committed to immediately transporting the patient to the operating room.

Over an 8-month period, between October 1999 and May 2000, 12 consecutive patients (67% male; mean age 60.5 years) with acute major, central pulmonary embolism underwent surgical pulmonary embolectomy. One patient had undergone pulmonary thromboendarterectomy 2 months earlier and presented with recurrent embolization from inferior venal caval thrombosis above his filter. In another patient, the source of emboli was tumor thrombus extending into the renal vein and inferior vena cava from a large, previously undiagnosed left renal cell carcinoma. A perfusion scan (5/12), spiral CT (6/12), pulmonary angiogram (2/12), and/or echocardiogram (4/10) confirmed the diagnosis. One patient was intubated on high-dose inotropic support. Most of the remaining patients had had a period of hypotension or syncope but responded well to volume or low-dose inotropic support. Despite the fact that one-half of the patients were transferred from outside hospitals, the mean time from diagnosis to arrival in the operating room was 1.6 h.

Four of the "hemodynamically stable" patients suffered a cardiac arrest in the operating room requiring emergent institution of cardiopulmonary bypass. Normothermic cardiopulmonary bypass without aortic cross-clamping was instituted. Transesophageal echocardiography was performed in all patients and four patients with right atrial or inferior vena caval thromboemboli underwent right atriotomy and clot extraction. Pulmonary clot extraction was performed under direct vision without any adjunctive maneuvers such as Fogarty balloon embolectomy. The patient with renal cell carcinoma underwent nephrectomy with en bloc inferior vena caval thrombectomy during a brief period of hypothermic circulatory arrest prior to pulmonary embolectomy. An IVC filter was placed before (3/12), during (5/12), or after surgery (2/12) in most patients.

All patients were successfully weaned from cardiopulmonary bypass and left the operating room in stable condition. One patient, a 49-year-old morbidly obese gentleman, who did not have an inferior vena caval filter, sustained multiple recurrent emboli on the first postoperative day. He ultimately succumbed to complications of heparin-induced thrombocytopenia despite repeat embolectomy, placement, and successful removal of a right ventricular assist device. The operative mortality was therefore 8.3%. The patient with the recurrent embolization after thromboendarterectomy was discharged from the hospital after a prolonged hospital course but died 2 months postoperatively of sepsis from *C. difficile* colitis. The remaining 10 patients were discharged from the hospital are doing well at home at a mean follow-up of 5 months.

VI. SUMMARY

Surgical pulmonary embolectomy has a definite role to play in the management of selected patients with acute, major pulmonary embolism. Rapid noninvasive diagnostic modalities allow proper patient selection based on anatomical location of the emboli, right ventricular function, and contraindications to thrombolysis. Operative results are a direct reflection of the preoperative hemodynamic status, the degree of underlying cardiopulmonary disease, and attention to minimizing surgical trauma and protecting the right heart. An operative mortality of 10% or less and excellent long-term outcomes can be expected if the procedure is performed, prior to cardiovascular collapse, as part of a multidisciplinary strategy that emphasizes careful patient selection, rapid diagnosis, triage, and transport.

REFERENCES

1. Ansari A. Acute and chronic pulmonary thromboembolism: current perspectives. Part I: Glossary of terms, historic evolution and prevalence. Clin Cardiol 1986; 9: 398–402.
2. Goldhaber SZ, Visani L, De Rosa M. Acute pulmonary embolism: clinical outcomes in the International Cooperative Pulmonary Embolism Registry (ICOPER). Lancet 1999; 353:1386–1389.
3. Peterson KL. Acute pulmonary thromboembolism: has its evolution been redefined? Circulation 1999; 99:1280–1283.
4. Surgery for pulmonary emboli? Lancet 1989; 1:198.
5. Beall AC, Jr. Pulmonary embolectomy. Ann Thorac Surg 1991; 51:179.
6. Pruszczyk P, Torbicki A, Pacho R, Chlebus M, Kuch-Wocial A, Pruszynski B, Gurba H. Noninvasive diagnosis of suspected severe pulmonary embolism: transesophageal echocardiography vs spiral CT. Chest 1997; 112:722–728.
7. Torbicki A, Pacho R, Jedrusik P, Pruszczyk P. Noninvasive diagnosis and treatment of a saddle pulmonary embolism. A case report in support of new trends in management of pulmonary embolism. Chest 1996; 109:1124–1126.
8. Kim KI, Muller NL, Mayo JR. Clinically suspected pulmonary embolism: utility of spiral CT. Radiology 1999; 210:693–697.
9. Trendelenburg F. Uber die operative behandlung der embolie derlungarterie. Arch Klin Chir 1998; 86:686–700.
10. Meyer JA. Friedrich Trendelenburg and the surgical approach to massive pulmonary embolism. Arch Surg 1990; 125:1202–1205.

11. Kirschner M. Ein durch die Trendelenburgsce Operation Geheilter Fall Embolic der Art. Pulmonalis 24;133:312–359.

12. Makey, AR and Bliss, BP. Pulmonary embolectomy. A review of five cases with three survivals. Lancet 1966; 2:1155–1158.

13. Steenburg RW, Warren R, Wilson RE, and Rudolf LE. A new look at pulmonary embolectomy. Surg Gynecol Obstet 1958; 107:214–220.

14. Romaine-Davis A. John Gibbon and his heart-lung machine. Philadelphia: University of Pennsylvania Press: 91.

15. Gibbon JH, Jr. Application of a mechanical heart and lung apparatus to cardiac surgery. Minn Med 1954; 37:171–180.

16. Kiser WJ. An experimental study of the effects of constriction on the great vessels. Surg Gynecol Obstet 1935; 51:765.

17. Sautter RD, Myers WO, Ray JF, III, Wenzel FJ. Pulmonary embolectomy: review and current status. Prog Cardiovasc Dis 1975; 17:371–389.

18. Allison PR, Dunhill MS, Marshall R. Pulmonary embolism. Thorax 1960; 15:273–283.

19. Sautter RD, Lawron BR, Magnin GE. Pulmonary embolectomy: A simplified technique. Wis Med J 1962; 61:309.

20. Vosschulte K. The surgical treatment of pulmonary embolism. J Cardiovasc Surg (Torino) 1965; (suppl):197–200.

21. Cross FS, Mowlem A. A survey of the current status of pulmonary embolectomy for massive pulmonary embolism. Circulation 1967; 35:186–191.

22. Clarke DB. Pulmonary embolectomy using normothermic venous inflow occlusion. Thorax 1968; 23:131–135.

23. Clarke DB, Abrams LD. Pulmonary embolectomy: a 25 year experience. J Thorac Cardiovasc Surg 1986; 92:442–445.

24. Kieny R, Charpentier A, Kieny MT. What is the place of pulmonary embolectomy today? J Cardiovasc Surg (Torino) 1991; 32:549–554.

25. Stulz P, Schlapfer R, Feer R, Habicht J, Gradel E. Decision making in the surgical treatment of massive pulmonary embolism. Eur J Cardiothorac Surg 1994; 8:188–193.

26. Bradley MN, Bennett AL, III, Lyons C. Successful unilateral pulmonary embolectomy without cardiopulmonary bypass. N Engl J Med 1964; 271:713.

27. Camishion RC, Pierucci L, Jr, Fishman NH, Fraimow W, Greening R. Pulmonary embolectomy without cardiopulmonary bypass. Indications, diagnostic criteria, and case report. Am J Surg 1966; 111:723–727.

28. O'Connell TJ, Schreiber JT. Selective pulmonary embolectomy without cardiopulmonary bypass. Ann Surg 1967; 165:466–469.

29. Yasargil EC. Simplified pulmonary embolectomy. J Cardiovasc Surg (Torino) 1967; 8:29–30.

30. Janke WH. Pulmonary embolectomy. Retrograde approach without use of a heart-lung bypass. JAMA 1968; 206:127–128.

31. Doane WA, McKittrick JE. Massive pulmonary emboli: ten-year review of cases and report of successful pulmonary embolectomy without cardiopulmonary bypass. Am Surg 1968; 34:762–767.

32. Borja AR, Lansing AM. Technique of selective pulmonary embolectomy without bypass. Surg Gynecol Obstet 1970; 130:1073–1076.

33. Nott DB. Pulmonary embolectomy using normothermic venous inflow occlusion. Med J Aust 1971; 1:1328–1331.

34. Senning A. Left anterior thoracotomy for pulmonary embolectomy with 29-year follow-up. Ann Thorac Surg 1998; 66:1420–1421.

35. Cooley DA, Beall AC, Jr, Alexander JK. Acute massive pulmonary embolism. Successful surgical treatment using temporary cardiopulmonary bypass. JAMA 1961; 177:283–286.

36. Sharp EH. Pulmonary embolectomy: successful removal of a massive pulmonary embolus with support of cardiopulmonary bypass. Ann Surg 1962; 156:1–4.

37. Donaldson GN, Willams L, Scannell G, Shaw R. A reappraisal of the application of the Trendelenburg operation to massive fatal embolism: report of successful pulmonary-artery thrombectomy using cardiopulmonary bypass. N Engl J Med 1963; 268:171–173.

38. Sautter RD. Massive pulmonary thromboembolism. Experience with 12 pulmonary embolectomies. JAMA 1965; 194:336–338.

39. Beall AC, Jr, Cooley DA. Current status of embolectomy for acute massive pulmonary embolism. Am J Cardiol 1965; 16:828–33.

40. Beall AC, Jr, Cooley DA. Experience with pulmonary embolectomy using temporary cardiopulmonary bypass. J Cardiovasc Surg (Torino) 1965; Suppl:201–206.

41. Barkin M, Finlayson DC, Wilson JK, Bailey P, Heslin DJ, Baker CB. Massive pulmonary embolism: successful surgical treatment using cardiopulmonary bypass. Can Med Assoc J 1965; 93:1128–1131.

42. Baker RR, Wagner HN, Jr. Pulmonary embolectomy in the treatment of massive pulmonary embolism. Surg Gynecol Obstet 1966; 122:513–516.

43. Stansel HC, Jr, Hume M, Glenn WL. Pulmonary embolectomy. Results in ten patients. N Engl J Med 1967; 276:717–721.

44. Sautter RD. The technique of pulmonary embolectomy with the use of cardiopulmonary bypass. J Thorac Cardiovasc Surg 1967; 53:268–274.

45. Cooley DA, Beall AC, Jr. Embolectomy for acute massive pulmonary embolism. Surg Gynecol Obstet 1968; 126:805–810.

46. Gentsch TO, Larsen PB, Daughtry DC, Chesney JG, Spear HC. Community-wide availability of pulmonary embolectomy with cardiopulmonary bypass. Ann Thorac Surg 1969; 7:97–103.

47. Heimbecker RO, Keon WJ, Richards KU. Massive pulmonary embolism. A new look at surgical management. Arch Surg 1973; 107:740–746.

48. Thomas DP. Treatment of pulmonary embolic disease. A critical review of some aspects of current therapy. N Engl J Med 1965; 273:885–892.

49. Daicoff GR, Rams JJ, Moulder PV. Pulmonary embolectomy. Surg Clin North Am 1966; 46:27–36.

50. Moulder PV, Daicoff GR, Rams JJ, Daily PO. The case for pulmonary embolectomy. Med Clin North Am 1967; 51:185–191.

51. Scannell JG. The surgical management of acute massive pulmonary embolism. Prog Cardiovasc Dis 1967; 9:488–494.

52. Keon WJ, Heimbecker RO. Massive pulmonary embolism: modern surgical management. Can J Surg 1969; 12:15–21.

53. Heimbecker RO, Keon WJ, Elliott G. Pulmonary embolectomy. Arch Surg 1967; 95:576–84.

54. Morrison MCT. Is pulmonary embolectomy obsolete. Br J Dis Chest 1963; 57:187.

55. Madsen CM, Buhl J. Fatal pulmonary embolism. Acta Chir Scand 1964; 128:721.

56. Meyerowitz BR. Pulmonary embolism in surgical patients: is embolectomy superior to prophylaxis? Surgery 1966; 60:521–535.

57. Berger RL. Pulmonary embolectomy with preoperative circulatory support. Ann Thorac Surg 1973; 16:217–227.

58. Sasahara AA, Barsamian EM. Another look at pulmonary embolectomy. Ann Thorac Surg 1973; 16:317–320.

59. Alpert JS, Smith RE, Ockene IS, Askenazi J, Dexter L, Dalen JE. Treatment of massive pulmonary embolism: the role of pulmonary embolectomy. Am Heart J 1975; 89:413–418.

60. Beall AC, Collins JJ, Jr. Editorial: What is the role of pulmonary embolectomy? Am Heart J 1975; 89:411–412.

61. Gray HH, Miller GA. Pulmonary embolectomy is still appropriate for a minority of patients with acute massive pulmonary embolism. Br J Hosp Med 1989; 41: 467–468.

62. Gray HH, Miller GA, Paneth M. Pulmonary embolectomy: its place in the management of pulmonary embolism. Lancet 1988; 1:1441–1445.

63. Clarke DB. Pulmonary embolectomy has a well-defined and valuable place. Br J Hosp Med 1989; 41:468–469.

64. Oakley CM. There is no place for acute pulmonary embolectomy. Br J Hosp Med 1989; 41:469.

65. Doerge H, Schoendube FA, Voss M, Seipelt R, Messmer BJ. Surgical therapy of fulminant pulmonary embolism: early and late results. Thorac Cardiovasc Surg 1999; 47:9–13.

66. Ullmann M, Hemmer W, Hannekum A. The urgent pulmonary embolectomy: mechanical resuscitation in the operating theatre determines the outcome. Thorac Cardiovasc Surg 1999; 47:5–8.

67. Doerge HC, Schoendube FA, Loeser H, Walter M, Messmer BJ. Pulmonary embolectomy: review of a 15-year experience and role in the age of thrombolytic therapy. Eur J Cardiothorac Surg 1996; 10:952–957.

68. Jakob H, Vahl C, Lange R, Micek M, Tanzeem A, Hagl S. Modified surgical concept for fulminant pulmonary embolism. Eur J Cardiothorac Surg 1995; 9:557–60; discussion 561.

69. Laas J, Schmid C, Albes JM, Borst HG. [Surgical aspects of fulminant pulmonary embolism]. Z Kardiol 1993; 82 (Suppl 2):25–28.

70. Meyns B, Sergeant P, Flameng W, Daenen W. Surgery for massive pulmonary embolism. Acta Cardiol 1992; 47:487–493.

71. Bauer EP, Laske A, von Segesser LK, Carrel T, Turina MI. Early and late results after surgery for massive pulmonary embolism. Thorac Cardiovasc Surg 1991; 39: 353–356.

72. Schmid C, Zietlow S, Wagner TO, Laas J, Borst HG. Fulminant pulmonary embo-

lism: symptoms, diagnostics, operative technique, and results. Ann Thorac Surg 1991; 52:1102–1105; discussion 1105–1107.

73. Meyer G, Tamisier D, Sors H, Stern M, Vouhe P, Makowski S, Neveux JY, Leca F, Even P. Pulmonary embolectomy: a 20-year experience at one center. Ann Thorac Surg 1991; 51:232–236.

74. Morshuis WJ, van Son JA, Vincent JG, Lacquet LK, Heystraten FM. [Surgical treatment of massive pulmonary embolism]. Ned Tijdschr Geneeskd 1990; 134: 1179–1183.

75. Gray HH, Morgan JM, Paneth M, Miller GA. Pulmonary embolectomy for acute massive pulmonary embolism: an analysis of 71 cases. Br Heart J 1988; 60:196–200.

76. Glassford DM, Jr, Alford WC, Jr, Burrus GR, Stoney WS, Thomas CS, Jr. Pulmonary embolectomy. Ann Thorac Surg 1981; 32:28–32.

77. Tschirkov A, Krause E, Elert O, Satter P. Surgical management of massive pulmonary embolism. J Thorac Cardiovasc Surg 1978; 75:730–733.

78. De Weese JA. The role of pulmonary embolectomy in venous thromboembolism. J Cardiovasc Surg (Torino) 1976; 17:348–53.

79. Mattox KL, Feldtman RW, Beall AC, Jr, DeBakey ME. Pulmonary embolectomy for acute massive pulmonary embolism. Ann Surg 1982; 195:726–731.

80. Shimokawa S, Watanabe S, Kobayashi A. Exsanguinating hemoptysis after pulmonary embolectomy. Ann Thorac Surg 1999; 68:2385–2386.

81. Wollman SB, Kushins LG. Survival following massive pulmonary hemorrhage complicating pulmonary embolectomy: a case report. Anesth Analg 1976; 55:182–184.

82. Makey AR, Bliss BP, Ikram H, Sutcliffe MM, Emery ER. Fatal intra-alveolar pulmonary bleeding complicating pulmonary embolectomy. Thorax 1971; 26:466–471.

83. Habicht JM, Hammerli R, Perruchoud A, Muller J, Stulz P. Long-term follow-up in pulmonary embolectomy: is NYHA (dyspnea) classification reliable? Eur J Cardiothorac Surg 1996; 10:32–37.

84. Soyer R, Brunet AP, Redonnet M, Borg JY, Hubscher, C, Letac B. Follow-up of surgically treated patients with massive pulmonary embolism—with reference to 12 operated patients. Thorac Cardiovasc Surg 1982; 30:103–108.

85. Lund O, Nielsen TT, Ronne K, Schifter S. Pulmonary embolism: long-term follow-up after treatment with full-dose heparin, streptokinase or embolectomy. Acta Med Scand 1987; 221:61–71.

86. Heit JA, Mohr DN, Silverstein MD, Petterson TM, O'Fallon WM, Melton LJ, III. Predictors of recurrence after deep vein thrombosis and pulmonary embolism: a population-based cohort study. Arch Intern Med 2000; 160:761–768.

87. Kasper W, Konstantinides S, Geibel A, Olschewski M, Heinrich F, Grosser KD, Rauber K, Iversen S, Redecker M, Kienast J. Management strategies and determinants of outcome in acute major pulmonary embolism: results of a multicenter registry. J Am Coll Cardiol 1997; 30:1165–1171.

88. Sasahara AA, Sharma GV, Barsamian EM, Schoolman M, Cella G. Pulmonary thromboembolism. Diagnosis and treatment. JAMA 1983; 249:2945–2950.

89. Kasper W, Konstantinides S, Geibel A, Tiede N, Krause T, Just H. Prognostic

significance of right ventricular afterload stress detected by echocardiography in patients with clinically suspected pulmonary embolism. Heart 1997; 77:346–349.

90. Chapoutot L, Nazeyrollas P, Metz D, Maes D, Maillier B, Jennesseaux C, Elaerts J. Floating right heart thrombi and pulmonary embolism: diagnosis, outcome and therapeutic management. Cardiology 1996; 87:169–174.

91. Casazza F, Bongarzoni A, Centonze F, Morpurgo M. Prevalence and prognostic significance of right-sided cardiac mobile thrombi in acute massive pulmonary embolism. Am J Cardiol 1997; 79:1433–1435.

92. Chartier L, Bera J, Delomez M, Asseman P, Beregi JP, Bauchart JJ, Warembourg H, Thery C. Free-floating thrombi in the right heart: diagnosis, management, and prognostic indexes in 38 consecutive patients. Circulation 1999; 99:2779–2783.

93. Goldhaber SZ. Optimal strategy for diagnosis and treatment of pulmonary embolism due to right atrial thrombus. Mayo Clin Proc 1988; 63:1261–1264.

94. Farfel Z, Shechter M, Vered Z, Rath S, Goor D, Gafni J. Review of echocardiographically diagnosed right heart entrapment of pulmonary emboli-in-transit with emphasis on management. Am Heart J 1987; 113:171–178.

95. Giannitsis E, Muller-Bardorff M, Kurowski V, Weidtmann B, Wiegand U, Kampmann M, Katus HA. Independent prognostic value of cardiac troponin T in patients with confirmed pulmonary embolism. Circulation 2000; 102:211–217.

96. Goldhaber SZ, Haire WD, Feldstein ML, Miller M, Toltzis R, Smith JL, Taveira da Silva AM, Come PC, Lee RT, Parker JA, et al. Alteplase versus heparin in acute pulmonary embolism: randomised trial assessing right-ventricular function and pulmonary perfusion. Lancet 1993; 341:507–511.

97. Konstantinides S, Tiede N, Geibel A, Olschewski M, Just H, Kasper W. Comparison of alteplase versus heparin for resolution of major pulmonary embolism. Am J Cardiol 1998; 82:966–970.

98. Konstantinides S, Geibel A, Olschewski M, Heinrich F, Grosser K, Rauber K, Iversen S, Redecker M, Kienast J, Just H, Kasper W. Association between thrombolytic treatment and the prognosis of hemodynamically stable patients with major pulmonary embolism: results of a multicenter registry. Circulation 1997; 96:882–888.

99. Torbicki A. Imaging venous thromboembolism with emphasis on ultrasound, chest CT, angiography and echocardiography. Thromb Haemost 1999; 82:907–912.

100. Blachere H, Latrabe V, Montaudon M, Valli N, Couffinhal T, Raherisson C, Leccia F, Laurent F. Pulmonary embolism revealed on helical CT angiography: comparison with ventilation-perfusion radionuclide lung scanning. Am J Roentgenol 2000; 174:1041–1047.

101. Torbicki A, Kurzyna M, Ciurzynski M, Pruszczyk P, Pacho R, Kuch-Wocial A, Szulc M. Proximal pulmonary emboli modify right ventricular ejection pattern. Eur Respir J 1999; 13:616–621.

102. Pruszczyk P, Torbicki A, Kuch-Wocial A, Chlebus M, Miskiewicz ZC, Jedrusik P. Transoesophageal echocardiography for definitive diagnosis of haemodynamically significant pulmonary embolism. Eur Heart J 1995; 16:534–538.

103. Zlotnick AY, Lennon PF, Goldhaber SZ, Aranki SF. Intraoperative detection of pulmonary thromboemboli with epicardial echocardiography. Chest 1999; 115: 1749–1751.

104. Gulba DC, Schmid C, Borst HG, Lichtlen P, Dietz R, Luft FC. Medical compared

with surgical treatment for massive pulmonary embolism. Lancet 1994; 343:576–577.

105. Jaumin P, Moriau M, el Gariani A, Rubay J, Baele P, Dautrebande J, Goenen M, Servaye-Kestens Y, Ponlot R. [Pulmonary embolectomy. Clinical experience]. Acta Chir Belg 1986; 86:123–125.

106. Stalpaert G, Suy R, Daenen W, Flameng W, Sergeant P, Nevelsteen A, Lauwers P, De Geest H, Van Elst F. Surgical treatment of acute, massive lung embolism. Results and follow-up. Acta Chir Belg 1986; 86:118–122.

Index

About the Editors

Samuel Z. Goldhaber is Associate Professor of Medicine, Harvard Medical School, and Staff Cardiologist in the Cardiovascular Division of Brigham and Women's Hospital (BWH), Boston, Massachusetts. He is Director of the BWH Cardiac Center's Anticoagulation Service and Director of the Venous Thromboembolism Research Group. He specializes in the epidemiology, diagnosis, treatment, and prevention of pulmonary embolism. Dr. Goldhaber is the author of more than 200 book chapters, original reports, and review articles. He is Editor-in-Chief of more than 40 books in the *Fundamental and Clinical Cardiology* book series (Marcel Dekker, Inc.). A Fellow of the American College of Chest Physicians and the American College of Cardiology, he received the A.B. degree (1972) from Harvard College, Cambridge, Massachusetts, and the M.D. degree (1976) from the Harvard Medical School, Boston, Massachusetts.

Paul M. Ridker is Director, Center for Cardiovascular Disease Prevention, Brigham and Women's Hospital, and Associate Professor, Harvard Medical School, Boston, Massachusetts. Dr. Ridker is the principal investigator of multiple federally funded grants targeting novel risk factors for thrombosis and thrombosis prevention and the recipient of the Established Investigator Award from the American Heart Association and the Distinguished Clinical Scientist Award from the Doris Duke Charitable Foundation. An elected member of the American Society for Clinical Investigation and the American Society for Epidemiology, Dr. Ridker received the B.S. degree (1981) from Brown University, Providence, Rhode Island, the M.D. degree (1986) from the Harvard Medical School, Boston, Massachusetts, and the M.P.H. degree (1992) from the Harvard School of Public Health, Boston, Massachusetts.

T - #0032 - 111024 - C0 - 229/152/22 - PB - 9780367396527 - Gloss Lamination